Measurement in Medicine
A Practical Guide

The success of the Apgar score demonstrates the astounding power of an appropriate clinical instrument. This down-to-earth book provides practical advice, underpinned by theoretical principles, on developing and evaluating measurement instruments in all fields of medicine. It equips you to choose the most appropriate instrument for specific purposes.

The book covers measurement theories, methods and criteria for evaluating and selecting instruments. It provides methods to assess measurement properties, such as reliability, validity and responsiveness, and to interpret the results. Worked examples and end-of-chapter assignments use real data and well-known instruments to build your skills at implementation and interpretation through hands-on analysis. This is a perfect course book for students and a perfect companion for professionals/researchers in the medical and health sciences who care about the quality and meaning of the measurements they perform.

- Focuses on the methodology of all measurements in medicine
- Provides a solid background in measurement evaluation theory
- Based on feedback from extensive classroom experience
- End-of-chapter assignments give students hands-on experience with real-life cases
- All data sets and solutions are available online

Practical Guides to Biostatistics and Epidemiology

Series advisors
Susan Ellenberg, *University of Pennsylvania School of Medicine*
Robert C. Elston, *Case Western Reserve University School of Medicine*
Brian Everitt, *Institute for Psychiatry, King's College London*
Frank Harrell, *Vanderbilt University Medical Center Tennessee*
Jos W.R. Twisk, *VU University Medical Center, Amsterdam*

This series of short and practical but authoritative books is for biomedical researchers, clinical investigators, public health researchers, epidemiologists, and non-academic and consulting biostatisticians who work with data from biomedical and epidemiological and genetic studies. Some books explore a modern statistical method and its applications, others may focus on a particular disease or condition and the statistical techniques most commonly used in studying it.

The series is for people who use statistics to answer specific research questions. Books will explain the application of techniques, specifically the use of computational tools, and emphasize the interpretation of results, not the underlying mathematical and statistical theory.

Published in the series
Applied Multilevel Analysis, by **Jos W.R. Twisk**
Secondary Data Sources for Public Health, by **Sarah Boslaugh**
Survival Analysis for Epidemiologic and Medical Research, by **Steve Selvin**
Statistical Learning for Biomedical Data, by **James D. Malley, Karen G. Malley and Sinisa Pajevic**

Measurement in Medicine

A Practical Guide

Henrica C. W. de Vet
Caroline B. Terwee
Lidwine B. Mokkink
Dirk L. Knol
Department of Epidemiology and Biostatistics
EMGO Institute for Health and Care Research
VU University Medical Center, Amsterdam

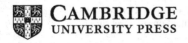

CAMBRIDGE
UNIVERSITY PRESS

University Printing House, Cambridge CB2 8BS, United Kingdom

One Liberty Plaza, 20th Floor, New York, NY 10006, USA

477 Williamstown Road, Port Melbourne, VIC 3207, Australia

314-321, 3rd Floor, Plot 3, Splendor Forum, Jasola District Centre, New Delhi - 110025, India

103 Penang Road, #05-06/07, Visioncrest Commercial, Singapore 238467

Cambridge University Press is part of the University of Cambridge.

It furthers the University's mission by disseminating knowledge in the pursuit of
education, learning and research at the highest international levels of excellence.

www.cambridge.org
Information on this title: www.cambridge.org/9780521133852

First published 2011
10th printing 2018

A catalogue record for this publication is available from the British Library

Library of Congress Cataloging in Publication data
  Measurement in medicine : a practical guide / Henrica C.W. de Vet ... [et al.].
    p. ; cm. – (Practical guides to biostatistics and epidemiology)
  Includes bibliographical references and index.
  ISBN 978-0-521-11820-0 (hardback) – ISBN 978-0-521-13385-2 (pbk.)
  1. Medical care–Evaluation–Methodology.   2. Clinical medicine–Statistical methods.   I. Vet,
  Henrica C. W. de.   II. Series: Practical guides to biostatistics and epidemiology.
  [DNLM: 1. Clinical Medicine–methods.   2. Diagnostic Techniques and
  Procedures.   3. Outcome Assessment (Health Care)   4. Psychometrics.   5. Statistics as Topic.
  WB 102]
  RA399.A1.M42 2011
  610.72'4–dc23   2011014907

ISBN 978-0-521-11820-0 Hardback
ISBN 978-0-521-13385-2 Paperback

Additional resources for this publication at www.clinimetrics.nl

Contents

Preface

Measuring is the cornerstone of medical research and clinical practice. Therefore, the quality of measurement instruments is crucial. This book offers tools to inform the choice of the best measurement instrument for a specific purpose, methods and criteria to support the development of new instruments, and ways to improve measurements and interpretation of their results.

With this book, we hope to show the reader, among other things,

- why it is usually a bad idea to develop a new measurement instrument
- that objective measures are not better than subjective measures
- that Cronbach's alpha has nothing to do with validity
- why valid instruments do not exist and
- how to improve the reliability of measurements

The book is applicable to all medical and health fields and not directed at a specific clinical discipline. We will not provide the reader with lists of the best measurement instruments for paediatrics, cancer, dementia and so on – but rather with methods for evaluating measurement instruments and criteria for choosing the best ones. So, the focus is on the evaluation of instrument measurement properties, and on the interpretation of their scores.

This book is unique in its integration of methods from different disciplines, such as psychometrics, clinimetrics and biostatistics, guiding researchers and clinicians to the most adequate methods to be used for the development and evaluation of measurements in medicine. It combines theory and practice, and provides numerous examples in the text and in the assignments. The assignments are often accompanied with complete data sets, where the reader can really practise the various analyses.

This book is aimed at master's students, researchers and interested practitioners in the medical and health sciences. Master's students on courses on measurements in medical and health sciences now finally have a textbook that delivers the content and methods taught in these courses. Researchers always have to choose adequate measurement instruments when designing a study. This book teaches them how to do that in a scientific way. Researchers who need to develop a new measurement instrument will also find adequate methods in this book. And finally, for medical students and clinicians interested in the quality of measurements they make every day and in their sound interpretation, this book gives guidelines for assessing the quality of the medical literature on measurement issues.

We hope that this book raises interest in and improves the quality of measurements in medicine. We also hope you all enjoy the book and like the examples and assignments. We appreciate feedback on this first edition and welcome suggestions for improvement.

The authors
December 2010

Introduction

1.1 Why this textbook on measurement in medicine?

Measurements are central to clinical practice and medical and health research. They form the basis of diagnosis, prognosis and evaluation of the results of medical interventions. Advances in diagnosis and care that were made possible, for example, by the widespread use of the Apgar scale and various imaging techniques, show the power of well-designed, appropriate measures. The key words here are 'well-designed' and 'appropriate'. A decision-maker must know that the measure used is adequate for its purpose, how it compares with similar measures and how to interpret the results it produces.

For every patient or population group, there are numerous instruments that can be used to measure clinical condition or health status, and new ones are still being developed. However, in the abundance of available instruments, many have been poorly or insufficiently validated. This book primarily serves as a guide to evaluate properties of existing measurement instruments in medicine, enabling researchers and clinicians to avoid using poorly validated ones or alerting them to the need for further validation.

When many measurement instruments are available, we face the challenge of choosing the most appropriate one in a given situation. This is the second purpose of this book. Researchers need systematic methods to compare the content and measurement properties of instruments. This book provides guidelines for researchers as they appraise and compare content and measurement properties.

Thirdly, if there is no adequate measurement instrument available, a new one will have to be developed, and it should naturally be of high quality. We describe the practical steps involved in developing new measurement instruments, together with the theoretical background. We want to help researchers who take the time and make the effort to develop an instrument that meets their specific needs.

Finally, evaluation of the quality of measurements is a core element of various scientific disciplines, such as psychometrics, epidemiology and biostatistics. Although methodology and terminology vary from discipline to discipline, their main objective is to assess and improve measurements. The fourth reason for this book is therefore to integrate knowledge from different disciplines, in order to provide researchers and clinicians with the best methods and ways to assess, appraise, and improve the methodological quality of their measurements.

1.2 Clinimetrics versus psychometrics

Psychometrics is a methodological discipline with its roots in psychological research. Within the field of psychometrics, various measurement theories have been generated, such as classical test theory and item response theory (Lord and Novick, 1968; Nunnally, 1978; Embretson and Reise, 2000). These theories will be further explained in Chapter 2. Cronbach and Spearman were two famous psychometricians. Psychometric methods are increasingly applied to other fields as well such as medicine and health.

The term 'clinimetrics' is indissolubly connected to Feinstein, who defined it as 'measurement of clinical phenomena'. He focused on the construction of clinical indexes, and promoted the use of clinical expertise, rather than statistical techniques, to develop measurement instruments (Feinstein, 1987).

However, in this book we avoid using the terms psychometrics and clinimetrics. Our basic viewpoint is that measurements in medicine should be performed using the most adequate methods. We do not label any of these as psychometric or clinimetric methods, but we do indicate which underlying theories, models and methods are applied.

1.3 Terminology and definitions

Literature on measurement can be confusing because of wide variation in names given to specific measurement properties and how they are defined. Often, many synonyms are used to identify the same measurement property.

For example, the measurement property reliability is also referred to as reproducibility, stability, repeatability and precision. Moreover, different definitions are used for the same property. For example, there are many definitions of responsiveness, which results in the use of different methods to evaluate responsiveness, and this may consequently lead to different conclusions (Terwee *et al.*, 2003).

This variation in terminology and definitions was one of the reasons to start an international Delphi study to achieve consensus based standards for the selection of health measurement instruments (the COSMIN study) (Mokkink *et al.*, 2010a). The COSMIN study aimed to reach consensus among approximately 50 experts, with a background in psychometrics, epidemiology, statistics, and clinical medicine, about which measurement properties are considered to be important, their most adequate terms and definitions and how they should be assessed in terms of study design and statistical methods.

We adhere to the COSMIN terminology throughout this book. Figure 1.1 presents the COSMIN taxonomy, showing terms for various measurement properties and their inter-relationships. In chapters focusing on measurement properties, we indicate other terms used in the literature for the same properties, and also present the COSMIN definitions.

1.4 Scope of measurements in medicine

The field of medicine is extremely diverse. There are so many different diseases, and we all know that health is not just the absence of disease. The World Health Organization (WHO) officially defined health as 'a state of complete physical, mental, and social well-being, not merely the absence of disease or infirmity'. Evaluating the effects of treatment or monitoring the disease course includes assessment of disease stages, severity of complaints and health-related quality of life. To broaden the scope further, measurements do not only include all outcome measurements, but also measurements performed to arrive at the correct diagnosis and those done to assess disease prognosis. Measurements are performed in clinical practice and for research purposes. This broad scope is also expressed in the types of measurements. Measurements vary from questions asked about symptoms during history-taking, to physical examinations and tests,

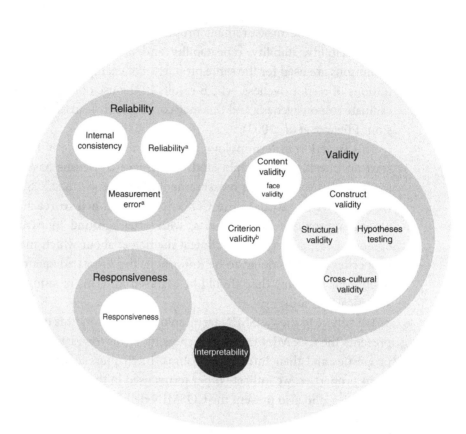

^a(test–retest, inter-rater, intra-rater); ^b(concurrent validity, predictive validity)

Figure 1.1   COSMIN taxonomy of relationships of measurement properties. Reprinted from Mokkink *et al.* (2010a), with permission from Elsevier.

laboratory tests, imaging techniques, self-report questionnaires, and so on. The methods described in this book apply to all measurements in the field of medicine.

1.5 For whom is this book written?

This book is for clinicians and researchers working in medical and health sciences. This includes those who want to develop or evaluate measurement instruments themselves, and those who want to read and interpret the literature on them, in order to select the most adequate ones.

We present the theoretical background for measurements and measurement properties, and we provide methods for evaluating and improving the quality of measurements in medicine and the health sciences.

A prerequisite for a correct understanding of all concepts and principles explained in this book is basic knowledge about study designs (i.e. cross-sectional and longitudinal), essentials of diagnostic testing and basic knowledge of biostatistics (i.e. familiarity with correlation coefficients, t-tests and analysis of variance).

This book is not directed at any specific clinical discipline and is applicable to all fields in medicine and health. As a consequence, the reader will not find a list of the best measurement instruments for paediatrics, cancer or dementia, etc., but a description of how measurement instruments should be developed, and how measurement properties should be assessed and can be improved.

1.6 Structure of the book

The book starts with introductory chapters focusing on measurement theories and models. In particular, Chapter 2 describes the essentials of the classical test theory and the item response theory. Chapter 3 describes the development of a measurement instrument.

Chapters 4–7 then focus on measurement properties. Each chapter describes the theoretical background of a measurement property, and shows how this property is assessed. The structure of a measurement instrument is discussed, and the principles of factor analysis and internal consistency are introduced in Chapter 4. Reliability and validity are presented in Chapters 5 and 6. In health care, changes in disease or health status over time are important, so responsiveness is discussed in Chapter 7.

Interpretation of the results of measurements deserves its own chapter. This aspect is often neglected, but is ultimately the main purpose of measurements. In Chapter 8 we discuss the interpretability of the scores and change scores on measurement instruments, paying special attention to minimal important changes within patients, and response shift.

Finally, Chapter 9 puts all the pieces together by describing how to perform a systematic review of measurement properties. This is a systematic review of the literature to identify instruments relevant for specific measurement situations and to assess the quality of their measurement properties.

1.7 Examples, data sets, software and assignments

We use real examples from research or clinical practice and, where possible, provide data sets for these examples. To enable readers to practise with the data and to see whether they can reproduce the results, data sets and syntaxes can be found on the website www.clinimetrics.nl.

For statistical analyses, we used the Statistical Package for the Social Sciences (SPSS). For analyses that cannot be performed in SPSS, we suggest alternative programs.

Each chapter ends with assignments related to the theories and examples covered in that chapter. Solutions to these assignments can also be found on the website www.clinimetrics.nl.

Concepts, theories and models, and types of measurements

2.1 Introduction

This chapter forms the backbone of the book. It deals with choices and decisions about *what* we measure and *how* we measure it. In other words, this chapter deals with the conceptual model behind the content of the measurements (*what*), and the methods of measurements and theories on which these are based (*how*). As described in Chapter 1, the scope of measurement in medicine is broad and covers many and quite different concepts. It is essential to define explicitly what we want to measure, as that is the 'beginning of wisdom'.

In this chapter, we will introduce many new terms. An overview of these terms and their explanations is provided in Table 2.1.

Different concepts and constructs require different methods of measurement. This concerns not only the type of measurement instrument, for example an X-ray, performance test or questionnaire, but also the measurement theory underlying the measurements. Many of you may have heard of classical test theory (CTT), and some may also be familiar with item response theory (IRT). Both are measurement theories. We will explain the essentials of different measurement theories and discuss the assumptions to be made.

2.2 Conceptual models

First, we will look at the concepts to be measured. Wilson and Cleary (1995) presented a conceptual model for measuring the concept health-related quality of life (HRQL). Studying this model in detail will allow us to distinguish

Table 2.1 Overview of terms used in this chapter

Term	Explanation
Concept	Global definition and demarcation of the subject of measurement.
Construct	A well-defined and precisely demarcated subject of measurement. By psychologists used for unobservable characteristics, such as intelligence, depression or health-related quality of life.
Conceptual model	Theoretical model of how different constructs within a concept are related (e.g. the Wilson and Cleary[a] model of health status).
Conceptual framework	A model representing the relationships between the items and the construct to be measured (e.g. reflective or formative model).
Measurement theory	A theory about how the scores generated by items represent the construct to be measured (e.g. classical test theory or item response theory).
Method of measurement	Method of data collection or type of measurement instrument used (e.g. imaging techniques, biochemical analyses, performance tests, interviews).
Patient-reported outcomes	A measurement of any aspect of a patient's health status that comes directly from the patient, without interpretation of the patient's responses by a physician or anyone else.
Non-patient-reported outcome measurement instruments	All other types of measurement instruments (e.g. clinician-based reports, imaging techniques, biochemical analyses or performance-based tests).
Health-related quality of life	An individual's perception of how an illness and its treatment affect the physical, mental and social aspects of his or her life.

[a] See Figure 2.1.

different levels of clinical and health measurements (Figure 2.1). The levels range from the molecular and cellular level to the impact of health or disease on individuals in their environment and their quality of life (QOL), which represents the level of a patient within his or her social environment.

We illustrate this conceptual model, using diabetes mellitus type 2 as an example. On the left-hand side, the physiological disturbances in cells, tissues or organ systems are described. These may lead to symptoms that subsequently affect the functional status of the patient. For example, in patients with diabetes the production of the hormone insulin is disturbed, leading to high levels of glucose in the blood. The patient's symptoms are tiredness or thirst. In the later phases of diabetes, there may be complications, such as retinopathy, which affects the patient's vision. Patients with diabetes are

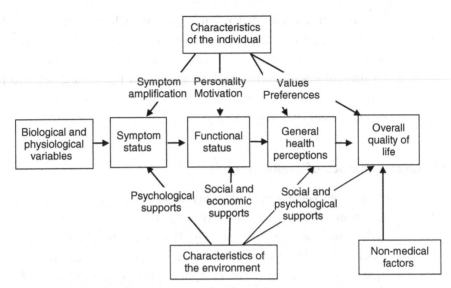

Figure 2.1   Relationships between measures of patient outcome in an HRQL conceptual model. Wilson and Cleary (1995), with permission. All rights reserved.

also more susceptible to depression. All these symptoms affect a patient's functioning. In the WHO definition of health, functioning encompasses all aspects of physical, psychological and social functioning. How patients perceive their health and how they deal with their limitations in functioning will depend on personal characteristics. Of course, the severity of the diabetes will affect the patient's functioning, but apart from that, a patient's coping behaviour is important. In addition, environmental characteristics play a role. For example, how demanding or stressful is the patient's job, and does the work situation allow the patient to adapt his or her activities to a new functional status? In HRQL, the factors we have described are integrated. Patients will weigh up all these aspects of their health status in their own way. Finally, in a patient's overall QOL, non-medical factors also play a role, such as financial situation or the country of residence. The Wilson and Cleary conceptual model illustrates how various aspects of health status are inter-related.

Wilson and Cleary developed their model not only to identify different levels of health, but also to hypothesize a causal pathway through which different factors influence HRQL. The arrows in the model indicate the most important flows of influence, but Wilson and Cleary acknowledge that there may be reciprocal relationships. For example, patients with diabetes may become depressed because of their functional limitations and poor HRQL. Distinguishing different levels ranging from the cellular level to the societal level, looking from left to right in Figure 2.1, allows to focus on several measurement characteristics.

2.3 Characteristics of measurements

From diagnosis to outcome measurements

When diagnosing a disease, we often focus on the left-hand side of the Wilson and Cleary model, while for the evaluation of outcomes of disease or treatment the levels on the right-hand side are more relevant. The diagnosis of many diseases is based on morphological changes in tissues, disturbances in physiological processes, or pathophysiological findings. For example, a high blood glucose level is a specific indicator of diabetes because it reflects a dysfunction in insulin production. Other diseases, such as migraine and depression, can only be diagnosed by their symptoms.

Functional status is frequently considered an outcome of a disease. However, physiotherapists and rehabilitation physicians may consider it a diagnosis, because their treatment focuses on improvement of functioning. Further to the right in the model, perceived health and HRQL are typically outcome measures. None the less, disease outcomes can also be assessed by parameters on the left-hand side. For example, the effect of cancer therapies on the progression of cancer growth is usually evaluated on the basis of morphological or biochemical parameters at tissue level. At the same time, symptoms that bother patients and affect their HRQL are of interest. This example shows that the outcome of cancer is assessed at different levels, ranging from biological parameters to HRQL. However, diagnoses are usually found on the left-hand side of the model.

From clinician-based to patient-based measurements

Measurements performed either by clinicians or by patients themselves have different locations in the Wilson and Cleary model. Measurements of aspects on the left-hand side of Figure 2.1, either for the purpose of diagnosis or for outcome assessment, are usually performed by clinicians. Signs may be observed by a clinician, for example a swelling in the neck, but symptoms such as pain or dizziness can only be reported by patients themselves. Functioning is assessed either by the clinician or patient. For example, physiotherapists often use standardized performance tests to assess physical functioning, but it can also be assessed by means of a questionnaire in which patients are asked about the extent to which they are able to perform indicated activities. If information is obtained directly from the patient, we refer to this as a patient-reported outcome (PRO). PROs are defined as any reports coming directly from patients about how they function or feel in relation to a health condition and its therapy, without interpretation of the patient's responses by a clinician or anyone else (Patrick *et al.* 2007). Symptoms, perceived health and HRQL are aspects of health status that can only be assessed by PROs, because they concern the patient's opinion and appraisal of his or her current health status. Therefore, the right-hand side of the Wilson and Cleary model consists exclusively of PROs.

From objective to subjective measurements

The terms objective and subjective are difficult to define, but the main issue is the involvement of personal judgement. In objective measurement, no personal judgement is involved, i.e. neither the person who measures nor the patient being measured can influence the outcome by personal judgement. In subjective measurement, either the patient being measured or the person performing the measurement is able to influence the measurement to some extent. The assessment of perceived health and HRQL requires subjective measurements, whereas laboratory tests are mostly objective measurements. Objective measurements are mainly found on the left-hand side of the Wilson and Cleary model, among the biological and physiological variables. Symptoms are, by definition, subjective measures. In medical jargon, a symptom is defined as a departure from normal function or feeling that is noticed by a patient, indicating the presence of disease or abnormality. A sign is an objective indication of some medical fact or characteristics that may be detected by a physician during physical examination of a patient (e.g. a swelling of the ankle). Moreover, the word 'sign' is also used as a synonym for 'indication'.

The distinction between objective and subjective measurements is not as sharp as it seems, however, and many measurements are incorrectly labelled as objective. Many imaging tests need a clinician or another expert to read and interpret the images. The degree of swelling in an ankle is also a subjective observation made by a clinician. Laboratory tests become less objective if, for example, the analyst has to judge the colour of a urine sample. These examples show that many test results have to be interpreted by looking, listening, smelling, etc., all of which make use of a clinician's organs of sense. All these measurements therefore have a subjective element. Instructions for a physical performance test need to be given by a physiotherapist, and the level of encouragement may vary greatly. In a cognitive or physical performance test the instructions and support given by the instructor may influence the motivation and concentration of the patient who is performing the test. Here the influence of the person instructing the measurement introduces a subjective element in these performance-based tests. Hence, we also find subjective measurements on the left-hand side of Figure 2.1. Objective measurements are often mistakenly considered better than subjective measurements. In later chapters, we will discuss this issue in much more detail.

From unidimensional to multidimensional characteristics

On the left-hand side of Figure 2.1 there are many examples of unidimensional characteristics (e.g. pain intensity, blood pressure or plasma albumin level). These characteristics represent only a single aspect of a disease. On the right-hand side, we find more complex characteristics, such as perceived health status or HRQL. These encompass not only physical aspects, but also psychological and social aspects of health, and because they cover more aspects, they are called multidimensional constructs. Therefore, the constructs on the right-hand side of the Wilson and Cleary model must be measured with instruments that cover all relevant aspects of the construct.

From observable to non-observable characteristics

Looking from left to right in Figure 2.1, the measurement of observable and non-observable characteristics can be distinguished. Many biological and physiological variables are obtained by direct measurement. For example, the size of a tumour is directly observable with an adequate imaging technique. However, among symptoms and in the functional status we already find non-observable characteristics, such as pain, fatigue and mental functioning. Health perception and QOL are all non-observable constructs. So, to measure these non-observable characteristics a new strategy must be found. Not surprisingly, psychologists have been very active in developing methods to measure unobservable characteristics, because these occur so often in their field. These non-observable characteristics are referred to as 'constructs' by psychologists. They developed CTT, a strategy that enabled them to measure these non-observable constructs indirectly: namely by measuring observable characteristics related to the non-observable constructs. This approach results in multi-item measurement instruments. However, not all multi-item measurement instruments function in this way, as we will explain in the next section. In this book, we use the term construct for a well-defined and precisely demarcated subject of measurement, and therefore not only for non-observable ones (see Table 2.1).

2.4 Conceptual framework: reflective and formative models

When working with multi-item measurement instruments, we need to know the underlying relationship between the items and the construct to be measured. This underlying relationship is what we mean by the term conceptual framework. The conceptual framework is important because it determines the measurement theory to be used in the development and evaluation of the instrument (Fayers *et al.*, 1997). Fayers *et al.* introduced the distinction between reflective and formative models in the field of QOL. In this section, we will first explain that distinction, and then discuss its consequences for measurement theories. However, implications for the development and evaluation of various measurement properties will be discussed in Chapters 3 and 4.

In its simplest form the relationships between constructs and items are represented by Figures 2.2a and 2.2b. In the conceptual framework depicted in Figure 2.2(a), the construct manifests itself in the items; in other words, the construct is reflected by these items. This model is called a reflective model (Edwards and Bagozzi, 2000), and the items are called effect indicators (Fayers *et al.*, 1997). An example of a reflective model is the measurement

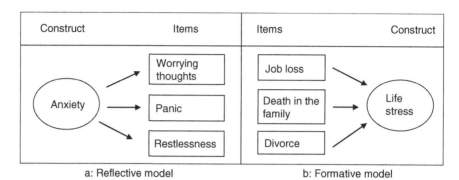

a: Reflective model   b: Formative model

Figure 2.2   Graphical representation of a reflective model (a) and formative model (b).

of anxiety. We know that anxious patients have some very specific feelings and characteristics, or specific behaviour. In patients who are very anxious, all these items will be manifest to a high degree, and in mildly anxious patients we will find these characteristics to a lesser degree. By observing or asking about these characteristics we can assess the presence and degree of anxiety.

In Figure 2.2(b) the construct is the result of the presented items. This model is called a formative model: the items 'form' or 'cause' the construct (Edwards and Bagozzi, 2000) and are called causal indicators (Fayers *et al.*, 1997) or causal variables. An example of a formative model is the measurement of life stress. We measure the amount of stress that a person experiences by measuring many items that all contain stress-evoking events. All events that will cause substantial stress should be represented by the items, so that all these items together will give an indication of the amount of stress that a person experiences.

How can we decide whether the relationship between items and construct is based on a reflective or a formative model? The easiest way to find out is to do a 'thought test': do we expect the items to change when the construct changes? This will be the case for anxiety, but not necessarily for life stress. For example, when a person loses his or her job, life stress will probably increase. However, when life stress increases, a person does not necessarily lose his or her job. If a change in the construct does not affect all items, the underlying model is probably formative. However, in the case of anxiety, if a patient becomes more anxious, we would expect the scores for all items to increase. This patient will panic more, become increasingly restless, and will also have more worrying thoughts. Thus, when change in the construct is expected to influence all items, the underlying model is reflective.

The distinction between formative and reflective models is not always clear-cut, as the following example will show. The Apgar score was developed by Apgar (1953) to rate the clinical condition of a newborn baby immediately after birth. It consists of five variables: colour (appearance), heart rate (pulse), reflex response to nose catheter (grimace), muscle tone (activity) and respiration, leading to the acronym Apgar. According to Feinstein (1987), the Apgar score is a typical example of a measurement instrument, in which the items refer to five different clinical signs that are not necessarily related to each other, i.e. corresponding to a formative model. However, it is questionable whether the Apgar score actually is based on a formative model. If we consider the Apgar score as an indication of a premature baby, then it may be based on a reflective model, because in premature babies, all the organ systems will be less well developed, and the baby may show signs of problems in all these systems. This example illustrates that, depending on the underlying hypothesized conceptual model, the Apgar score can be considered to be based on a formative or reflective model. The example again emphasizes the importance of specifying the underlying conceptual model.

Complex constructs, such as QOL, may combine reflective and formative elements. For example, Fayers and Hand (1997) depicted a hypothetical conceptual framework of the construct of QOL in patients with cancer. In the lower part of Figure 2.3 there are a number of treatment-related symptoms, which result in a lower QOL. The relationship between these symptoms (represented by the rectangles) and the construct of QOL is based on a formative model. On the left-hand side, we can see the symptom 'pain', which may be disease- or treatment-related, but which also affects QOL, based on a formative model. The same holds for the relationship on the right-hand side, where we see how the consequences of chemotherapy affect QOL. At the top of the figure, we see that a low QOL leads to psychological distress, which manifests itself in the symptoms presented at the top of the figure. This part forms a reflective model.

The chronology of the Wilson and Cleary model can help us to some extent to determine the conceptual framework. Measurement of symptoms and functional limitations that are consequences of the disease will follow

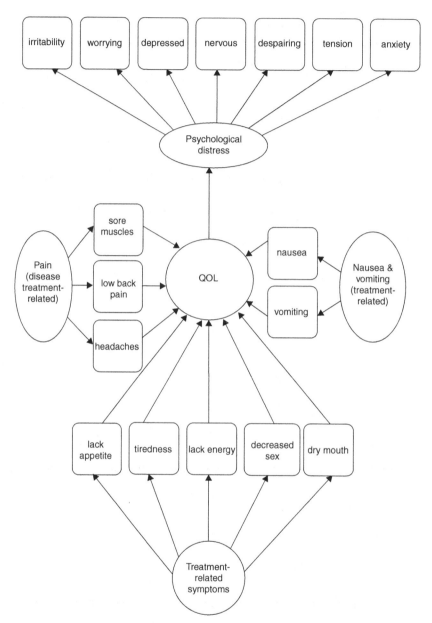

Figure 2.3   Overview of the relationships between various factors with the construct of QOL. The squares represent the items and the circles represent the constructs. Arrows running from constructs to items represent reflective models and arrows running from items to construct represent formative models. Fayers and Hand (1997), with kind permission from Springer Science+Business Media.

a reflective model, while measurement of the effects these symptoms and functional limitations have on general perceived health or HRQL usually follows a formative model.

2.5 Measurement theories

A measurement theory is a theory about how the scores generated by items represent the construct to be measured (Edwards and Bagozzi, 2000). This definition suggests that measurement theories only apply to multi-item instruments. This is true: for single-item instruments no measurement theory is required. However, it should be emphasized that measurement theories are not necessary for all multi-item measurement instruments. Only unobservable constructs require a measurement theory. For observable characteristics, it is usually obvious how the items contribute to the construct being measured and no measurement theory is required. We illustrate this with a few examples. Physical activity can be characterized by frequency, type of activity and intensity. To obtain the total energy expenditure we know how to combine these items. Moreover, for some research questions we are only interested in certain types of physical activity or only in the frequency of physical activity. To assess the severity of diarrhoea, a clear example of an observable characteristic, faecal output can be characterized by frequency, amount and consistency. Another example concerns comorbidity, which is characterized by the number of accompanying diseases, the type of diseases or organ systems involved, and the disease severity or the disability or burden they cause. However, if we talk about comorbidity burden, we move in the direction of unobservable constructs.

It is a challenge to measure unobservable constructs. Such constructs are often encountered in the psychological and psychiatric disciplines, but also when assessing PROs in other medical disciplines. These constructs are usually measured indirectly using multiple observable items. In Section 2.4, we saw that these multi-item instruments need a conceptual framework that describes the relationship between the items and the construct to be measured. Furthermore, when using multi-item instruments, we also need measurement theories to describe the statistical relationships between the items and the construct. Therefore, we introduce the basic statistical representations of the reflective and formative models in Figure 2.4. The circle

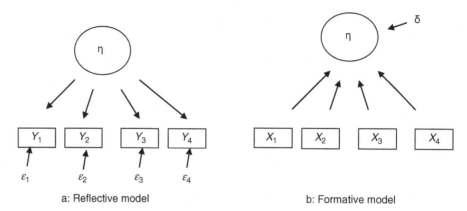

a: Reflective model   b: Formative model

Figure 2.4   Conceptual frameworks representing a reflective model (a) and a formative model (b).

represents the unobservable construct, indicated by the Greek letter η (eta). The rectangles represent the observable items (e.g. the items in a questionnaire). In the reflective model these are indicated with a Y, because they are the consequences of η, whereas in a formative model the rectangles are the determinants of η, and are indicated with an X. This convention corresponds to Y as the typical notation for dependent variables and X for independent variables. We also see in Figure 2.4 that each Y is accompanied by an error term ε (the Greek letter epsilon), while in the formative model there is only one error term δ (the Greek letter delta), often called the disturbance term.

A measurement theory about how the scores generated by the items represent the construct to be measured is thus based on the relationships between the Xs and η, or between the Ys and η. There are two well-known measurement theories: CTT and IRT. Both apply to reflective models. They will be further explained in Sections 2.5.1 and 2.5.2.

For multi-item measurement instruments based on a formative model, there are no well-known measurement theories. This does not mean that there is no theory at all underlying formative models, but rather that the theories are less well developed (Edwards and Bagozzi, 2000). Therefore, development of multi-item instruments based on a formative model is merely based on common sense. Feinstein (1987) suggested the term 'sensibility' in this respect, which he defined as 'enlightened common sense' or 'a mixture of ordinary common sense with a reasonable knowledge of pathophysiology and clinical reality'. However, we do not adopt this term, because it would falsely suggest that the development and evaluation of measurement instruments based on CTT and IRT require no common sense or clinical knowledge.

2.5.1 Classical test theory

We have mentioned CTT as a strategy to measure constructs that are not directly observable. CTT was developed in the early twentieth century by psychologists such as Spearman and Cronbach (Lord and Novick, 1968). Information about an unobservable construct is obtained by measuring items that are manifestations of the construct, because these are much easier to capture. Thus, CTT is suitable for the measurement of constructs that follow a reflective model. The basic formula of the CTT (Lord and Novick, 1968) is

$$Y_i = \eta + \varepsilon_i$$

in which Y_i is the observed score of the item i, η is the 'true' score of the construct to be measured and ε_i is the error term for item i. 'True' in this context refers to the average score that would be obtained if the instrument was given an infinite number of times. It refers only to the consistency of the score, and not to its validity (Streiner and Norman, 2008). The formula expresses that a patient's item score (the observed score Y_i) is the sum of the score of the unobservable construct (η) plus the associated unobservable measurement error (ε_i). Sometimes the symbol T, referring to 'true score', is used in this formula instead of η.

Suppose we want to measure the degree of somatization in a patient who visits a general practitioner. To measure the degree of somatization we use the 'somatization' questionnaire, which is part of the four-dimensional symptom questionnaire (4DSQ) (Terluin et al., 2006). This self-reported questionnaire consists of 16 items. If a patient scores the first item Y_1 of the questionnaire, it will give an indication of the degree of somatization of this patient, but not a perfect indication. This means that it will be accompanied by an error term ε_1. The observed score for the second item Y_2 can again be subdivided into the true score (η) and an error term ε_2. All items in the questionnaire can be seen as repeated measurements of η.

The CTT requires a number of assumptions. Essential assumptions are that each item is an indicator of the construct to be measured (reflective model), and that the construct is unidimensional. In our example, all items should reflect the patient's degree of somatization. Another assumption is that the error terms are not correlated with the true score, and are not correlated with each other. This implies that the average value of the measurement errors (ε_i's) approaches 0. These are all very important assumptions. If they hold, it means that if we take the average value of Y_i over many items we approach the true score η. It also implies that the items will correlate to some degree with each other and with the total score of the measurement instrument.

Measurement instruments that satisfy conditions of the CTT model have a number of characteristics that are advantageous for the evaluation of their measurement properties, as will be shown in later chapters. More details about CTT can be found in classical textbooks written by Lord and Novick (1968) and Nunnally (1978), and in a recent overview by DeVellis (2006).

2.5.2 Item response theory

IRT is also a measurement theory that can be applied when the underlying model is reflective. IRT was developed in the 1950s, by among others the psychologist Birnbaum. Lord and Novick's book (1968) contains a few chapters on IRT, written by Birnbaum. In IRT, constructs were originally called latent traits. Latent means 'hidden' and the term 'trait' finds its origin in psychology. IRT is also frequently applied in education, where the unobservable constructs are often called 'latent ability'. IRT models are typically used to measure a patient's ability, for example, physical ability or cognitive ability. The construct (i.e. 'ability') is usually denoted with the Greek letter θ (theta) in an IRT model, whereas it is denoted by η in CTT. This is just another notation and name for the same construct.

Take as an example the walking ability of a group of patients. We assume that this is a unidimensional construct, which might range from 'unable to walk' to 'no limitations at all'. Each patient has a location on this continuum of walking ability. This location is called the patient location (or ability or endorsement). IRT models make it possible to estimate the locations (θ) of patients from their scores on a set of items. Typical of IRT is that the items also have a location on the same scale of walking ability. This location is called the item location (or item difficulty). Measurements based on the IRT

Table 2.2 Items of a 'Walking ability' scale with responses of seven patients

Walking ability	Patients						
	A	B	C	D	E	F	G
Stand	1	1	1	1	1	1	0
Walking, indoors with help	1	1	1	1	1	0	0
Walking, indoors without help	1	1	1	1	0	0	0
Walking, outdoors 5 min	1	1	1	0	0	0	0
Walking, outdoors 20 min	1	1	0	0	0	0	0
Running, 5 min	1	0	0	0	0	0	0

model therefore enable us to obtain information about both the location of the patient and the location of the items (Embretson and Reise, 2000; Hays *et al.*, 2000).

Before we explain IRT further, we will describe Guttman scales, because these form the theoretical background of IRT. A Guttman scale consists of multiple items measuring a unidimensional construct. The items are chosen in such a way that they have a hierarchical order of difficulty. Table 2.2 gives an example of a number of items concerning walking ability. The six items in Table 2.2 are formulated as 'are you able to stand?', 'are you able to walk indoors with help?', and so on. The answers are dichotomous; *yes* is coded as 1, and *no* is coded as 0. The answers of seven patients (A–G) are shown in Table 2.2. The questions are ranked from easy at the top (an activity almost everybody is able to do), to difficult at the bottom (an activity almost nobody is able to do). Patient A has the highest walking ability and patient G the lowest.

The principle is that if a patient scores 1 for an item, this patient will score 1 for all items that are easier, and vice versa, a patient who scores 0 for an item will score 0 for all items that are more difficult. Such a Guttman scale is called a deterministic scale. If there are no misclassifications, the sum-scores of a patient provide direct information about the patient's walking ability. Of course, in practice, some misclassifications will occur. Such a hierarchical scale also forms the basis of IRT, but in IRT more misclassifications are allowed. Therefore, IRT is based on probabilities.

Although IRT models are often used to measure some type of 'ability', other concepts can also be measured with an IRT model. For example,

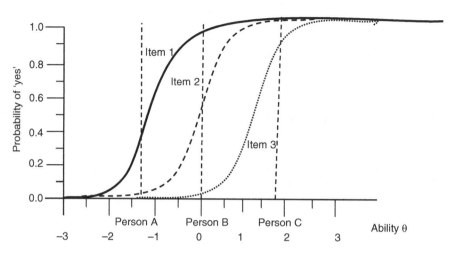

Figure 2.5   Item characteristic curves for three items with equal discrimination but different levels of difficulty.

severity of depression may range from 'absent' to 'present with a high severity'. The degree of difficulty when we are measuring 'ability' is easily translated into the degree of endorsement of an item (i.e. how often patients have a positive score for an item) when we are measuring the severity of depression. Items that are only present in patients with very severe depression will be endorsed by a few patients. Items that are already present in patients with mild depression will be endorsed by almost all patients.

IRT methods describe the association between a respondent's underlying level of ability or severity (θ) and the probability of a particular response to the item. Every item is characterized by an item characteristic curve. The item characteristic curve shows the relationship between the position of the item on the scale of abilities (x-axis) and the probability that patients will have a positive score for this item (y-axis). The item characteristic curve usually is a non-linear monotonic function. Figure 2.5 shows an example of three items with a dichotomous outcome, measuring physical ability.

On the x-axis, there are three patients (A, B and C) with different levels of physical ability. The curves for the items 'sitting on a chair' (item 1), 'walking without a stick' (item 2) and 'walking at high speed' (item 3) should be interpreted as follows. Patients with the same physical ability as patient B (i.e. with a trait level θ of 0) have a probability of more than 90% to answer item 1 (sitting on a chair) with *yes*. Patients such as patient B have a probability of about 50% to answer item 2 (walking without a stick) with *yes*, and will most likely answer item 3 (walking at high speed) with *no*, because the probability that they will answer *yes* is less than 5%. For patients such as patient A there is only a probability of about 30% that they are able to sit on a chair, and they are probably not able to walk without a stick or walk at high speed (probability of a positive answer for the latter items is less than 5%), while patients with a physical ability such as patient C are very likely to be able to sit on a chair and walk without a stick, and there is a probability of about 90% that they are able to walk at high speed. Item 3 (walking at high speed) is the most difficult item, and item 1 is the easiest item. The most difficult items are found on the right-hand side of the figure, and the easiest on the left-hand side. Taking a good look at what patient A and patient C can and can not do, it is clear that patients with little ability (i.e. severely disabled) are found on the left-hand side of the *x*-axis, and they are probably able to do most of the easy items. On the right-hand side, we find patients with high abilities (i.e. only slightly disabled). They are able to do the easy items and there is some probability that they can also do the difficult items. Thus, patient B is more disabled than patient C, and item 1 is the easiest item, while item 3 is the most difficult one.

With this example we have shown how item difficulty and patient ability are linked to each other in IRT models: the higher the ability of a patient, the *more likely* it is that the patient gives a positive answer to any relevant item. The more difficult the item, the *less likely* it is that an item is answered positively by any relevant patient.

Figure 2.5 represents a Rasch model. The Rasch model is the simplest IRT model. It is a one-parameter logistic model in which all the curves have the same shape (see Figure 2.5). The item characteristic curves are based on the following formula:

$$P_i(\theta) = \frac{e^{\theta - b_i}}{1 + e^{\theta - b_i}},$$

where $P_i(\theta)$ represents the proportion of patients with a certain degree of ability or severity of the construct under study, expressed as θ, who will answer the item (i) positively. The parameter b_i is called the difficulty or threshold parameter. This is the only parameter that is relevant in a Rasch model. For each value of θ, $P(\theta)$ can be calculated if the value of b for that item is known. Suppose $\theta = 1$, and $b = 1$, then the value of the numerator becomes e^0, which equals 1, and the denominator obtains the value $1 + e^0$, which amounts to 2. Thus, $P(\theta)$ is 0.5. This calculation shows that, in more general terms, $P(\theta)$ will be 0.5 when $b = \theta$. In other words, the value of b_i determines the values of θ at which the probability of answering this item positively and negatively is equal. The items are ordered on the x-axis according to their difficulty. Readers familiar with logistic regression analysis may recognize this type of formula and the shape of the curves.

In a two-parameter IRT model, apart from the difficulty parameter b_i, a discrimination parameter a_i appears in the formula to indicate that the slopes of the item characteristic curves vary. The Birnbaum model is an example of a two-parameter model for dichotomous outcomes. The formula of the Birnbaum model is:

$$P_i(\theta) = \frac{e^{a_i(\theta - b_i)}}{1 + e^{a_i(\theta - b_i)}}.$$

Now, the parameters a_i and b_i determine the relationship between the ability of θ and $P(\theta)$, i.e. the probability of answering these items positively. The parameters a_i and b_i thus determine the location and form of the item characteristic curves. Higher values of a_i result in steeper curves. A few examples of items in the Birnbaum model are shown in Figure 2.6.

The value of discrimination parameter a of item 2 is greater than the value for a of item 1. This results in a steeper curve for item 2. The difficulty parameter b of both items is about the same, because the items reach the $P(\theta) = 0.5$ at about the same value of θ.

Item 1 increases slowly, and patients with a broad range of ability are likely to score this item positively. For patients such as patient A with only little ability (e.g. $\theta = -1$), there is already a probability of 10% that they will score this item positively, and for patients with a trait level like patient B who have a high ability, there is still a probability of 10% that they will score this item negatively. A flat curve means that a certain score on the item gives less information about the position of a patient on the x-axis than a steep curve. In other words, items with a steep curve are better able to discriminate between patients with low ability and those with high ability. Figure 2.6 also shows that the item characteristic curves of item 1 and 2 cross. This

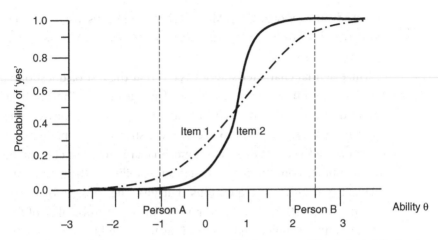

Figure 2.6   Item characteristic curves for two items with the same difficulty but differing in discrimination.

means that for patients with ability like patient A, item 2 is the most diffi-cult, and for patients with ability like patient B, item 1 is the most difficult. Crossing item characteristic curves are not desirable, because they imply that we cannot state in general which item is the most difficult. Whether item 1 is more difficult than item 2 depends on the trait level. Crossing items hamper the interpretation of the scores.

This section provides only a short introduction to the simplest IRT mod-els. First, there is a non-parametric variant of IRT analysis, called Mokken analysis. For parametric analysis, there are many different IRT models. For polytomous answer categories, the Graded Response Model or the Generalised Partial Credit Model can be used, and there are also multidi-mensional models. For a detailed overview of all these models, we refer to Embretson and Reise (2000). In this book, we only describe these models as far as they are relevant for the assessment of the measurement properties of measurement instruments. As most of these models require specialized software, we will often describe the potentials of IRT, without providing data sets with which to perform these analyses.

Like CTT, IRT can only be applied to measurement instruments based on a reflective model. The extra assumption for IRT models is that the items can, to some extent, be ordered according to difficulty. If variables can be ordered well there is a greater chance that an IRT model will fit. IRT has many advantages over CTT. Most of these will be discussed in later chapters; here we will introduce computer adaptive testing (CAT), one of its important applications.

The essential characteristic of CAT is that the test or questionnaire is tailored to the 'ability' of the individual. This means that the items chosen correspond to the ability of each individual respondent. For example, when it appears from the answers to the first questions that a patient cannot walk outdoors, all the questions about items that are more difficult will be omitted. The computer continuously calculates the ability of the patient and chooses relevant questions. The questions that give the most information about a patient are questions to which the patient has a probability of 0.5 to give a positive answer. Tailoring the questions to the ability of patients implies that the set of items may be different for each patient. Nevertheless, on the basis of the test results the position of the patient on the x-axis of Figures 2.5 and 2.6 can be estimated. This means that it is possible to compare the patient scores, despite the different items in each test. For these continuous calculations and the choice of relevant items, a computer is necessary. It has been found that CAT tests usually include fewer items than the corresponding regular tests, which is also a major advantage.

2.6 Summary

Medicine is a broad field, covering both somatic and psychological disorders. Conceptual models help us to decide which aspects of a disease we are interested in. These models distinguish several levels of measurement, ranging from the cellular level to the functioning of a patient in his or her social environment. There are measurements used for diagnosis, for evaluating treatment- and clinician-based outcomes and PROs, objective and subjective measurements, and unidimensional and multidimensional measurement instruments. We explained that the distinction between observable and non-observable characteristics is most important, because it has consequences for the measurement theory to be used. To measure unobservable constructs, indirect measurement with multi-item instruments is often indicated. These multi-item instruments can be based on reflective models or formative models, depending on whether the items reflect or form the construct, respectively.

Most measurements in medicine concern observable variables, which are assessed by direct measurements. In addition, there are some indirect measurements using multiple items, which are based on formative models. However, the measurement theories, CTT and IRT, are only applicable for measurements with multi-item instruments based on reflective models. These measurement theories offer some tools and advantages in the development and evaluation of such measurement instruments, as we will see in Chapters 3 and 4. These are very welcome though, because unobservable constructs are difficult to measure. The measurement theories do not, however, replace 'proper' thinking about the content of measurements. The development and evaluation of all measurement instruments, either direct or indirect, require specific expertise of the discipline one is working in (e.g. imaging techniques, microbiology, genetics, biochemistry, psychology and so on). In the following chapters it will also become clear that all measurements in medicine, irrespective of the type and theory used, should be evaluated for their properties, such as validity, reliability and responsiveness.

Assignments

1. Outcome measures in a randomized clinical trial

In a randomized clinical trial on the effectiveness of Tai Chi Chuan for the prevention of falls in elderly people, a large number of outcome measures were used (Logghe *et al.*, 2009). The primary outcome was the number of falls over 12 months. Secondary outcomes were balance, fear of falling, blood pressure, heart rate at rest, forced expiratory volume during the first second, peak expiratory flow, physical activity and functional status.

Allocate these outcome measures to the different levels in the Wilson and Cleary conceptual model.

2. What is the construct?

Bolton and Humphreys (2002) developed the Neck Bournemouth Questionnaire (see Table 2.3). The authors describe the instrument as a comprehensive outcome measure reflecting the multidimensionality of the musculoskeletal illness model. At the same time, the questionnaire is short and practical enough for repeated use in both clinic-based and research-based settings.

Table 2.3 The Neck Bournemouth Questionnaire. Bolton and Humphreys (2002), with permission

The following scales have been designed to find out about your neck pain and how it is affecting you. Please answer ALL the scales by circling ONE number on EACH scale that best describes how you feel:

1. Over the past week, on average how would you rate your neck pain?

   No pain   Worst pain possible

   0   1   2   3   4   5   6   7   8   9   10

2. Over the past week, how much has your neck pain interfered with your daily activities (housework, washing, dressing, lifting, reading, driving)?

   No interference   Unable to carry out activities

   0   1   2   3   4   5   6   7   8   9   10

3. Over the past week, how much has your neck pain interfered with your ability to take part in recreational, social, and family activities?

   No interference   Unable to carry out activities

   0   1   2   3   4   5   6   7   8   9   10

4. Over the past week, how anxious (tense, uptight, irritable, difficulty in concentrating/relaxing) have you been feeling?

   Not at all anxious   Extremely anxious

   0   1   2   3   4   5   6   7   8   9   10

5. Over the past week, how depressed (down-in-the-dumps, sad, in low spirits, pessimistic, unhappy) have you been feeling?

   Not at all depressed   Extremely depressed

   0   1   2   3   4   5   6   7   8   9   10

6. Over the past week, how have you felt your work (both inside and outside the home) has affected (or would affect) your neck pain?

   Have made it no worse   Have made it much worse

   0   1   2   3   4   5   6   7   8   9   10

7. Over the past week, how much have you been able to control (reduce/help) your neck pain on your own?

   Completely control it   No control whatsoever

   0   1   2   3   4   5   6   7   8   9   10

After reading the 7 items in this questionnaire:

(a) Try to allocate the items in this questionnaire to the levels of the Wilson and Cleary model.

(b) Can you decide from examining the content of this questionnaire, whether it is based on a reflective or a formative model?

3. Item response theory

In Section 2.5.2, the formula for the IRT two-parameter model was presented. We stated that when parameters a and b for an item are known, it is possible to calculate $P(\theta)$ (i.e. the probability of a confirmative answer) at different values of θ. Suppose we have two items:

item A with $b = 1.0$ and $a = 0.7$
item B with $b = 0.5$ and $a = 1.2$

(a) Which item is the most difficult?
(b) Which item discriminates best?
(c) Calculate $P(\theta)$ for the following values of θ: $-3, -2, -1, 0, 1, 2, 3$.
(d) Try to draw the items in a figure with θ on the x-axis and $P(\theta)$ on the y-axis.
(e) Do the items cross?
(f) You don't want the items to cross. If they do cross, which one would you delete?

Development of a measurement instrument

3.1 Introduction

Technical developments and advances in medical knowledge mean that new measurement instruments are still appearing in all fields of medicine. Think about recent developments such as functional MRI and DNA microarrays. Furthermore, existing instruments are continuously being refined and existing technologies are being applied beyond their original domains. The current attention to patient-oriented medicine has shifted interest from pathophysiological measurements to impact on functioning, perceived health and quality of life (QOL). Patient-reported outcomes (PROs) have therefore gained importance in medical research.

It is clear that the measurement instruments used in various medical disciplines differ greatly from each other. Therefore, it is evident that details of the development of measurement instruments must be specific to each discipline. However, from a methodological viewpoint, the basic steps in the development of all these measurement instruments are the same. Moreover, basic requirements with regard to measurement properties, which have to be considered in evaluating the adequacy of a new instrument, are similar for all measurement instruments. Chapters 3 and 4 are written from the viewpoint of developers of measurement instruments. When describing the different steps we have the development of PROs in mind. However, at various points in this chapter we will give examples to show analogies with other measurement instruments in medicine.

Before deciding to develop a new measurement instrument, a systematic literature review of the properties of all existing instruments intended to measure the specific characteristic or concept is indispensable. Such a

Table 3.1 Six steps in the development of a measurement instrument

Step 1	Definition and elaboration of the construct intended to be measured
Step 2	Choice of measurement method
Step 3	Selecting and formulating items
Step 4	Scoring issues
Step 5	Pilot-testing
Step 6	Field-testing

literature review is important for three reasons. First, searching for existing instruments prevents the development of new ones in fields where many already exist. In this situation, an additional instrument would yield results incomparable with studies that used other instruments, and this would only add confusion. A second reason for such a review is to get ideas about what a new instrument should or should not look like. Instruments that are not applicable, or are of insufficient quality can still provide a lot of information, if only about failures that you want to avoid. Thirdly, it saves a lot of time and effort if you find a measurement instrument that can be translated or adapted to your own specific needs. Thus, only if no instrument is available, should a new measurement instrument be developed.

Developing a measurement instrument is not something to be done on a rainy Sunday afternoon. If it is done properly, it may take years. It takes time because the process is iterative. During the development process, we have to check regularly whether it is going well. The development of a measurement instrument can be divided into six steps, as shown in Table 3.1.

In practice, these steps are intertwined, and one goes back and forth between these steps, as indicated in Figure 3.1, in a continuous process of evaluation and adaptation. The last steps in the development process consist of pilot-testing and field-testing. These steps are essential parts of the development phase, because in this phase the final selection of items takes place. Moreover, if the measurement instrument does not perform well it has to be adapted, evaluated again, and so on. In Table 3.1 and Figure 3.1, the pilot test is placed before field-testing. However, if field-testing is intended, among other things, to reduce the number of items, the pilot test may be conducted

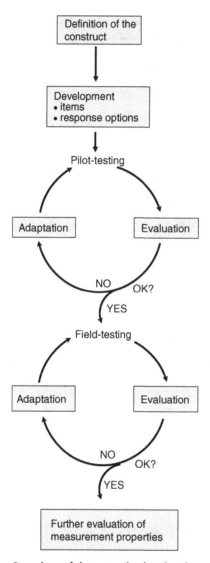

Figure 3.1   Overview of the steps in the development and evaluation of a measurement instrument.

after field-testing (i.e. when the measurement instrument has, more or less, its definite form and size).

The first five steps are dealt with in this chapter, which ends with pilot-testing as a preliminary evaluation. Field-testing will be described in Chapter 4.

3.2 Definition and elaboration of the construct to be measured

The most essential questions that must be answered are 'what do we want to measure?', in 'which target population?' and for 'which purpose?'. The construct should be defined in as much detail as possible. In addition, the target population and the purpose of measurement must be considered.

3.2.1 Construct

Definition of the construct starts with a decision concerning its level in the conceptual model and considerations about potential aspects of the construct, as discussed in Chapter 2. Suppose we want to measure the severity of diabetes. Then the first question is: do we want to measure the pathophysiological process, the symptoms that persons with diabetes perceive or the impact on their functioning or QOL? In other words, which level in the conceptual model (see Section 2.4) are we interested in? Suppose we want to measure the symptoms. Symptoms can be measured by checking whether they are present or absent, but we might also choose to measure the severity of each symptom separately. Suppose that one of the symptoms we are interested in is fatigue. Are we then interested only in physical fatigue, or mental fatigue as well? Note that by answering these questions we are specifying in more detail what we want to measure.

If a construct has different aspects, and we want to measure all these aspects, the measurement instrument should anticipate this multidimensionality. Thinking about multidimensionality in this phase is primarily conceptual, and not yet statistical. For example, in the development of the Multidimensional Fatigue Inventory (MFI), which is a multi-item questionnaire to assess fatigue (Smets *et al.*, 1995), the developers postulated beforehand that they wanted to cover five aspects of fatigue: general fatigue, physical fatigue, mental fatigue, reduced motivation and reduced activity. They developed the questionnaire in such a way that all of these aspects were covered. It is of utmost importance that before actually constructing a measurement instrument, we decide which aspects we want to include. This has to be done in the conceptual phase, preferably based on a conceptual model, rather than by finding out post hoc (e.g. by factor analysis; see Chapter 4) which aspects turn out to be covered by the instrument.

3.2.2 Target population

The measurement instrument should be tailored to the target population and so this must be defined. The following examples will illustrate its importance.

Age, gender and severity of disease determine to a large extent the content and type of instrument that can be used. Very young children are not able to answer questions about symptoms, so pain in newborns is measured by structured observation (Van Dijk *et al.*, 2005). For the same reason, pain observation scales have also been developed for patients with severe dementia (Zwakhalen *et al.*, 2006).

Physical functioning is an important issue in many diseases, but different measurements may be required for different diseases. Instruments to measure physical functioning in patients with spinal cord lesions, cardiovascular disease, cerebrovascular disease or multiple sclerosis will all have a substantially different content.

The severity of a disease is also important, because pathophysiological findings and symptoms will differ with severity, as will functioning and perceived health status. A screening questionnaire used in general practice to identify persons with mild depression will differ from a questionnaire that aims to differentiate between the severe stages of depression.

Other characteristics of the target population may also be important, for example, whether or not there is much comorbidity, or other circumstances/conditions that influence the outcome of the measurements.

There is no universal answer to the question concerning which characteristics of the target population should be considered, but the examples given above indicate how a measurement instrument should be tailored to its target population.

3.2.3 Purpose of measurement

Three important objectives of measurement in medicine are diagnosis, evaluation of therapy and prediction of future course. Guyatt *et al.* (1992) stated that for diagnostic purposes we need discriminative instruments that are able to discriminate between persons at a single point in time. To evaluate the effects of treatment or other longitudinal changes in health status, we need evaluative instruments able to measure change over time. A third class of instruments is aimed at the prediction of outcomes. Predictive measurements aim to classify individuals according to their prognosis (i.e. the future course of their disease). Nowadays, prediction models are used to define a set of variables that best predict this future course. These are usually referred to as prediction models or prediction rules, rather than measurement instruments, because they usually contain a number of different constructs and variables. For the development of such 'instruments', we refer to a handbook about predictive modelling by Steyerberg (2009). In our opinion, it is better to speak of discriminative, evaluative or predictive applications than of instruments, because the same instrument can be used for different purposes. As we saw in Chapter 2, the purpose of the measurement clearly has bearing on the choice of construct to be measured, and it also has consequences for the development of the instrument, as we will see in Section 3.4.3.

3.3 Choice of measurement method

The type of measurement instrument should correspond closely to the construct to be measured. Some constructs form an indissoluble alliance with a measurement instrument (e.g. body temperature is measured with a thermometer and a sphygmomanometer is usually used to assess blood pressure in clinical practice). The options are therefore limited in these cases, but in other situations, many possibilities may be available. Physical functioning provides a nice example of the interplay between the construct to be measured and the most adequate type of measurement instrument. Suppose we aim to assess physical functioning in patients who have had a cerebrovascular accident. We can measure what patients *can do* when they are invited to (i.e. the construct 'capacity'), or what they *think they can do* (i.e. the construct 'perceived ability'), or what they *actually do* (i.e. the construct 'physical activity', which is sometimes used as a proxy for physical functioning). Note that capacity, perceived ability and physical activity are different constructs. When deciding on the type of measurement instrument, we have to define exactly which of these we want to measure. To obtain information about what patients *can do*, we can choose between asking them or testing their physical function in performance tests, such as the 'timed stand up and go' test. To assess what patients perceive that they can do, we must ask them what they can do, either by interview or questionnaire, because perception always requires direct information from patients. To assess what patients actually do, we might choose to ask them, by interview or questionnaire, or we might assess their physical activity with activity monitors, such as accelerometers.

When designing a PRO instrument, we next must decide whether a multi-item measurement instrument is needed, or whether a single-item instrument will suffice. This evokes an interesting discussion, with arguments concerning reliability and the definition of the construct. The reliability issue is particularly important for unidimensional constructs. For example, physical fatigue can be measured by multiple items, which are all reflections of being physically fatigued. A multi-item instrument will be more reliable than a single-item instrument. The explanation will be given in Chapter 5.

The other issue concerns the definition of the construct: do patients consider the same aspects of fatigue as the developers had in mind, and does the construct 'fatigue' have the same meaning for all patients? In a multi-item measurement instrument the content of the items is often more specific, and multidimensional instruments include all the dimensions considered to be relevant for the construct. This not only makes it easier for patients to understand these items, but we now know that the same construct is being measured for all patients. For example, with a single-item instrument we leave it to the patient to define the meaning of fatigue. One patient might, for example, feel physically exhausted but mentally alert, while another patient feels mentally tired but physically fit. So, a single question excludes the possibility of a detailed description of the fatigue experienced by the patients, and it hampers the interpretation of the score. In particular, if more aspects are involved, multi-item instruments, in which multiple dimensions can be distinguished are more informative, because they provide subscores for each domain.

However, after having considered these arguments, what do we choose? The prevailing opinion is that complex constructs are best measured with multi-item measurement instruments, but there might be situations in which a single-item instrument is preferable (Sloan *et al.*, 2002). A single-item instrument might be attractive when a construct is not the main issue of interest in a study, because it is simple and short and thus reduces the burden of administration. One may also choose to use a single question when the global opinion of the patient is of specific interest. Single items are usually formulated in quite general terms. For example, 'If you consider all aspects, how would you rate your fatigue?'. With regard to measurement properties, it is not always the case that multi-item instruments are more valid than when the same construct is assessed with a single item (Sloan *et al.*, 2002). In a multi-item measurement instrument, it is easy and worthwhile to add one global question about the construct. As we will see later, this addition might also help in the interpretation and validation of the measurement instrument. For further reading on single-item versus multi-item instruments we refer to Sloan *et al.* (2002) and Fayers and Machin (2007).

3.4 Selecting items

This chapter focuses on multi-item measurement instruments, because they are the most interesting from a methodological point of view. When talking about multi-item instruments, one immediately thinks of questionnaires, but performance tests also contain different tasks and the assessment of an electrocardiogram or MRI requires the scoring of different aspects that can be considered as items. For reasons of convenience, we focus on questionnaires. However, examples throughout the chapter will show that the basic methodological principles can be applied to other measurement instruments as well, such as imaging techniques or physical tests.

3.4.1 Getting input for the items of a questionnaire: literature and experts

3.4.1.1 Literature

Examining similar instruments in the literature might help not only to clarify the constructs we want to measure, but also to provide a set of potentially relevant items. We seldom have to start from scratch. This is only the case with new diseases. The discovery of AIDS in the 1980s posed the challenge of finding out which signs and symptoms were characteristic expressions of AIDS, and which specific pathophysiological changes in the immune system were typical of patients with AIDS. This made it possible to develop a conceptual model (comparable with a Wilson and Cleary model), as new knowledge about AIDS became available. To develop a questionnaire to assess health-related quality of life (HRQL) in patients with AIDS, it was necessary to find out what the important symptoms were, and how these affected HRQL in the physical, social and psychological domains. Among the important domains for these patients were the impact of fatigue, body image and forgiveness. Fatigue could be assessed with existing measurement instruments, but the constructs impact of body image and forgiveness had to be developed entirely from scratch (The WHOQOL HIV Group, 2003).

Nowadays there are 'item banks' for specific topics. An item bank contains a large collection of questions about a particular construct, but it is more than just a collection. We call it an item bank if the item characteristic curves of the items that measure a specific construct have been determined by item response theory (IRT) analysis. Item banks form the basis for computer adaptive testing, which was described in Section 2.5.2. One example of an item bank is the PROMIS (Patient-Reported Outcomes Measurement Information System), initiated by the National Institutes of Health (www. nihpromis.org) in the USA (Cella *et al.*, 2007). PROMIS has developed item banks for, among other things, the following constructs: pain, fatigue, emotional distress and physical functioning. The items were derived from existing questionnaires, and subsequently tested for their item characteristics. Item banks are an extremely rich source of items that can be used to develop new measurement instruments (e.g. to develop a disease-specific instrument to measure physical functioning in patients with Parkinson's disease or rheumatoid arthritis).

3.4.1.2 Experts

Clinicians who have treated large numbers of patients with the target condition have extensive expertise on characteristic signs, typical characteristics and consequences of the disease. Instruments to measure these constructs should therefore be developed in close cooperation with these experts. At the level of symptoms, functioning and perceived health, the patients themselves are the key experts. Therefore, patients should be involved in the development of measurement instruments when their sensations, experiences and perceptions are at stake. For the development of performance tests to assess physical functioning, patients can also indicate which activities cause them the most problems. The best way to obtain information from clinicians or patients about relevant items is through focus groups or in-depth interviews (Morgan, 1998; Krueger, 2000). Developers need to have an exact picture in mind of the construct to be measured; otherwise, it is impossible to instruct the focus groups adequately and to extract the relevant data from the enormous yield of information.

3.4.1.3 An example of item selection for a patient-reported outcomes instrument

DuBeau *et al.* (1998) organized focus groups to obtain responses from patients with urge urinary incontinence (UI), about how UI affected their HRQL. They first invited patients to describe their UI in their own words. Subsequently, they asked them open-ended questions about which aspects of their daily lives were most affected by their UI. Patients were also asked open-ended questions about the influence of UI on specific areas of their physical health, self-care, work, household activities, social activities and hobbies. The discussion was driven mainly by the patients' responses. They were also asked to share advice about strategies for coping with UI with other focus group members. Qualitative content analysis of the focus group transcripts was used to determine relevant items. These were compared with previously described UI-related QOL items obtained from the literature. Of the 32 items identified by the focus groups as HRQL items, more than half were distinct from items obtained from the literature or from clinical experts. Examples of these were 'interruption of activities' and 'lack of self-control'. Patient-defined items focused more on coping with embarrassment and interference than on avoidance of actual activity performance. This example illustrates the value of involving patients as key experts on what is important for their HRQL. However, it also shows the need to have a clear definition in mind of the construct 'impact on HRQL', because some of the items identified by the patients, particularly those concerning coping strategies, have questionable impact on QOL. For details about focus groups, see the handbooks written by Morgan (1998) and Krueger (2000).

3.4.1.4 An example of item selection for a non-patient-reported outcomes instrument

Let us take a look at MRI findings in the diagnosis of Alzheimer's disease (AD). AD is a degenerative disease characterized by cerebral atrophy with changes in cortical and subcortical grey matter. These changes can be visualized by MRI as signal hyperintensities. In the 1990s, the involvement of white matter was under debate, and at that time conflicting results were attributed to a possible heterogeneous population or to a suboptimal rating scale.

Table 3.2 Visual rating of signal hyperintensities observed on MRI

Periventricular hyperintensities (PVH 0–6)			
Caps	occipital	0/1/2	0 = absent
	frontal	0/1/2	1 = ≤5 mm
Bands	lateral ventricles	0/1/2	2 = >5 mm and <10 mm
White matter hyperintensities (WMH 0–24)			
Frontal		0/1/2/3/4/5/6	0 = na
Parietal		0/1/2/3/4/5/6	1 = <3 mm, $n \leq 5$
Occipital		0/1/2/3/4/5/6	2 = <3 mm, $n > 6$
Temporal		0/1/2/3/4/5/6	3 = 4–10 mm, $n \leq 5$
			4 = 4 mm, $n > 6$
			5 = >11 mm, $n > 1$
			6 = confluent
Basal ganglia hyperintensities (BG 0–30)			
Caudate nucleus		0/1/2/3/4/5/6	
Putamen		0/1/2/3/4/5/6	
Globus pallidus		0/1/2/3/4/5/6	
Thalamus		0/1/2/3/4/5/6	
Internal capsule		0/1/2/3/4/5/6	
Infra-tentorial foci of hyperintensity (ITF 0–24)			
Cerebellum		0/1/2/3/4/5/6	
Mesencephalon		0/1/2/3/4/5/6	
Pons		0/1/2/3/4/5/6	
Medulla		0/1/2/3/4/5/6	

Semi-quantitative rating of signal hyperintensities in separate regions, with the range of the scale, between brackets.

n, number of lesions; na, no abnormalities.

Source: Scheltens *et al.* (1993), with permission.

Scheltens *et al.* (1993) developed a rating scale to quantify the presence and severity of abnormalities on MRI. In this scale (see Table 3.2), periventricular (grey matter) and white matter hyperintensities were rated separately, and semi-quantitative regional scores were obtained by taking into account the size and anatomical distribution of the high signal abnormalities.

Using this rating scale, the researchers found that there was white matter involvement in late onset AD, but not in patients with pre-senile onset AD. These groups did not differ regarding grey matter involvement on MRI.

This example shows that for these types of measurements too one has to find out (e.g. by comparing patient groups), which characteristics are typical of the disease and how these can best be quantified.

3.4.2 Formulating items: first draft

All the sources mentioned above may provide input for items. However, some new formulations or reformulations should always occur, because the information obtained from experts and from the literature must be transformed into adequate items. Furthermore, a new measurement instrument is seldom based completely on existing items, so brand new items should also be formulated. The formulation of adequate items is a challenging task, but there are a number of basic rules (Bradburn *et al.*, 2004).

- Items should be comprehensible to the total target population, independent of their level of education. This means that difficult words and complex sentences should be avoided. It is often recommended that the items should be written in such simple language that anyone over 12 years of age can understand them (Streiner and Norman, 2008).
- Terms that have multiple meanings should be avoided. For example, the word 'fair' can mean 'pretty good, not bad', 'honest', 'according to the rules' and 'plain', and the word 'just' can mean 'precisely', 'closely' and 'barely'. Respondents may interpret these questions using these words differently, but they will not indicate that the words are difficult.
- Items should be specific. For example, in a question about 'severity of pain' it should be specified whether the patient has to fill in the average pain or the worst pain. Moreover, it should be clear to which period of time the question refers. Should the patient rate current pain, pain during the previous 24 hours, or pain during the previous week?
- Each item should contain only one question instead of two or more. The words 'and' and 'or' in a question may point to a 'two-in-one question'. Take for example, the item 'When I have pain I feel terrible, and I feel that it's all too much for me'. Some patients may indeed feel terrible, but patients who don't have the feeling that it's all too much for them will find it very hard to respond to this item.
- Negative wording in questions should be avoided, because this makes them difficult to answer. For example, the item 'I have no pain when

walking slowly' should be answered with 'no' by patients who do have pain when walking slowly.

These are only a few examples of requirements in formulating adequate items. In scientific disciplines with a long tradition in survey methodology, such as sociology and psychology, there are many handbooks on the formulation of items for questionnaires. To read more about the essentials for adequate formulation of questions and answers we therefore refer to handbooks on survey methodology (e.g. Bradburn *et al.*, 2004).

The first draft of a questionnaire should contain as many items as possible. In this phase, creativity should dominate rigor because, as we will see in Chapter 4, there will be ample opportunities for evaluation, item reduction and reconsideration in subsequent phases. However, it is good to keep a number of issues in mind while selecting and formulating the items.

3.4.3 Things to keep in mind

Having decided that you are, indeed, going to develop a multi-item measurement instrument it is time to think about the conceptual framework, i.e. the direction of the arrows between the potential items and the construct (see Section 2.4). We should realize in this phase whether we are dealing with a formative or a reflective model (recall Figure 2.2), because the type of model has important consequences for the selection of items for the multi-item measurement instrument.

In a reflective model, the items are manifestations (indicators) of the construct. This implies that the items will correlate with each other, and also that they may replace each other (i.e. they are interchangeable). For that reason, it is not disastrous to miss some items that are also good indicators of the construct. In the developmental phase, the challenge is to come up with as many items as possible. Even items that are almost the same are allowed. In practice a large number of items are selected, but these will later be reduced by special item reduction techniques, such as factor analysis and examination of item characteristics (as will be described in Chapter 4).

In a formative model, each item contributes a part of the construct, and together the items form the whole construct. Here the challenge is to find *all* items that contribute substantially to the construct. In formative models, items do not necessarily correlate with each other, and thus are not inter-changeable; one item cannot be replaced by another. Therefore, missing an important item inevitably means that the construct is not measured com-prehensively. In a questionnaire to measure the construct 'life stress', all items that cause considerable stress should be included in the questionnaire, even if some are endorsed by only a small proportion of the population. For example, the death of a close family member is very stressful, but only a small proportion of the population will answer this item positively. For formative models, the items together should cover the whole construct, and important items must not be missed. This is an important issue that must be kept in mind during item generation. However, the assessment of import-ance and the elimination of less important items should take place during field-testing (see Chapter 4). Note that factor analysis does not play a role in item reduction in formative models.

Can the researcher choose freely between reflective and formative mod-els? In the developmental stage, the answer is 'to some extent'. However, some constructs lend themselves better to be measured with reflective models and others with formative models. Socio-economic status (SES) is usually meas-ured with a formative model, based on the items 'level of education', 'income' and 'profession', but one can try to find reflective items for SES. Examples of such questions are: 'How high up are you on the social ladder?' and 'How do you rate your socio-economic status?'.

In Chapter 2, Figure 2.2(b) showed that life stress could be measured based on a formative model. The items in that measurement instrument comprised events that all cause stress. These are presented on the left-hand side of Figure 3.2. However, one can also think of a measurement instrument consisting of items that are reflections of stress. We know that stress results in a number of symptoms, such as 'troubling thoughts about the future' and 'sleep disturbances', some of which are presented on the right-hand side of Figure 3.2. So, in the case of the measurement of stress a researcher can choose between a formative and a reflective model.

Another issue to keep in mind is the difficulty of the items. Note that this not only holds when we are going to use IRT analysis (i.e. considering the hierarchy of items). In classical test theory (CTT) the total range of easy and difficult items relevant for our target population should also be covered. For instance, in our example concerning the severity of depression, if the target

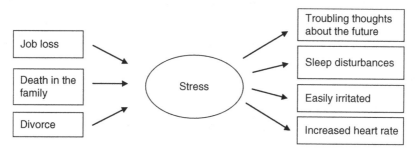

Figure 3.2 Conceptual framework for the measurement of stress. The left-hand side depicts a formative model, the right-hand side a reflective model.

population consists of patients with all levels of depression, we have to think about items characteristic of mild depression, as well as those indicative of moderate and severe depression. Therefore, the difficulty of items in relation to the target population is another thing that must be kept in mind while selecting items. We will discuss this in more detail in Chapter 4.

According to Guyatt *et al.* (1992), measurement instruments with a discriminative purpose require items that have a discriminating function, and these items do not necessarily have the ability to measure changes in the health status of an individual patient. When composing an evaluative instrument, the answers to the items should change when the patient's health status improves. However, this distinction is less pronounced than Guyatt and colleagues have suggested. Let us consider a questionnaire to assess the construct 'severity of depression'. Assuming a reflective model, the questionnaire consists of items that are all reflections of depression. If the severity of the depression changes, the responses to all items will also change. This is an implicit assumption of a reflective model. The questionnaire therefore meets the requirements for an evaluative measurement instrument. Nevertheless, it will also be able to discriminate between various stages of depression. It can be assumed that patients with severe depression have already gone through states of mild and moderate depression. Therefore, if the instrument is able to distinguish between these stages longitudinally (within an individual), it will also be able to distinguish between them cross-sectionally (between individuals). Given that we are measuring the same construct, there will be very little difference between the

Table 3.3 Things to keep in mind in the selection and formulation of items

---

Construct
Target population
Purpose of measurement
Reflective or formative model
Difficulty of the items
Application in research or clinical practice
Correspondence with response options

---

requirements for items for discriminative purposes and those for evaluative purposes.

This does not mean that we can forget the purpose of the measurement. It does still have some influence on the composition of the measurement instrument, i.e. in the choice of items. Let us return to the example concerning the construct 'severity of depression' that we want to measure. Suppose that we want to identify cases of mild depression in general practice by means of a screening questionnaire. This is a discriminative purpose, in which case we have to be sure to include a large number of items in the range of the borderline between no depression and mild depression. The result of the measurements are dichotomized best as either no depression or depression. However, if we want to measure the degree of depression in patients visiting general practice, we want to have items covering the whole range of the depression scale. The ultimate result of the measurement may be a variable with several categories, ranging from no depression to very severe depression, or may even be expressed as a distribution of continuous scores.

Furthermore, in the development of a measurement instrument, application in research or in clinical practice must be kept in mind. In clinical practice, the instruments are usually shorter, due to time constraints. Moreover, fewer distinctions may be made (e.g. in grade of severity), because only classifications that have consequences for clinical management are relevant.

Last but not least, while writing the items, one should keep the response options in mind. The statements or questions contained in the items must correspond exactly with the response options. Table 3.3 provides an overview of things to keep in mind during the item selection phase.

3.5 Scores for items

3.5.1 Scoring options

Every measurement leads to a result, either a classification or a quantification of a response. The response to a single item can be expressed at nominal level, at ordinal level and at interval or ratio level.

The *nominal level* consists of a number of classes that lack an order. Often the number of classes is only two: the characteristic white mass on a mammogram, for example, is present or absent. The item is then called dichotomous. Sometimes, however, there are more categories. An example is cause of death, which has a large number of classes, with no logical order. The system of the International Classification of Functioning (ICF) (WHO, 2001), which contains classes such as sleeping, function, walking and body structure, is also a nominal level.

The *ordinal level* also consists of classes, but now an order is observable. Severity of disease can be measured on an ordinal scale. One can speak of mild, moderate or severe diabetes, and the colour of the big toe in patients with diabetes can be pink, red, purple or black. If numbers are assigned to the classes of foot ulcers in patients with diabetes, we know that 2 (red) is worse than 1 (pink), and 4 (black) is worse than 3 (purple). However, the 'distance' between 1 and 2 and between 3 and 4 in terms of degree of severity is unknown, and is not necessarily the same. Figure 3.3 shows an example of an ordinal scale designed by the COOP-WONCA Dartmouth project team (Nelson *et al.*, 1987). Both the words and the drawings can be used to express the degree to which the patient has been bothered by emotional problems. These drawings are sometimes used for children, older people or patients who have difficulty in reading or understanding the words.

We have to mention Likert items when dealing with measurements at an ordinal level. Originally, the Likert items consisted of statements about opinions, feelings or attitudes, for which there is no right or wrong or no favourable answer. The response options are bipolar, and consist of three, five or seven classes with, conventionally, strongly disagree on the left-hand side and strongly agree on the right-hand side, and the middle category being a neutral score. If we want to force respondents to choose positive or negative answers, four or six classes can be used. All classes may be given a

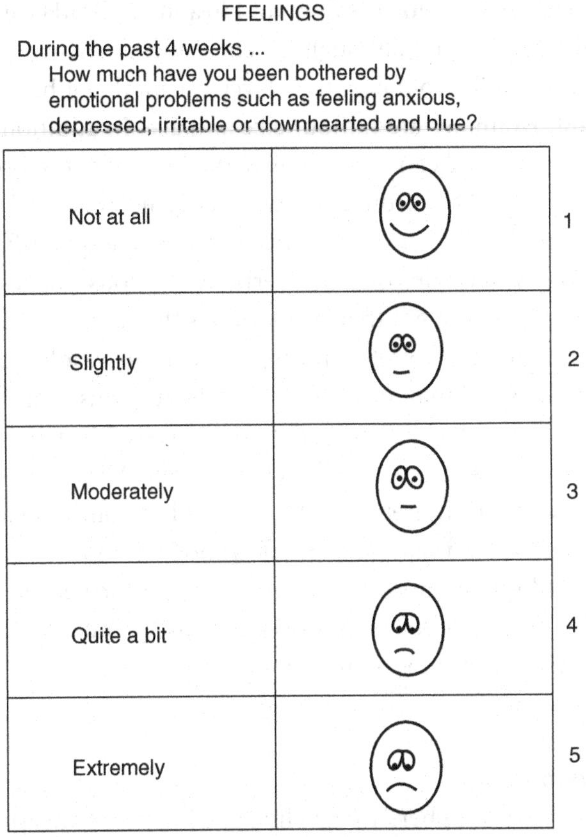

FEELINGS

During the past 4 weeks ...
    How much have you been bothered by
    emotional problems such as feeling anxious,
    depressed, irritable or downhearted and blue?

Not at all		1
Slightly		2
Moderately		3
Quite a bit		4
Extremely		5

Figure 3.3   Example of different types of scales to grade emotional feelings. Nelson *et al.*
(1987), with permission.

verbal description, but this is not always the case. Nowadays, items scored
at ordinal level are often called Likert items even when they do not refer to
opinions or attitudes, such as 'I am able to get out of bed without help', with
the following response options: totally disagree, somewhat disagree, don't
disagree, don't agree, somewhat agree, strongly agree. Even items with other
response categories are called Likert items.

At the *interval level*, the scores of measurements are expressed in numbers
to quantify the measurement results. Examples are body temperature, plasma
glucose level and blood pressure. In these cases, the distances between the
scores are known, and we can start adding and subtracting. For example, the

distances between systolic blood pressures of 140 and 150 mmHg and between 150 and 160 mmHg are equal, although the consequences may differ.

The *ratio level* is similar to the interval level, except that it has an absolute (true) zero point. Examples are tumour size and age. In addition to adding and subtracting scores, we can also calculate the ratio of two scores.

Both the nominal and the ordinal levels use classifications and are known as categorical variables. Interval and ratio levels enable quantification and are known as continuous variables. The term 'continuous' suggests that the variable can take all values, but this is not always the case. For example, the pulse rate per minute has counts, and is expressed as whole numbers. In other examples the scale may not allow finer distinctions – although they exist – and the results of a measurement are expressed in whole numbers (e.g. body height is usually expressed in centimetres). Variables that cannot take all values are called discrete variables instead of continuous variables. The order of nominal, ordinal, interval and ratio level allows progressively more sophisticated quantitative procedures to be performed on the measurements. In this book, we focus only on the consequences for assessment of the measurement properties of instruments.

3.5.2 Which option to choose?

To what extent can researchers freely choose the level of measurement of the responses? If a measurement is at interval scale, it is always possible to choose a lower level of measurement. For example, the glucose level of patients with diabetes is expressed in mmol/l (interval level), but one might choose to make a response scale at ordinal level with categories of normal, moderately elevated, substantially elevated and extremely elevated. A nominal scale in this example would consist of two categories: not elevated and elevated. However, by choosing a lower level of measurement, information is lost: knowing the exact plasma glucose level is more informative than knowing only whether or not it is elevated.

Nominal variables, such as blood group or gender, cannot be measured on an ordinal scale or an interval scale. However, intensity of pain, for example, is sometimes measured at ordinal level and sometimes at interval level. At ordinal level, for example, the following categories are used: no pain, mild pain, moderate pain and severe pain. To measure pain at interval level, we

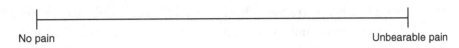

No pain   Unbearable pain

Figure 3.4   A visual analogue scale (VAS) to measure pain intensity.

ask patients to score the intensity of their pain on a visual analogue scale (VAS). A VAS is a horizontal line with a length of 100 millimetres (mm), with an anchor point at the left indicating 'no pain', and an anchor point on the right indicating 'unbearable pain', and no demarcations or verbal expressions in between (see Figure 3.4). The patient is asked to indicate the intensity of his or her pain on this 100-mm line. The intensity of the pain is now expressed in mm, and it has become a continuous variable.

The question is, however, do we obtain more information by choosing an interval scale rather than an ordinal scale? That depends on whether patients are able to grade their amount of pain in such detail. Patients cannot reliably discriminate between 47 mm and 48 mm of pain on a 0–100 mm VAS, and it is questionable whether they can distinguish, for example, 55 mm from 47 mm.

The same issue is of concern when setting the number of categories in an ordinal scale. For measurements in medicine, the answer is not only based on how many degrees of the characteristic can be distinguished by clinicians or patients, but it is primarily determined by how many categories are relevant. The number may differ for research and clinical practice. If the doctor has only two options to choose from (e.g. treatment or no treatment) then two categories might suffice. So, it depends on the number of categories that are clinically relevant for the doctor. In research, we often want to have many options, in order to obtain more detailed distinctions or a more responsive measure. Miller (1956) found that seven categories are about the maximum number of distinctions that people are able to make from a psycho-physiological perspective. Whether or not all the categories used are informative can be examined by IRT analysis (Chapter 4).

3.6 Scores for scales and indexes

Now that we have seen how the individual items in a multi-item measurement instrument are scored, we will discuss how sum-scores or overall scores can be obtained. We will first discuss how this works for unidimensional multi-item instruments based on reflective models, which we call scales, and then for multi-item measurements that contain different dimensions, i.e. based on formative models, which we call indexes. Be aware that scales and indexes are defined differently by different authors (Sloan *et al.*, 2002). In this book, we follow Fayers and Machin (2007), by defining scales, such as the somatization scale of the four-dimensional symptom questionnaire (4DSQ; Terluin *et al.* 2006). We encountered these in Chapter 2, as representing multiple items measuring a single construct, and indexes such as the Apgar score summarizing items representing multiple aspects or dimensions.

3.6.1 Summarizing scores in reflective models

How do we obtain scale scores? Usually the item scores are just summed up. An example is the Roland–Morris Disability Questionnaire (RDQ; Roland and Morris, 1983), which consists of 24 items asking patients whether or not they have difficulty in performing 24 activities because of their low back pain. Each 'yes' scores one point, so the total score ranges from 0 to 24. If items are scored on an ordinal level, summation also takes place. For example, the somatization subscale of the 4DSQ had 16 items, scored on a three-point scale: 0 for symptom 'not present', 1 for symptom 'sometimes present' and 2 for symptom 'regularly present', 'often', 'very often or constantly'. This scale with 16 items (each scored 0, 1 or 2) can have values in the range of 0–32. Instead of the sum-scores of scales, the average score might also be taken. Average scores may be easier to understand because their values are in the same range as the item scores themselves, i.e. if item scores range from 0 to 2 points the average score is also within this range.

The Guttman scale was introduced in Chapter 2 as a basis for IRT scales. The items concerning walking ability had a nice hierarchical order of difficulty. Just adding the item scores (1 or 0) is an adequate way in which to obtain a sum-score for a person's walking ability. In addition, this sum-score conveys a lot of information about the patient's walking ability. For example, in the case of a perfect Guttman scale (i.e. with no misclassifications), a patient with a sum-score of 2 (like person E in Table 2.2) has no problems with standing and is able to walk indoors with help, but is not able to walk indoors without help and outdoors.

Summing up with or without using weights

In IRT models, in order to calculate an overall score the item scores are also often summed up. For Rasch models (i.e. IRT models in which all items have the same discrimination parameter a; see Chapter 2), the sum of the items (ΣY_i) is taken. In a two-parameter IRT model, in which the items have different discrimination parameters, the items are weighted with the value of a, the discrimination parameter: sum-score $= \Sigma a_i Y_i$ (Embretson and Reise, 2000).

We have just seen that some IRT models with different discrimination parameters require weighing with the discrimination parameter a as a weight. In reflective models using CTT, the scores of the items in multi-item instruments are sometimes weighted as well. For that purpose, weights obtained from factor analysis can be used (Hawthorne *et al.*, 2007). However, a weighted score is not necessarily better. First, it should be recognized that a weighted score will show a high correlation with an unweighted score, because (under CTT) all items are correlated, and secondly, the weights apply to the populations in which the weights were assessed, and not necessarily to other populations. Therefore, the item scores are usually summed up without weights.

3.6.2 Summarizing scores in formative models

As shown in Table 3.4, multidimensional constructs can be measured by indexes, in which each item represents a different dimension. These are based on formative models. The term index is used for an instrument consisting of multiple dimensions, which are summarized in one score. The term profile is used for a multidimensional construct that consists of different dimensions for which a score is presented for each dimension. Each dimension may consist of either a single item, or a number of items representing a unidimensional scale. In the latter case, the profile is a combination of a reflective and a formative model. Some examples will illustrate the distinction between indexes and profiles.

There are various comorbidity indexes (De Groot *et al.*, 2003), and most of these use a weighing system to summarize the number of comorbid diseases and their severity or impact. Whelan *et al.* (2004) assessed the severity of diarrhoea by scoring using a stool chart. The stool chart consisted

Table 3.4 Overview of terms for multi-item measurement instruments

Terms for multi-item measurement instruments	Unidimensional or multidimensional	Scores
Scale	Unidimensional: set of items measuring one dimension	Sum-scores based on a reflective model
Index	Multidimensional: set of items measuring different dimensions	Sum-score based on a formative model or observable constructs
Profile	Multidimensional	A score per dimension

of a visual presentation of three characteristics of the faecal output: the amount/weight (<100 g, 100–200 g, >200 g), the consistency (hard and formed, soft and formed, loose and unformed, liquid) and the frequency. They developed a scoring system to combine these three characteristics into a daily faecal score, which makes it an index.

The Multi-dimensional Fatigue Inventory (MFI; Smets *et al.*, 1995) consists of a number of scales based on a reflective model. The scores on these unidimensional scales are presented separately, i.e. the different dimensions are not summed. The results of the MFI are therefore expressed as a profile. For cancer staging, the TNM system is used, which expresses whether or not there is a tumour (T), whether or not there are positive nodules (N) and whether or not there are metastases (M). These three characteristics are always presented separately and never summed or summarized in another way. Therefore, we call it a profile.

Before we elaborate on how sum-scores for instruments containing different dimensions should be calculated, we first discuss whether they should be combined at all. There is no simple yes or no answer to this question. From a theoretical point of view, it is incorrect to combine them, because we know that we are comparing apples with oranges when summing up items from multidimensional constructs. Thus, summing loses information about the underlying separate dimensions. For theoretical reasons, presenting one score per domain (i.e. a profile) is preferable (Feinstein, 1987; Fayers and Machin, 2007). However, for practical reasons one overall score is sometimes used. One sum-score is much easier to work with, and in the end we usually want to have one answer as to whether or not, for example, overall fatigue has improved. However, if we want to intervene in a patient with fatigue in clinical practice, we have to know which domain is most affected. This is in analogy with school marks. Of course, we want to assess the performance of pupils with regard to their languages, mathematics, geography and so on, but in the end we have to determine whether the pupils will pass or fail their exams. In that case, a summarization of the scores is needed. This may be a sum-score or an average score, but the example of exam scoring also suggests other algorithms that may be applied (e.g. when failing an exam it is, in particular, the lowest scores that are important).

3.6.3 Weighted scores

In indexes, in which every item represents a different dimension, each item is often given the same weight. There are various diagnostic criteria, based on a number of signs and/or symptoms, which are indicative of a certain disease. For example, to diagnose complex regional pain syndrome type 1 in one of the extremities (e.g. the right foot), five criteria are postulated: the presence of unexplained diffuse pain; colour changes in the right foot compared with the left foot; swelling; differences in body temperature in the right foot compared with the left foot; and a limited active range of motion in the right foot. If four of these five criteria are satisfied, the patient is considered to have complex regional pain syndrome type 1 (Veldman *et al.*, 1993). In this case, the criteria have equal weights.

There are also examples of indexes in which items receive different weights. The visual rating scale of hyperintensities observed on MRI for the diagnosis of AD (see Table 3.2) is an example of the use of different weights, with a maximum score of 6 for periventrical hyperintensities and a maximum score of 30 for basal ganglia hyperintensities.

3.6.3.1 How and by who are weights assigned

When it is decided that the different dimensions should be given different weights, the important questions are 'who chooses the weighting scheme?' and 'how is this accomplished?'. Factor analysis is not an option here, because in formative models correlation between the items or dimensions is not expected. The weights may be decided upon by the researchers or the patients. Empirical evidence may guide the weighting, but the weights are often chosen by subjective judgements. Note that by just summing up or averaging the scores, equal weights are implicitly assigned to each domain.

Judgemental weights

For PRO instruments, it is sensible to let patients weigh the importance of the various dimensions. For this purpose, weights are sometimes decided upon in a consensus procedure involving patients. The resulting weights are then considered to be applicable to the 'average' patient. However, it is known that patients can differ considerably with regard to what they consider as important, and this may even change in different stages of their disease, as was observed in terminally ill cancer patients (Westerman *et al.*, 2007). Therefore, some measurement instruments that have been developed use an individual weighting (Wright, 2000).

For example, the SEIQOL-DW (Schedule for Evaluation of Individual Quality Of Life with Direct Weighting (Browne *et al.*, 1997) is a QOL measurement instrument, in which the individual patient determines the importance of the various domains. For this purpose the total HRQL is represented by a circle. The patient mentions the five areas of life that are most important to him/her. For the direct weighting the patient, with help from the researcher, divides the circle into five pie segments according to the relative importance of these five areas of life, with percentages that add up to 100%. Then the patient rates the quality of these five areas on a vertical 0–100 VAS. The ultimate SEIQOL-DW score is calculated as the sum of the score for each of the five areas multiplied by the percentage of relative importance of that area.

Empirical weights

There are different methods that can be used to assign weights to the dimensions, based on empirical evidence. As can be deduced from Figure 2.4, in a formative model the relationship between the construct η and the items X_i can be represented as follows:

$$\eta = \beta_1 X_1 + \beta_2 X_2 + \beta_3 X_3 + \beta_4 X_4 + \cdots + \beta_k X_k + \delta.$$

This formula resembles a regression equation. In regression analysis, we have data about k independent variables X_i, and a dependent variable Y, which are all directly measurable. However, in the formula above we face a problem: we have an unobservable construct η instead of Y. So, although we know that η is a composition of the Xs, we cannot calculate how it is determined by the Xs because we cannot measure η. We need an external criterion to obtain an independent assessment of η. Sometimes only one item is used to ask about the global rating of the construct. That is why we remarked earlier in this chapter (Section 3.3) that it is wise to include such a global item.

A more satisfying approach is to use more than one item to estimate η. We have seen that latent constructs can best be estimated by several reflective items. This observation leads to a model with multiple indicator (reflective) items and multiple causal (formative) items. Such a model is called a MIMIC model, i.e. a model with multiple indicators and multiple causes (see Figure 3.5). The upper part of this model (i.e. the relationship between Ys and η) is a reflective model, and the lower part (i.e. the relationship between Xs and η) is a formative model. Now the construct η is

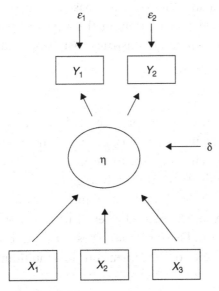

Figure 3.5   MIMIC model.

estimated by both Y_1 and Y_2 and by X_1, X_2 and X_3. Here we enter the field of structural equation modelling.

For example, we know that SES, represented by the construct η in Figure 3.5, is composed of education level, income and profession, represented by the Xs. However, we cannot perform a regression analysis until we know the values of SES (construct η). We might therefore formulate items that try to measure SES via a reflective model, represented by the items Y_1 and Y_2. Examples of such questions are: 'How high up are you on the social ladder?' and 'How do you rate your socio-economic status?'. Structural equation modelling is used to estimate the βs corresponding to the Xs. For a gentle introduction to structural equation modelling we refer to Streiner (2006).

This MIMIC model is not yet widely used within medicine, but it may be a useful strategy to calculate sum-scores or to obtain more information about the relative importance of the various determinants (Xs). At the same time, some comments have to be made. First, we are assuming that we have all the important components (Xs) in our analyses. Secondly, we have to realize that there is circular reasoning in this model: we are using suboptimal items (Ys) to find a way to measure the construct η with the use of Xs. And thirdly, which measurement of construct η do we prefer: the formative part in which we define the construct, based on its components now that we know the relative contribution, or the reflective part, which is based on questions about our total construct (Atkinson and Lennox, 2006)?

3.6.3.2 Preference weighting or utility analysis

Patient preferences and the relative importance of different aspects of a construct are often assessed by utility analysis, a method that is taken from economics. In these analysis choices have to be made between different resources, based on the individual valuation of these goods. Typical methods used to measure utilities are standard gamble and time trade-off techniques (Drummond *et al.*, 2005). Another method to elicit patient preferences is called conjoint analysis (Ryan and Farrar, 2000). These methods can be used to analyse the relative importance of the dimensions in a multidimensional instrument.

Table 3.5 Overview of strategies for the weighting of domains in formative models

Method of weighting	Who determines the weights?
Judgemental	Patient groups
	Individual patients
	Researchers
Empirical	Structural equation modelling
	Preference analysis or utility analysis

3.6.3.3 Alternative methods

In some situations, neither simple summations nor weighted sums appear to be justified, and in some areas it is questionable whether domains can be summed at all. In the case of HRQL, there are several variables that may each individually lead to a low QOL, such as severe pain or severe depression. In these situations the construct (e.g. QOL) is mainly determined by the domain with the lowest score, and other domains will be given less weight. Another example is the burden of pain. If patients who have pain in more than one location in their body have to rate the overall burden of their pain, the most serious location will overrule all the others, and the others will add only little or nothing to the burden. However, as soon as pain in the most serious location disappears, the pain in other locations gains more weight. In such examples the overall score will be equal to the maximum (or minimum) value of the Xs, expressed as max (or min) $(X_1, X_2, X_3, \cdots, X_k) \equiv X$. Note that such a strategy to calculate scores also applies to school exams.

Table 3.5 presents an overview of the methods of weighing informative models.

3.7 Pilot-testing

The development of a measurement instrument progresses through a number of test phases, as shown in Figure 3.1 depicting the iterative process. The first draft of the measurement instrument is tested in a small sample of patients (e.g. 15–30 persons), after which adaptations will follow. This pilot-testing is intended to test the comprehensibility, relevance, and acceptability and feasibility of the measurement instrument. Pilot-testing is necessary not only for questionnaires, but also for other newly developed measurement instruments. We will first describe the aim of pilot-testing the PRO instruments, followed by pilot-testing the non-PRO instruments.

3.7.1 Pilot-testing of patient-reported outcomes instruments

For PRO instruments, comprehensibility is of major importance. Asking students or colleagues to fill in the questionnaire, or asking persons who do not suffer from the disease can be a very useful first step. It is a fast and cheap method that can immediately reveal a number of problems (Collins, 2003). However, it is not sufficient. After adaptations, the target population must be involved in the pilot-testing, because only the target population can judge comprehensibility, relevance and completeness. With regard to comprehensibility, for example, only patients with a fluctuating intensity of pain experience difficulties in answering the question about 'severity of pain during the past 24 hours', and will ask for further specification about whether average pain or maximum pain is meant. With regard to relevance, for example, the question 'relaxation therapy reduces my pain' contains the implicit assumption that everybody in the target population has had experience with relaxation therapy. If 'not applicable' is not one of the response options for this item, patients who have never received relaxation therapy will answer no, or give a neutral answer, or leave this item open, resulting in a missing value. To test for completeness, it is wise to ask at the end of the list of questions whether patients feel that items they consider relevant are missing from the list, and because participants in the pilot-testing are from the relevant study population, this is an easy way to ensure that no important items have been left out.

In the pilot-testing, after participants have completed the questionnaire, they should be asked about their experience. This should go deeper than simply asking whether the questions were comprehensible or whether they had any problems with the response categories. Two well-known methods are 'think aloud' and 'probing'. Using the 'think aloud' method, patients are invited to say exactly what they are thinking when filling in the questionnaire. How do they interpret the various terms? How do they choose their answers? What context do they use to answer the questions? Do they think about their most serious episodes, or do they take some kind of average? In the 'probing' method, patients are questioned in detail by a researcher about the perceived content and interpretation of the items. The interviewer can ask how they interpreted specific words, and why they chose a specific response category. It might be interesting to ask, for example, which reference the patients used to rate their QOL. Did they compare themselves to other people of the same age or to the situation before they became ill, or do they have some other point of reference? Patients may differ in this respect (Fayers *et al.*, 2007). The Three Step Test Interview (Van der Veer *et al.*, 2003) combines the think aloud and the probing methods, and is therefore a very powerful tool with which to establish whether the patients understand the questions or tasks, whether they do so in a consistent way, and in the way the researcher intended. We used this method to evaluate the TAMPA Scale of Kinesiophobia, an existing questionnaire that was considered to be well validated. It emerged that patients had difficulties with some of the wording, and that some items contained implicit assumptions (Pool *et al.*, 2009).

Acceptability refers to the question of whether or not patients are willing to do something, and feasibility refers to whether or not they are able to do it. We might question whether patients are willing to keep a food diary in which they register the amounts of all the foods they eat during a period of 3 days, or whether they are willing to fill in questionnaires when this takes more than half an hour, i.e. acceptability. Whether or not patients are able to fill in the questionnaire themselves or whether an interview would be more adequate are examples of feasibility. Feasibility will depend on the difficulty of the questionnaire and the age and capacities of the patients. In some situations 'proxy' respondents may be needed, for example, family members or care-givers who answer if patients themselves are not able to do so. Furthermore, the length of the questionnaire is important. This can be assessed in the pilot-testing: how long does it take the respondents to complete the questionnaire? When a questionnaire is too long patients may lose concentration or motivation before the end of the questionnaire. Note that in research, the individual measurement instruments may be quite short, but a battery of 10 fairly short questionnaires may add up to a 60-min questionnaire. What is acceptable and feasible depends heavily on the age, fitness and capabilities of the patients.

3.7.2 Pilot-testing of non-patient-reported outcomes instruments

In this chapter, we have focused on questionnaires, but several issues are also relevant for other newly developed measurement instruments. For many tests in which the patients are actively involved, such as mental tests or physical capacity or performance tests, it is necessary to check whether the instructions to patients are unambiguous and well understood by patients. This concerns comprehensibility.

The measurement instrument has to be acceptable to patients. For non-PRO instruments, important questions are, for example, whether patients are willing to carry an accelerometer for a number of days, or whether they want to participate in a performance test when their knees are still rather painful. With imaging techniques, other considerations play a role, i.e. radiation load or other invasive aspects of some tests.

The terms acceptability and feasibility apply to both patients undergoing the tests and researchers performing the tests. For example, from the researcher's point of view, a test that takes 30 min may not be feasible, whereas it may be acceptable for the patients.

It goes without saying that if the measurement instrument undergoes substantial adaptations after the pilot-testing, the revised instrument should be tested again in a new sample of the target population.

3.8 Summary

Researchers have a tendency to develop new measurement instruments. However, so many measurement instruments are already available in all fields that investigators should justify their reasons for developing any new instrument. Nevertheless, although in general we discourage the development of new instruments, we have still explained 'how to do it', because we know that people will do it anyway. We also acknowledge that in some situations it is necessary, because no suitable measurement instrument is available.

There are a number of important points that we want to repeat at the end of this chapter. First of all, a detailed definition of the construct to be measured is indispensable. Secondly, expertise about the content of a field is essential. This holds for all measurements. Methodologically sound strategies cannot replace good content. Thirdly, during the construction of a measurement instrument (e.g. item selection) the future application of the measurement instrument (target population, purpose, research or practice) should be kept in mind. Fourthly, development is an iterative process, i.e. a continuous process of evaluation and adaptation. The pilot-testing should be rigorous and adequate time should be reserved for adaptations and retesting.

We have discussed some consequences of the type of measurement model in the development of measurement instruments: when dealing with reflective models, items may replace each other, while using a formative model all relevant items should be included. Moreover, in unidimensional scales the scores for the items can easily be added together or averaged. In constructs with several dimensions, or indexes, it is more difficult to calculate an overall score, and profile scores are often preferred over total scores. As a consequence, unidimensional or narrow constructs are much easier to interpret than complex multidimensional constructs, which is why the former are preferred. Methods to deal with formative models are under development, for example in the field of marketing research, but applications in clinical and health research are still scarce.

The first draft of a measurement instrument should undergo pilot-testing, to establish whether patients can understand the questions or tasks, whether they do so in a consistent way, and in the way the researcher intended. In addition, a measurement instrument should be tested for its acceptability and feasibility. If it has been adapted substantially, it is wise to repeat the pilot-testing in a new sample of the target population.

Assignments

1. Definition of a construct

Suppose you want to increase the physical activity of sedentary office workers. How would you define the construct physical activity in this context? Take into account the following considerations:

(a) Why do you want to increase their physical activity?
(b) What kind of physical activity do you want to measure?

(c) Which different aspects of physical activity do you want to measure?

(d) How does the purpose of the measurement affect what you want to measure?

2. Choice between objective and subjective measurements

(a) Suppose you want to measure walking ability in elderly patients, 6 months after a hip replacement because of osteoarthritis. Can you give an example of a subjective and objective measurement instrument to assess walking ability?

(b) Which one would you prefer?

(c) Give an example of a research question for which an objective measurement would be the most appropriate, and an example of a research question that would require a subjective measurement.

3. Choice between a reflective and a formative model

Juniper *et al.* (1997) developed an Asthma Quality of Life Questionnaire (AQLQ). They based this on 152 items that are, as they say in the abstract of their paper, 'potentially troublesome to patients with asthma'. In addition to outcome measures, which focused on symptoms, their aim was to develop a questionnaire to assess the impact of the symptoms and other aspects of the disease on the patient's life. Examples of such items were: 'How often during the past 2 weeks did you feel afraid of getting out of breath?', 'In general, how often during the last 2 weeks have you felt concerned about having asthma?', 'How often during the past 2 weeks has your asthma interfered with getting a good night's sleep?', and 'How often during the past 2 weeks did you feel concerned about the need to take medication for your asthma?'.

From this set of 152 items, they wanted to select certain items for inclusion in the AQLQ. They decided to compare two strategies to achieve this goal: one based on a reflective model and the other based on a formative model.

(a) What do you think of their plan to compare these two strategies for item selection?

(b) Which model would you prefer in this situation?

4. Cross-cultural adaptation of an item

In the Netherlands, almost everybody has a bicycle, which is used to travel short distances (e.g. going to school, to work or for trips within town). If persons are no longer able to use their bicycle, because of some kind of physical disability, this might limit their social participation.

A typical item in a Dutch questionnaire is: 'I am able to ride my bike', with response options: 'strongly disagree' (0) to 'strongly agree' (4).

Suppose you have to cross-culturally adapt this item for use in a research project in the USA. You expect that over 50% of the respondents will answer: 'not applicable' to this item. How would you deal with that item if you know that:

(a) The item is one of 10 items in a scale to assess physical functioning, assuming a reflective model.

(b) The item is one of 10 items in a scale to assess physical functioning, based on IRT, and therefore assuming a hierarchy in the difficulty of the items.

(c) The item is one of 10 items in an index concerning social participation, assuming a formative model.

5. Use of sum-scores

(a) In Assignment 2 of Chapter 2 we introduced the Neck Bournemouth Questionnaire, and concluded that this questionnaire included several different constructs. The authors calculate an overall score of the seven items. Do you agree with this decision?

(b) Some of the Neck Disability Index (NDI) items are presented in Table 3.6. Do these items correspond with a reflective model or a formative model?

(c) Would you calculate a sum-score for this questionnaire?

Table 3.6 Some items of the Neck Disability Index

---

(1) Pain intensity
- ☐ I have no pain at the moment
- ☐ The pain is very mild at the moment
- ☐ The pain is moderate at the moment
- ☐ The pain is fairly severe at the moment
- ☐ The pain is very severe at the moment
- ☐ The pain is the worst imaginable at the moment

(2) Personal care (washing, dressing, etc.)
- ☐ I can look after myself normally without causing extra pain
- ☐ I can look after myself normally but it causes extra pain
- ☐ It is painful to look after myself and I am slow and careful
- ☐ I need some help but manage most of my personal care
- ☐ I need help every day in most aspects of self-care
- ☐ I do not get dressed, I wash with difficulty and stay in bed

(3) Lifting
- ☐ I can lift heavy weights without extra pain.
- ☐ I can lift heavy weights but it gives extra pain.
- ☐ Pain prevents me from lifting heavy weights off the floor, but I could manage if they are conveniently positioned, for example on a table.
- ☐ Pain prevents me from lifting heavy weights, but I can manage light to medium weights if they are conveniently positioned
- ☐ I can lift very light weights.
- ☐ I cannot lift or carry anything at all.

(4) Reading
- ☐ I can read as much as I want to with no pain in my neck.
- ☐ I can read as much as I want to with slight pain in my neck.
- ☐ I can read as much as I want with moderate pain in my neck.
- ☐ I can't read as much as I want because of moderate pain in my neck.
- ☐ I can hardly read at all because of severe pain in my neck.
- ☐ I cannot read at all.

(5) Headaches
- ☐ I have no headaches at all.
- ☐ I have slight headaches, which come infrequently.
- ☐ I have moderate headaches, which come infrequently.
- ☐ I have moderate headaches, which come frequently.
- ☐ I have severe headaches, which come frequently.
- ☐ I have headaches almost all the time.

Field-testing: item reduction and data structure

4.1 Introduction

Field-testing of the measurement instrument is still part of the development phase. When a measurement instrument is considered to be satisfactory after one or more rounds of pilot-testing, it has to be applied to a large sample of the target population. The aims of this field-testing are item reduction and obtaining insight into the structure of the data, i.e. examining the dimensionality and then deciding on the definitive selection of items per dimension. These issues are only relevant for multi-item instruments that are used to measure unobservable constructs. Therefore, the focus of this chapter is purely on these measurement instruments. Other newly developed measurement instruments (e.g. single-item patient-reported outcomes (PROs)) and instruments to measure observable constructs go straight from the phase of pilot-testing to the assessment of validity, responsiveness and reliability (see Figure 3.1).

It is important to distinguish between pilot-testing and field-testing. Broadly speaking, pilot-testing entails an intensive qualitative analysis of the items in a relatively small number of representatives of the target population, and field-testing entails a quantitative analysis. Some of these quantitative techniques, such as factor analysis (FA) and the item response theory (IRT), require data from a large number of representatives of the target population. This means that for adequate field-testing a few hundred patients are required.

In this chapter, the various steps to be taken in field-testing are described in chronological order. We start to examine the responses to the individual items. In multi-item instruments based on a formative model (see

Sections 2.5 and 3.4.3), item reduction is based on the importance of the items. Therefore, the importance of the items has to be judged by the patients in order to decide which items should be retained in the instrument. In the case of reflective models, FA is one of the methods used for item reduction, and at the same time, this is a method to decide on the number of relevant dimensions. After the identification of various dimensions, the items within each dimension are examined in more detail. Note that in all these phases, item reduction and adaptation of the measurement instrument may take place.

4.2 Examining the item scores

The example in this section concerns a multi-item questionnaire to assess the coping behaviour of patients with hearing impairments: the Communication Profile of the Hearing Impaired (CPHI). There is evidence that coping behaviour is a more relevant indicator of psychosocial problems in people with hearing impairment than the degree and nature of the hearing impairment (Mokkink *et al.*, 2009). The CPHI questionnaire was derived from a more extensive US questionnaire. In this example, we focus on the dimension of maladaptive behaviour. The eight items of this scale are presented in Table 4.1. Consecutive patients ($n = 408$) in an audiological centre completed the questionnaire. The items were scored on a Likert scale (score 0–4), ranging from 'usually' or 'almost always' (category 0) to 'rarely' or 'almost never' (category 4). Table 4.1 shows the percentage of missing scores for each item and the distribution of the population over the response categories. From these data, a number of important characteristics of the items can be derived. This holds for instruments based on formative models as well as on reflective models.

4.2.1 Missing scores

Missing scores and patterns of missing scores may point to various problems. If scores are often missing for some items, we have to take a closer look at the formulation of these items. Possible explanations for incidental missing scores are that the patients do not understand these items, the items are not applicable to them, or the patients' answers do not fit the response options. Missing scores might also occur when patients don't know the answer or

Table 4.1 Presentation of missing scores and distribution of the responding population ($n = 408$) over the response categories of the CPHI – 'maladaptive behaviour' scale

Item	Content of the items	Missing scores (% of 408)	Distribution of responding population (%) over the response options				
			0	1	2	3	4
19	One way I get people to repeat what they said is by ignoring them	1.2	0.7	2.2	5.5	26.3	65.3
32	I tend to dominate conversations so I won't have to listen to others	1.0	2.2	6.7	7.2	22.5	61.4
37	If someone seems irritated at having to repeat, I stop asking them to do so and pretend to understand	1.7	9.5	15.7	8.5	34.6	31.7
38	I tend to avoid social situations where I think I'll have problems hearing	1.7	8.2	18.5	14.2	22.7	36.4
41	I avoid conversing with others because of my hearing loss	0.7	4.0	7.7	9.1	32.0	47.2
44	When I don't understand what someone said, I pretend that I understood it	0	2.0	8.8	8.6	46.1	34.5
48	I avoid talking to strangers because of my hearing loss	0.2	4.9	7.1	8.9	26.8	52.3
58	When I don't understand what someone has said, I ignore them	0.2	5.4	7.9	8.8	36.9	41.0

don't want to give the answer. The latter might be the case, for example, for items about sexual activity or about income. After an appropriate pilot study, all these reasons for missing scores should have already been identified and remedied. Many missing scores at the end of the questionnaire may point to loss of concentration or motivation of the patients. In Table 4.1, we see that for the items of the CPHI subscale 'maladaptive behaviour' there were incidental missing scores, but less than 2% per item.

It is difficult to say what percentage of missing scores is acceptable. One should consider deleting incidental items with a large percentage of missing scores, and try to replace them with items for which less missing values are expected. The decision should be based on the weighting between percentage of missing scores and the importance of that specific item. It is quite arbitrary where the border between 'acceptable' and 'not acceptable' lies, but in our opinion, in most cases less than 3% is acceptable, and more than 15% is not acceptable.

4.2.2 Distribution of item scores

It is important to inspect the distribution of the score at item level in order to check whether all response options are informative, and to check whether there are items for which a large part of the population has the same score.

To check whether all response options are informative, using classical test theory (CTT), we can determine to what extent the response options are used. If there are too many response options in an ordinal scale, there may be categories that are seldom used. In that case, combining these options might be considered. For example, if on a seven-point ordinal scale the extreme categories are not frequently used, combining the categories 1 and 2, and categories 6 and 7 might be an option.

In IRT analysis, it is possible to draw per item response curves for each response option on the ordinal scale. These response curves present the probability of choosing that option, given a certain level of the trait. We have seen such response curves in Figure 2.5, in which three dichotomous items were presented. Items with ordinal response options result in multiple curves per item. The response curve of item 58 of the CPHI is presented in Figure 4.1. At the lower trait levels, patients most probably score in category 0, and at the highest trait level, category 4 is the most probable score.

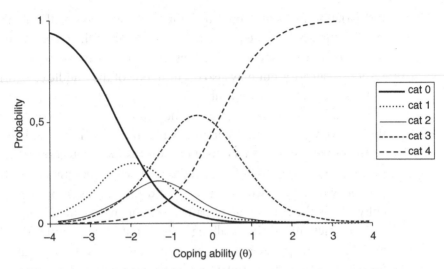

Figure 4.1   Response curves for the five response options of item 58 of the CPHI.

At trait level 0, category 3 will most probably be chosen as the response option. We see that there is no position on the trait level where category 2 has the highest probability to be scored. So, for item 58, category 2 does not add much information. When items have many response options, there is a higher chance that some are non-informative. If in a questionnaire one specific response category provides little information for almost all items, one may decide to delete this category.

The distribution of the population over the response categories also provides information about the discriminative power of an item. Items for which a large part of the population has a similar score are barely able to discriminate between patients, and therefore contain less information. The distribution of the population over the response categories can easily be seen from frequency tables, as shown in Table 4.1. For items scored on a continuous scale (e.g. a visual analogue scale), the mean item score and the standard deviation (SD) provide information about the distribution. Very high or very low mean item scores represent items on which almost everybody agrees or disagrees, or, if items assess ability, very easy items that almost everybody is able to do or difficult items that almost nobody is able to do. Item variance is expressed in the SD of the item scores. Items with a small SD, indicating that the variation in population scores for this item is low, will contribute little to discrimination of the population. Clustering of the scores of all patients into one or two response categories often occurs in the highest or lowest response category, but may also occur in one of the middle categories.

With regard to the CPHI subscale 'maladaptive behaviour', in Table 4.1 we see that for all items the majority of the population scored 3 or 4. This means that on average the patients do not exhibit much 'maladaptive behaviour'.

The distribution of the population over response categories also provides information about the difficulty of items. For this analysis, we only use the patients who responded. In the case of dichotomous responses, item difficulty equals the percentage of patients endorsing the item. For example, in an instrument measuring 'walking ability', an item containing an activity that only 10% of the population scores positive, is more difficult than an activity for which 95% of the population scores positive. The difficulty of the items can also be judged in an ordinal scale with a small number of categories. Table 4.1 shows that the eight items of the maladaptive behaviour scale have about the same degree of 'difficulty'. In the context of behaviour, 'easy items' reflect behaviour that patients with slight maladaptive behaviour will already exhibit, while 'difficult' items reflect behaviour that is typical for patients with severe maladaptive behaviour. What this means for the use of the scale will be discussed in Section 4.6, after we have examined the structure of the data and identified which scales can be distinguished. We will first discuss item reduction in instruments based on formative models.

4.3 Importance of the items

The issue of importance of the items is most relevant for formative models. As explained in Chapter 3 (Section 3.4.3), the strategy for the development of multi-item instruments based on formative models (indexes) differs from the strategy for the development of multi-item instruments based on reflective models (scales). As stated in Section 3.4.3, FA has no role in instruments based on formative models. In these instruments the most important items should all be represented. This implies that for the decision with regard to which items should be included we need a rating of their importance. These ratings of importance can be obtained from focus groups or interviews with patients, but they are usually determined during field-testing. For example, Juniper *et al.*

(1992) used such a method for the development of the Asthma Quality of Life Questionnaire (see Assignment 3, Chapter 3). They had a set of 152 potential items to measure several domains of quality of life impairment that are important to adult patients with asthma. Domains of quality of life impairment included asthma symptoms, emotional problems caused by asthma, troublesome environmental stimuli, problems associated with the avoidance of environmental stimuli, activities limited by asthma and practical problems. In a structured interview, 150 adults with asthma were asked which of the 152 items had been troublesome for them at any time during the past year. In addition, they were asked to indicate the importance of each of the identified items on a five-point scale, ranging from 'not very important' to 'extremely important'. For each item the percentage that labelled the item as troublesome (frequency), and the mean importance score of those labelling the items as troublesome were multiplied, resulting in a mean impact score between 0 and 5. For example, 92% reported 'shortness of breath' as troublesome, and the importance of this item was, on average, rated as 3.60, resulting in a mean impact score of 3.31 (0.92 × 3.60). The item 'keeping surroundings dust-free' was rated as troublesome by 51% of the population, with a mean importance score of 3.96, resulting in a mean impact score of 2.02 (0.51 × 3.96). Within each domain, Juniper et al. (1992) chose the items with the highest mean impact score for their instrument. Additional criteria were adequate representation of both physical and emotional function and a minimum of four items per domain.

Performing item reduction in this way implies that items with low mean impact scores are not included in the measurement instrument. The reason for this is that these items are either not troublesome or not important for most of the patients. In this way, the final selection of items for the instrument is made.

For measurement instruments based on reflective models, the importance of the items for the patients is a less relevant criterion for item reduction. For these models, specific statistical techniques are available to guide item reduction. These will be discussed in the remainder of this chapter.

4.4 Examining the dimensionality of the data: factor analysis

Identification of dimensions is important for the scoring of items (as we saw in Section 3.6), but also for the interpretation of the results (as will be discussed in Chapter 8). FA is the most used method to examine the dimensionality of the data. FA is an extension of CTT, and is based on item correlations. The basic principle is that items that correlate highly with each other are clustered in one factor, while items within one factor preferably show a low correlation with items belonging to other factors. The goal of FA is to examine how many meaningful dimensions can be distinguished in a construct. In addition, FA serves item reduction, because items that have no contribution or an unclear contribution to the factors can be deleted.

Within FA, exploratory FA (EFA) and confirmatory FA (CFA) can be distinguished. When there are no clear-cut ideas about the number of dimensions, the factor structure of an instrument can best be investigated with EFA. If previous hypotheses about dimensions of the construct are available, based on theory or previous analyses, CFA is more appropriate: it tests whether the data fit a predetermined factor structure. For that reason, EFA is usually applied in the development phase of the instrument. CFA is mainly used to assess construct validity, and will be discussed in Chapter 6, which focuses on validity.

In this chapter, we describe EFA. Within EFA, principal components analysis (PCA) and common FA can be distinguished. Although the theoretical principles of PCA and common FA differ, the results are usually quite similar. In practice, PCA is most often used because, statistically, it is the simplest method. For details about the choice between various methods of FA we refer to a paper written by Floyd and Widaman (1995). We are not going to elaborate in detail on the statistical background of FA, but we will describe the principles and various steps that must be taken. We use an example to illustrate the procedure and interpretation. For introductory information about FA we refer to books written by Fayers and Machin (2007: Chapter 6) and Streiner and Norman (2008: Appendix C).

4.4.1 Principles of exploratory factor analysis

FA is based on item correlations. Items that correlate highly with each other are clustered in one factor, and these items share variance which is explained by the underlying dimension. With FA, we try to identify these factors, and

Table 4.2 Correlation matrix^a of Y_i with F_j, representing factor loadings (λ_{ij}), and explained variances of factors and items

Variable	Factor loadings					Communalities = explained variance (R^2)
	Factor 1	Factor 2	Factor 3	...	Factor m	
Y_1	0.658	0.048	−0.324	...	...	$\Sigma \lambda_{1j}^2 =$ explained variance of Y_1 by $F_1 \dots F_m$
Y_2	0.595	0.035	−0.527	...	...	$\Sigma \lambda_{2j}^2 =$ explained variance of Y_2 by $F_1 \dots F_m$
Y_3	0.671	−0.116	0.154	...	...	
...	...	...	...	...	...	
Y_{k-1}	0.511	0.500	−0.085	...	...	
Y_k	0.459	0.441	−0.185	...	...	$\Sigma \lambda_{kj}^2 =$ explained variance of Y_k by $F_1 \dots F_m$
Eigenvalue	$\Sigma \lambda_{i1}^2$	$\Sigma \lambda_{i2}^2$	$\Sigma \lambda_{i3}^2$	...	$\Sigma \lambda_{im}^2$	$\Sigma \Sigma \lambda_{ij}^2 =$ explained variance of $Y_1 \dots Y_k$ by $F_1 \dots F_m$

^{a} The term 'Component loading matrix' is used in SPSS.

explain as much as possible of the variance with a minimal number of factors. This is done by solving the following set of equations, which look like a series of regression equations:

$$Y_1 = \lambda_{11}F_1 + \lambda_{12}F_2 + \cdots + \lambda_{1m}F_m + \varepsilon_1,$$
$$Y_2 = \lambda_{21}F_1 + \lambda_{22}F_2 + \cdots + \lambda_{2m}F_m + \varepsilon_2,$$
$$\dots\dots\dots\dots\dots\dots\dots\dots\dots\dots\dots\dots\dots\dots$$
$$Y_k = \lambda_{k1}F_1 + \lambda_{k2}F_2 + \cdots + \lambda_{km}F_m + \varepsilon_k.$$

(4.1)

In these equations, Y_i are the observed values of the k items, F_j are the m factors and λ_{ij} represent the loadings of items Y on the respective factors. Each of the factors contributes to some extent to the different items, as can be seen in Formula 4.1. We prefer items that load high on one factor and low on the others. The factors F_1 to F_m are uncorrelated. When both F_j and Y_i are standardized (mean = 0; variance = 1) then λ_{ij} can be considered as standardized regression coefficients, based on the correlation matrix of Y with F, as presented in Table 4.2.

As illustration, some (fictive) factor loadings are presented in Table 4.2. We see that items Y_1 and Y_2 both load high on factor F_1, and low on factor F_2. This means that they both contribute considerably to the measurement of the dimension represented by factor F_1, and less to the dimension represented by factor F_2. The items Y_{k-1} and Y_k contribute to the dimensions represented by factors F_1 and F_2.

Several parameters in Table 4.2 need to be explained. The term λ_{ij}^2 is the square of the factor loading, and represents the percentage of variance of the item i that is explained by the factor j. For each factor, looking at the columns in Table 4.2, the sum of the squared factor loadings represents the total amount of variance in the data set that is explained by this factor and this is referred to as the eigenvalue of the factor. These eigenvalues are presented in the last row of Table 4.2. The eigenvalue divided by the number of items in the questionnaire is the percentage of variance in the data explained by the factor. For each item, looking at the rows in the table, the sum of the squared factor loadings represents the amount of explained variance of this item via all factors. This is called the communality.

PCA aims to explain as much as possible of the total variance in the instrument, with a minimal number of factors: $\Sigma \Sigma \lambda_{ij}^2$ is maximized. In PCA, the first factor F_1 explains the maximum variation $\Sigma \lambda_{i1}^2$, then F_2, uncorrelated with F_1, explains the maximum amount of the remaining variance $\Sigma \lambda_{i2}^2$, and so on.

4.4.2 Determining the number of factors

As an example, we examine the factor structure of a questionnaire to assess the physical workload of employees with musculoskeletal complaints (Bot *et al.*, 2004a). From the 'workload section' of the Dutch Musculoskeletal Questionnaire (Hildebrandt *et al.*, 2001) they selected only items that expressed force, dynamic and static load, repetitive load, (uncomfortable) postures, sitting, standing and walking. These 26 items formed the starting point of the FA. Response options were 0, 1, 2 or 3, corresponding to 'seldom or never', 'sometimes', 'often' and '(almost) always', thereby estimating the frequencies of postures, movements and tasks. The goal of their FA was to obtain a small number of factors that measure different dimensions of the construct 'physical workload'. We describe here the main steps and results of the analysis of data from 406 employees with complaints of the upper extremities. For the data set and syntax, we refer to the website www.clinimetrics.nl. This enables you to perform the analysis yourselves.

4.4.2.1 Step 1: correlation of items

A FA starts by examining the inter-item correlation matrix, presenting the correlation of all items with each other. Items that do not correlate with any of the others (< 0.2) can immediately be deleted, and items that show a very high correlation (> 0.9) must be considered carefully. If there are items that are almost identical, one of them may be deleted. Variables negatively correlated with the others may need a reverse score to facilitate interpretation at a later stage.

4.4.2.2 Step 2: the number of factors to be extracted

Table 4.3 shows the first 10 factors (called components in PCA) with their eigenvalues for the physical workload questionnaire. Looking at the column of the cumulative percentage of explained variances, we see that the first two factors explain 48.7% of the variance in the data set, the first six factors explain 68.0% and the first 10 factors explain 79.5%. Thus, the other 16 factors (there were 26 items and therefore a maximum of 26 factors) explain the remaining 20.5%.

Several criteria are used to decide how many factors are relevant. One criterion is to retain only those factors with an eigenvalue larger than 1. In the example (Table 4.3), that would be six factors. Another criterion to consider is the relative contribution of each additional factor. This can be judged from the 'elbow' in the scree plot (see Figure 4.2), in which the eigenvalue is plotted against the factors (components). Scree is a term given to an accumulation of broken rock fragments at the base of cliffs or mountains. This figure shows that the first two factors explain most of the variance, and a third factor adds very little extra information (the slope is almost flat). This corresponds with the observation in Table 4.3 that the percentages of variance explained by components 3–6 are relatively low.

Furthermore, it is important to check the cumulative percentage of explained variance after each factor. If the cumulative explained variance is low, more factors might be retained to provide a better account of the variance. Bot *et al.* (2004a) decided to retain six factors at this stage.

Table 4.3 Output PCA of 26-item 'physical workload' questionnaire showing the eigenvalues and percentages of variance explained by the factors

Total variance explained

| Component | Initial eigenvalues | | |
	Total	% of Variance	Cumulative %
1	8.966	34.484	34.484
2	3.701	14.236	48.721
3	1.575	6.058	54.779
4	1.349	5.189	59.967
5	1.077	4.141	64.108
6	1.014	3.898	68.006
7	0.872	3.355	71.361
8	0.797	3.067	74.428
9	0.718	2.763	77.191
10	0.588	2.261	79.452
...	...	...	...
25	0.164	0.632	99.470
26	0.138	0.530	100.000

Extraction method: principal components analysis.

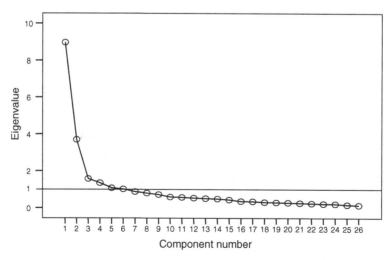

Figure 4.2   Scree plot of the eigenvalues of the 'physical workload' questionnaire. Reproduced from Bot *et al.* (2004a), with permission from BMJ Publishing Group, Ltd.

4.4.3 Rotation and interpreting the factors

4.4.3.1 Step 3: rotation

Rotation facilitates the interpretation of the factors: it results in factor load-ings that are closer to 1 or closer to 0. The communalities (i.e. the explained variance of Y_i), remain the same, but the percentage of variance explained by each factor might change. There are various rotation methods. Orthogonal rotation (e.g. Varimax) is often chosen, as we did in this example. This led to the rotated component matrix (shown on the website www.clinimetrics.nl).

4.4.3.2 Step 4: interpretation of the factors

It is important to note at this point that EFA is a statistical technique that requires the researcher to make subjective choices at several points. They should give 'labels' to the factors. This means that they should examine which items load on the same factor, decide what the common 'thing' is that these items measure, and give the factor a name that reflects the meaning of these items.

The decision with regard to how many factors should be retained is also quite arbitrary. The content of the factors and their interpretability often have a decisive role, because we don't want an instrument with factors with an unclear content. This choice is then supported by one or more of the other criteria: eigenvalue > 1 or scree plot. In our example there were six factors with eigenvalue > 1, but the scree plot showed that after two factors the slope flattened substantially. Bot *et al.* (2004a) could not find a meaning-ful interpretation for six factors. As their goal was to obtain a small number of factors, they decided to repeat the FA choosing only two factors, as sug-gested by the scree plot.

By repeating PCA with a two-factor model and applying orthogonal rota-tion (Varimax), the factor loadings depicted in Table 4.4 appeared. We see that most items load on either one of the two factors. Taking a closer look at the items, we see that factor 1 contains items related to 'heavy physical work' and factor 2 contains items that reflect 'long-lasting postures and repetitive movements'. These two factors could be interpreted in a meaningful way.

4.4.4 Optimizing the dimensionality

For item reduction, we examine the factor loadings in Table 4.4 in detail. Items that hardly load at all on any of the factors can be deleted. A min-imum loading of 0.5 (Nunnally and Bernstein, 1994; p. 536) is usually taken

Table 4.4 Factor loadings for two factors after Varimax rotation. Bot *et al.* (2004a), with permission

		Factor 1	Factor 2
1	Standing	**0.71**	0.08
2	Sitting	−0.77	0.16
3	Video display unit work	−0.72	0.25
4	Walking	**0.67**	−0.01
5	Kneeling/squatting	**0.72**	0.09
6	Repetitive movement	0.09	**0.77**
7	Twisted posture	0.35	**0.57**
8	Neck bent forward	0.14	**0.71**
9	Turning/bending neck	0.15	**0.71**
10	Wrists bent or twisted	0.15	**0.73**
11	Hands above shoulders	**0.65**	0.27
12	Hands below knees	**0.68**	0.22
13	Moving loads (> 5 kg)	**0.77**	0.19
14	Moving loads (> 25 kg)	**0.62**	0.19
15	Exerting force with arms	**0.82**	0.29
16	Maximal force exertions	**0.77**	0.34
17	Physical hard work	**0.77**	0.29
18	Static posture	−0.20	**0.78**
19	Uncomfortable posture	**0.50**	**0.55**
20	Working with vibrating tools	0.36	0.27
21	Handling pedals with feet	0.15	0.11
22	Climbing stairs	0.38	0.00
23	Often squatting	**0.69**	0.22
24	Walking on irregular surfaces	0.40	−0.02
25	Sitting/moving on knees	**0.54**	0.05
26	Repetitive tasks with arms/hands	−0.10	**0.77**
Eigenvalue		8.97	3.70
Variance explained before rotation[a]		34.5%	14.2%
Variance explained after rotation[a]		30.8%	17.9%
Total variance explained		48.7%	

Factor loadings ≥ 0.5 are in bold print.

Eigenvalues refer to the total variance explained by each factor.

[a] Percentage of the variance explained by each factor before and after Varimax rotation.

as threshold. With > 0.5 as threshold, the items 20, 21, 22 and 24 are problematic. These items apparently do not measure one of the aspects of the construct workload, and were therefore deleted from the measurement instrument. They should be deleted one by one, because the deletion of one item may change the loadings of the other items. Therefore, PCA should be performed again, after the deletion of each item.

Items that load substantially (> 0.3) on more than one factor also need consideration (Nunnally and Bernstein, 1994; p. 536). Although these items do measure aspects of workload, they are sometimes deleted because they hamper a clear interpretation. Moreover, in scoring they would add to more than one dimension. The decision with regard to whether or not to retain these items in the instrument will depend on how important they are for the construct under study. Items 7 and 19 were deleted for this reason. Bot *et al.* (2004a) also deleted the two items 'sitting' and 'video display unit work' at this point, because of their negative loading. In our example, we keep these items in to see what happens. So, based on the FA, we retain 20 of the original 26 items: 14 items contributing to factor 1 representing 'heavy physical work', and six items contributing to factor 2 representing 'long-lasting postures and repetitive movements'.

Selecting new items is still an option in this phase. When performing FA we might find a factor that consists of only a few items. If this factor represents a relevant aspect of the construct under study, we might consider formulating extra items for this dimension. In the example of 'physical workload', the items 'sitting' and 'video display unit work' might have resulted in a separate factor if there had been more items representing this same aspect. If the authors had considered this to be a relevant aspect, they could have formulated extra items to obtain a stronger factor. Ideally, there should be a minimum of three items contributing to one factor. Note that a new field study is required to examine the consequences of adding extra items to the factor structure (reflecting the iterative process represented in Figure 3.1).

4.4.5 Some remarks on factor analysis

First of all, we should note that when the conceptual phase of the development of a measurement instrument has been well thought out (i.e. there is a conceptual model), and an extensive examination of the literature has taken place, CFA could immediately be applied. In fact, it is strange that one would still have to explore the dimensions of the construct. For item reduction (i.e. deleting items that do not clearly load on one of the dimensions), EFA is well justified.

In our example, we used SPSS. The item correlations are calculated with Pearson's correlation coefficients, which assume normal distributions of the responses to the items. However, in the case of dichotomous response categories, FA should be based on tetrachoric correlations, and in the case of ordinal data polychoric correlations can be calculated. The program Mplus is suitable for these analyses.

A substantial number of patients are required to perform FA: rules of thumb vary from four to 10 patients per item with a minimum of 100 patients (Kline, 2000, p. 142). Other methods can be applied for smaller sample sizes.

4.4.6 Other methods to examine the dimensionality

One of the methods used to assess multidimensionality, applicable with smaller numbers, is multifactor or multidimensional inventories (Streiner and Norman, 2008, p. 96). According to theory or by examining inter-item correlations, items are clustered into a number of scales. Then, for each item, correlations with its own scale and the other scales are calculated. An item is said to belong to a subscale when the correlation with its own scale is high and the correlation with other scales is low. This method is far less powerful than FA.

Within IRT analysis, certain methods can be used to examine the dimensionality of a measurement instrument. However, these are quite complex, and seldom used for this purpose (Embretson and Reise, 2000). The number of dimensions is usually determined by FA. Subsequently, items in each dimension are examined in more detail by IRT analysis.

When FA or other methods have shown which items cluster into one dimension, we proceed to examine the functioning of items within such a unidimensional scale. We start by describing the principles of internal consistency based on CTT, followed by an illustration of examination of item characteristics with IRT techniques.

4.5 Internal consistency

Internal consistency is defined by the COSMIN panel as the degree of interrelatedness among the items (Mokkink *et al.*, 2010a). In a unidimensional (sub)scale of a multi-item instrument, internal consistency is a measure of the extent to which items assess the same construct. If there is one item that measures something else, this item will have a lower item-total correlation than the other items. If the assessment of internal consistency follows FA, as it should, it is obvious that the items within one factor will correlate. However, maybe one wants an instrument to be as short as possible. In that case, examination of the internal consistency is aimed at item reduction. It indicates which items can best be deleted, and also how many items can be deleted. First, we will examine inter-item and item-total correlations, and then assess and discuss Cronbach's alpha as a parameter of internal consistency.

4.5.1 Inter-item and item-total correlations

Inter-item correlations and item-total correlations indicate whether or not the item is part of the scale. We already had a look at the inter-item correlation matrix as the first step in FA, described in Section 4.4.2.1. After FA, the inter-item correlations found for items within one dimension should be between 0.2 and 0.5. If the correlation of two items is higher than 0.7, they measure almost the same thing, and one of them could be deleted. The range 0.2–0.5 is quite wide, but is dependent on the broadness of the construct to be measured. For example, 'extraversion' is a broad concept, expecting lower inter-item correlations within one scale, compared with a scale for 'talkativeness', which is a rather narrow concept.

The item-total correlation is a kind of discrimination parameter, i.e. it gives an indication of whether the items discriminate patients on the construct under study. For example, patients with a high score on a depression scale must have a higher score for each item than patients with a low score on the depression scale. If an item shows an item-total correlation of less than 0.3 (Nunnally and Bernstein, 1994), it does not contribute much to the distinction between mildly and highly depressed patients, and is a candidate for deletion.

4.5.2 Cronbach's alpha

Cronbach's alpha is a parameter often used to assess the internal consistency of a scale that has been shown to be unidimensional by FA. The basic

Table 4.5 Item total statistics

	Scale mean if item deleted	Scale variance if item deleted	Corrected item-total correlation	Squared multiple correlation	Cronbach's alpha if item deleted
1	23.35	37.953	0.511	0.607	0.749
2	23.43	56.801	−0.610	0.698	0.858
3	23.74	54.811	−0.523	0.531	0.848
4	23.56	39.167	0.491	0.462	0.751
5	24.19	40.637	0.636	0.595	0.745
11	24.05	40.392	0.583	0.465	0.747
12	24.21	40.535	0.648	0.582	0.744
13	23.69	37.034	0.756	0.705	0.725
14	24.20	40.379	0.606	0.614	0.746
15	23.57	35.425	0.811	0.769	0.715
16	23.97	37.691	0.786	0.773	0.726
17	23.85	36.971	0.743	0.674	0.726
23	23.76	38.618	0.650	0.525	0.738
25	24.47	43.670	0.455	0.352	0.762

principle of examining the internal consistency of a scale is to split the items in half and see whether the scores of two half-scales correlate. A scale can be split in half in many different ways. The correlation is calculated for each half-split. Cronbach's alpha represents a kind of mean value of these correlations, adjusted for test length. Cronbach's alpha is the best known parameter for assessing the internal consistency of a scale.

We continue with the example of the 'physical workload' questionnaire (Bot *et al.*, 2004a); see website www.clinimetrics.nl. In Sections 4.4.3 and 4.4.4 we identified a factor 'heavy physical work', which consisted of 14 items. Cronbach's alpha is 0.78 for this factor. In SPSS, using the option 'Cronbach's alpha if item deleted', one can see what the value of Cronbach's alpha would be if that item was deleted (Table 4.5). It appears that Cronbach's alpha increases most if item 2 is deleted (i.e. the item with the highest value in the last column); in the next step, after running a new analysis without item 2, deletion of item 3 would increase Cronbach's alpha most. This comes as no surprise, because these were the two items that showed negative correlations with the factor. Without these two items, Cronbach's alpha becomes 0.92 for a 12-item scale (see website www.clinimetrics.nl).

For reasons of efficiency, one might want to further reduce the number of items. A well-accepted guideline for the value of Cronbach's alpha is between 0.70 and 0.90. A value of 0.98, for example, indicates that there is a redundancy of items, and we might therefore want to delete some of the items. Again, the option 'Cronbach's alpha if item deleted' helps us to choose which item(s) to delete (i.e. the item with the highest value in the last column after running a new analysis). If we want an instrument with a limited number of items (e.g. to save time on a performance test), we can delete items until Cronbach's alpha starts to decrease below acceptable levels. As the 'physical workload' questionnaire was already short and easy to fill in, Bot *et al.* (2004a) decided not to reduce the number of items any further.

4.5.3 Interpretation of Cronbach's alpha

The internal consistency of a scale is often assessed, merely because it is so easy to calculate Cronbach's alpha. It requires only one measurement in a study population, and then 'one click on the button'. However, this α coefficient is very often interpreted incorrectly. As a warning against misinterpretation, we will now describe what Cronbach's alpha does *not* measure. For further details about this issue we refer to a paper written by Cortina (1993).

First, Cronbach's alpha is *not* a measure of the unidimensionality of a scale. When a construct consists of two or three different dimensions, then a reasonably high value for Cronbach's alpha can still be obtained for all items. In our example of the 'physical workload' questionnaire (Bot *et al.*, 2004a) we identified two factors: the 'heavy physical work' factor consisting of 12 items with a Cronbach's alpha of 0.92, and the 'long-lasting postures and repetitive movements' factor, consisting of six items with a Cronbach's alpha of 0.86. However, if we calculate Cronbach's alpha for all 20 items in the instrument, the value is 0.90. This is a high value for Cronbach's alpha, and does not reveal that there are two dimensions in this instrument. This shows that unidimensionality cannot be assessed with Cronbach's alpha.

Secondly, Cronbach's alpha does *not* assess whether the model is reflective or formative. It occurs quite often that only when a low Cronbach's alpha is observed, one starts to question whether one would expect the items in a measurement instrument to correlate (i.e. whether the measurement instrument is really based on a reflective model). But it is not as easy as simply stating that when Cronbach's alpha is low, it probably *is* a formative model. An alternative explanation for a low Cronbach's alpha is that the construct may be based on a reflective model, but the items are poorly chosen. So, Cronbach's alpha should not be used as a diagnostic parameter to distinguish between reflective and formative models.

Thirdly, it is sometimes argued that Cronbach's alpha is a parameter of validity. Cortina (1993) stated quite convincingly that this is a deceiving thought, because an adequate Cronbach's alpha (notwithstanding the number of items) suggests only that, on average, items in the scale are highly correlated. They apparently measure the same construct, but this provides no evidence as to whether or not the items measure the construct that they claim to measure. In other words, the items measure something consistently, but what *that* is, remains unknown. So, internal consistency is not a parameter of validity.

The value of Cronbach's alpha is highly dependent on the number of items in the scale. We used that principle for item reduction: when Cronbach's alpha is high we can afford to delete items to make the instrument more efficient. Reversely, when the value of Cronbach's alpha is too low, we can increase the value by formulating new items, which are manifestations of the same construct. This principle also implies that with a large number of items in a scale, Cronbach's alpha may have a high value, despite rather low inter-item correlations.

As can be seen in the COSMIN taxonomy (Figure 1.1), the measurement property 'internal consistency' is an aspect of reliability, which is the topic of Chapter 5. There we will explain why Cronbach's alpha is expected to be higher in instruments with a larger number of items.

4.6 Examining the items in a scale with item response theory

After we have illustrated how the dimensions in a construct are determined, and how the scales can be optimized by FA and further item-deletion based on calculations of Cronbach's alpha, we will show which additional analyses can be performed when the data fit an IRT model. As we already saw in Chapter 2 (Section 2.5.2) IRT can be used to examine item functioning characteristics, such as item difficulty and item discrimination. In addition, it can be used to estimate the location of the individual items on the level of the trait. Therefore, it is a powerful method with which to examine the distribution of the items over the scale in more detail. However, these characteristics can only be examined if the data fit an IRT model.

To illustrate the examination of items in relation to their scale, we will use data on the Roland–Morris Disability Questionnaire (RDQ), a 24-item self-report instrument to assess disability due to low back pain, with a dichotomous response option: *yes* or *no*. As the RDQ was originally not developed by means of IRT analysis, an explanation of why we use this example is justified. First of all, instruments with dichotomous response options are very illustrative of what happens in IRT analysis, and not many newly developed multi-item scales use dichotomous response options; secondly, the basic principles and their interpretations are similar in existing and newly developed scales. Note that many new scales use items from already existing scales.

The RDQ was completed by 372 patients suffering from chronic low back pain (own data). For all items, we present a frequency distribution. The percentage of patients who answered *yes* to each item, and the discrimination and difficulty parameters of all items on the RDQ are presented in Table 4.6. For dichotomous items, the frequency of endorsement is an indication of the item difficulty. Therefore, it is not surprising that the Pearson correlation coefficient between the percentage of patients answering *yes* and the difficulty parameter was 0.966 in this example.

4.6.1 Fit of an item response theory model

For IRT analysis, we first have to choose one of the available IRT models. The RDQ is an already existing questionnaire, so we therefore examined which IRT model showed the best fit with the RDQ data in the study population: the one-parameter Rasch model or the two-parameter Birnbaum model. If we are developing a new instrument (i.e. selecting and formulating new items), we can do it the other way around: first choose a model and then select only items that fit this model. For example, a researcher may try to develop an instrument that fits a one-parameter Rasch model, i.e. all items should have the same slope of the item characteristic curve. When testing a large number of items, only items with a high and similar discrimination parameter (i.e. with steep item characteristic curves) are selected. Items with item characteristic curves that deviate too much are deleted. So, in that case

Table 4.6 Frequency distribution, item difficulty and discrimination parameters for 24 items of the Roland–Morris Disability Questionnaire (RDQ)

	Items of the RDQ	% yes	Dicrimination parameter a	Difficulty parameter b
1	I stay at home most of the time because of my back	57.5	1.338	0.304
2	I change position frequently to try and get my back comfortable	5.1	1.349	−2.722
3	I walk more slowly than usual because of my back	25.3	2.142	−0.831
4	Because of my back, I am not doing any of the jobs that I usually do around the house	28.2	1.311	−0.927
5	Because of my back, I use a handrail to get upstairs	34.4	1.325	−0.637
6	Because of my back, I lie down to rest more often	29.8	1.361	−0.830
7	Because of my back, I have to hold onto something to get out of an easy chair	37.1	1.752	−0.448
8	Because of my back, I try to get other people to do things for me	58.6	0.748	0.524
9	I get dressed more slowly than usual because of my back	34.4	2.220	−0.492
10	I only stand up for short periods of time because of my back	44.9	0.576	−0.383
11	Because of my back, I try not to bend or kneel down	35.5	1.149	−0.647
12	I find it difficult to get out of a chair because of my back	36.8	1.402	−0.516
13	My back is painful almost all the time	18.8	0.921	−1.839
14	I find it difficult to turn over in bed because of my back	38.4	1.684	−0.408
15	My appetite is not very good because of my back pain	92.7	0.755	3.687
16	I have trouble putting on my socks (or stockings) because of the pain in my back	29.6	1.434	−0.816
17	I only walk short distances because of my back pain	39.0	1.126	−0.492
18	I sleep less well because of my back	47.6	0.785	−0.138
19	Because of my back pain, I get dressed with help from someone else	93.5	1.628	2.245
20	I sit down for most of the day because of my back	79.8	0.482	2.991
21	I avoid heavy jobs around the house because of my back	11.8	1.238	−2.025
22	Because of my back pain, I am more irritable and bad tempered with people than usual	61.8	0.422	1.190
23	Because of my back, I go upstairs more slowly than usual	28.0	2.533	−0.683
24	I stay in bed most of the time because of my back	96.8	1.471	2.946

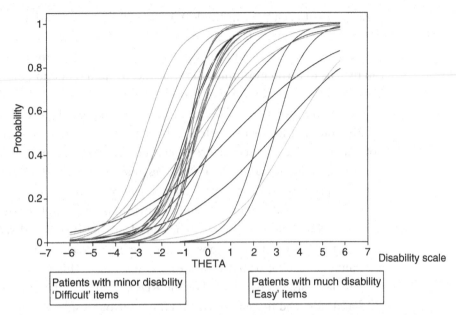

Figure 4.3   Item characteristic curves of the 24 items of the RDQ in the Birnbaum model.

the items are selected or adapted to fit the model, knowing that the measurement instrument is better if the items fit a strict IRT model. Thus, from the standpoint of the developer, the model determines the data, and from the standpoint of the evaluator, the data determine the model.

The item characteristic curves of the 24 items in the Birnbaum model are presented in Figure 4.3. We see that the slopes of the items differ, which means that items do not have the same discrimination parameter. This can also be seen in Table 4.6, on which Figure 4.3 is based. Remember that the Birnbaum model allows the items to have different discrimination parameters (see Section 2.5.2). Therefore, it is not surprising that the Birnbaum model fits the data better than the Rasch model (analysis performed in Mplus: -2 log likelihood ratio $= -2[(-4406.930 - (-4335.224))] = 143.4$, df $= 23$; $P < 0.001$).

We continue with the Birnbaum model and keep all items in the model.

4.6.2 Distribution of items over the scale

The distribution of items can be seen in Figure 4.3, and the corresponding Table 4.6 enables us to take a closer look at the difficulty and discrimination parameters of each item in the RDQ. We will first repeat what was said in Chapter 2 about the interpretation of these item characteristic curves, and then discuss how examination of the distribution of the items over the scale can help us to further optimize the scale (i.e. by item reduction or by formulating new items in certain ranges of the scale).

For the interpretation of Figure 4.3, we look back at Figure 2.5 (Section 2.5.2). Note that in the example in Chapter 2 the question was whether or not patients were able to perform a certain activity: a *yes* answer indicates 'more ability'. Note that in the RDQ a *yes* answer indicates 'more disability'. For example, a *yes* answer to item 24 'I stay in bed most of the time because of my back' indicates much disability; this item has a high positive value (i.e. $\theta = 2.946$) and can therefore be found on the right-hand side of the scale. Item 21 'I avoid heavy jobs around the house because of my back' has a θ value of -2.025, which indicates less disability. This item is found on the left-hand side of the scale. For the RDQ, the 'difficult' items are on the left-hand side, and the 'easy' items on the right-hand side.

Examination of the distribution of the items over the scale can guide further item reduction. For item reduction, we look at items with low discrimination parameters, and also at the locations of the items. Item 22 'because of my back pain I am more irritable and bad tempered with people than usual' has a flat curve, i.e. a low discrimination parameter (see Table 4.6). This means that patients with varying amounts of disability have about the same probability to answer this question with *yes*. When developing a measurement instrument to assess disability, one would not select items with a low discrimination parameter, because they discriminate poorly between patients with low and high disability. When adapting an existing instrument, items with low discrimination parameters are the first candidates to be deleted.

Figure 4.3 shows approximately 10–14 items located quite close to each other. If we wanted to reduce items from the RDQ, we might choose to remove some of the items with almost the same difficulty parameter. It is best to keep the items with the highest discrimination parameter and delete those with a lower discrimination parameter. However, the content of the items may also play a role, so we should take into account the type of activities involved. For example, items 7 and 12 both concern 'getting out of a chair', and the difficulty parameters of both items (-0.448 and -0.516) are about the same.

Their discrimination parameters differ (1.752 and 1.402), and therefore item 7, with the highest discrimination parameter, is preferred.

We also see that there are more items at the lower end (left-hand side) of the 'ability' scale, considering that $\theta = 0$ represents the mean ability of the population. This means that the RDQ is better able to discriminate patients with a low disability than patients with a high disability. If items are to be removed, items with a slightly negative difficulty parameter are the first candidates.

The location of the items should be considered against the background of the purpose of the instrument. An equal distribution is desired if the instrument has to discriminate between patients at various ranges on the scale. However, if the instrument is used to discriminate between patients with mild low back pain and severe low back pain (i.e. used as a diagnostic test), the large number of items at the range that forms the border between mild and severe low back may be very useful, as the test gives the most information about this range.

Examination of the distribution of the items over the scale shows whether there is a scarceness of items (i.e. gaps at certain locations on the scale). As the field study is still part of the development process, one might choose to formulate extra items that cover that part of the trait level.

When the distances between the items on the 'ability' scale are about equal, the sum-scores of the instrument can be considered to be an interval scale. By calculating sum-scores of the RDQ items, we assume that the distance from one item to the other is the same. We can see in Figure 4.3 though that this is not the case. If there is a scarceness of items on some parts of the range, this means that if the ability of patients changes over this range of ability, the sum-score of the RDQ will hardly change. If the ability of a patient changes from $\theta = 0$ to $\theta = -2$, the RDQ sum-score will probably change a lot, because, as can be seen in Figure 4.3, a large number of items probably change from 0 to 1 in this range. So, if patient trait levels change from 0 to –2 due to therapy (i.e. they become less disabled), their probability that they will answer *yes* on these items (meaning have difficulty with these items) changes from a very high probability to a very low probability. IRT fans claim that only IRT measurements, and those preferably based on the Rasch model, are real measurements, with the best estimate of the trait level (Wright and Linacre, 1989). However, the correlation between CTT-based and IRT-based scores is usually far above 0.95.

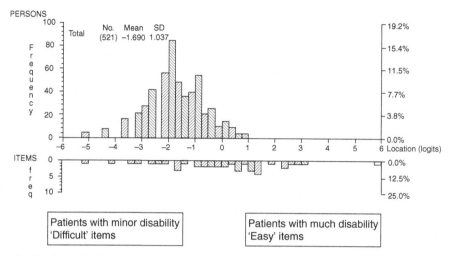

Figure 4.4   Distribution of subjects and item difficulties on the eight-item Neck Pain Disability Index on a logit scale. Van der Velde *et al.* (2009), with permission.

With IRT it is possible to make an overview of the items and the population depicted at the same trait level. Figure 4.4 shows such a graph for the Neck Disability Index, which has been evaluated with Rasch analysis, using the partial credit model, by Van der Velde *et al.* (2009). The Neck Disability Index is a 10-item instrument that can be used to assess how neck pain affects the patient's ability to manage everyday activities, such as personal care, lifting, concentration, sleeping and work. The response options range from 0 (indicating 'no trouble') to 5 (indicating 'can't do, or heavily impaired'). Of the 10 items, eight items appeared to form a unidimensional scale (Van der Velde *et al.*, 2009).

The upper part of Figure 4.4 shows the distribution of the population. The population does not seem to be greatly affected by neck pain, because the majority of patients' scores do not experience much difficulty with the items.

The lower part of Figure 4.4 shows the location of items on the trait level, using the partial credit model. As each item has six response classes, there are five difficulty parameters (thresholds) per item. The first difficulty parameter of an item represents the point at the trait level at which the probability of scoring 1 is higher than the probability of scoring 0. The second difficulty parameter represents the point at the trait level at which the probability of scoring 2 is higher than the probability of scoring 1, etc. For these eight items, a total of 40 difficulty parameters is presented.

In Figure 4.4, the difficulty parameters of the items are nicely spread over the trait level, with a few items on the left-hand side of the trait level (representing difficult items) and only one difficulty parameter with a θ above 3.5 (representing very easy items). In the development phase, it is very useful to make such a figure, because it clearly shows whether there are sufficient items at the locations where most of the patients are. When there are a lot of patients on locations of the scale where there are insufficient items, this is a sign that more items should be generated in this range of the scale. This can easily be done in the developmental phase of a questionnaire.

4.6.3 Floor and ceiling effects

Sparseness of items is often observed at the upper and lower end of a scale. This may cause floor and ceiling effects. However, the adequacy of the distribution of the items over the scale is dependent on the distribution of the population over the trait level. When there are hardly any patients with scores at the ends of the scale, then not many items are needed there; however, when a large proportion of the patients is found at either the higher or the lower end of the scale, then more items are needed to discriminate between these patients. Graphs of the distribution of items and the distribution of the population on the same trait axis, as in Figure 4.4, give the information needed to assess floor or ceiling effects. Floor and ceiling effects can occur if more than 15% of the patients achieve the lowest or highest possible score, respectively (McHorney and Tarlov, 1995).

By generating extra items, floor and ceiling effects can be prevented in the developmental phase of measurement instruments. However, floor and ceiling effects often occur when existing measurements are applied to another population, which is less or more severely diseased than the population for which the instrument was originally developed. As we will see in Chapters 7 and 8, floor and ceiling effects also have consequences for the responsiveness and interpretability of a measurement instrument.

4.7 Field-testing as part of a clinical study

Field-testing is definitely part of the developmental phase. Thus, if the measurement instrument does not meet certain requirements in this field test, it can still be adapted. Ideally, this process of evaluation and adaptation should be completed before an instrument is applied in clinical research or practice. However, there is usually insufficient time and funds for proper field-testing and the further adaptation and re-evaluation of a measurement instrument. What often happens is that it will be further evaluated during use. This has some serious drawbacks. Researchers who evaluate the measurement instrument alongside an empirical study will often be reluctant to conclude that it is not performing well, because this invalidates the conclusions of their own research. They might also be reluctant to propose changes to the measurement instrument, because they realize that this will lead to a different version than the one used in their study. And, of course, the decision to delete some items is easier to make than the decision to add new items. They would only propose to adapt the instrument, if it is performing really badly. In summary, if a measurement instrument is evaluated alongside another study, researchers are usually less critical, and the threshold for adaptation of the instrument will be higher.

The instrument is often published in too early a stage; sometimes even immediately after pilot-testing. When further adaptations are necessary, either after field-testing or during further evaluation, different versions of the instruments will appear, thus adding to the abundance of existing measurement instruments. Therefore, journal editors should be reluctant to accept a publication concerning a measurement instrument that is not evaluated as satisfactory by its developers.

4.8 Summary

Developing a measurement instrument is an iterative process in which the creative activity of development is alternated with thorough evaluation. After the instrument has been found to be performing satisfactorily with regard to comprehensibility, relevance and acceptability during pilot-testing, it should be subjected to field-testing. The aim of field-testing is item reduction, examination of the dimensionality, and then deciding on the definitive selection of items per dimension. The first step is to examine the distribution of scores for each item. Items with too many missing values and items over which there is a too homogeneous distribution of the study population could be deleted. For a formative model, the level of endorsement and experienced importance of items form the basis of the decision about which items are retained and which items are deleted from the instrument. For reflective models, FA is indicated as the basis on which to decide on the number of relevant dimensions (scales). Items that do not belong to any of these scales can be deleted. After FA, the scales are further optimized. Some scales may need extra items, but this step is usually aimed at further item reduction. Cronbach's alpha can be used to reduce the number of items, while maintaining an acceptable internal consistency. Furthermore, it is important to consider the distribution of the items over the scale in relation to its purpose: discriminating patients on all ranges of the scale or at certain locations, but also in relation to the distribution of the population over the trait level. This can be performed with CTT techniques, but IRT is a more powerful method with which to examine the item functioning within a scale.

Assignments

1. Methods of item selection

In Chapter 3, Assignment 3 concerned the paper by Juniper *et al.* (1997) on the development of the Asthma Quality of Life Questionnaire (AQLQ). This questionnaire aims to assess the impact of symptoms and other aspects of the disease on the patient's life. For the development of this questionnaire, Juniper *et al.* (1997) departed from 152 items that are, as they define in the abstract of their paper, 'potentially troublesome to patients with asthma'. They compared the impact method (see Section 4.3) with FA (labelled as a psychometric method by the authors) for the selection of relevant items for the AQLQ.

(a) Explain the elementary difference between item selection via FA and via the impact method.

(b) There are a number of items that would have been included in the questionnaire if FA had been used, but not using the impact method, and vice versa. An example of an item selected by the impact method, and not by FA is: 'how often during the past 2 weeks did you experience asthma symptoms as a result of being exposed to cigarette smoke?'. An example of an item selected by FA, and not by the impact method is 'feeling irritable'. Explain why these items were selected by one specific method and not by the other method.

(c) How could one make use of both methods?

2. Interpretation of items in a factor analysis

This assignment is based on the example of the physical workload questionnaire, described in Sections 4.4 and 4.5. In Table 4.4, items 2 and 3 have strong negative factor loadings.

(a) Explain why items 2 and 3 ('sitting' and 'video display unit work') load on the same factor as items 1 and 4 (standing and walking).

(b) We saw in Section 4.5.2 that items 2 and 3 were the first items to be deleted when trying to improve Cronbach's alpha. Explain why that would be the case.

(c) How can these negative factor loadings be avoided?

(d) Can you explain why item 19 (uncomfortable posture) loads on two factors? Is it appropriate to keep item 19 in the questionnaire? What are the consequences?

3. Factor analyses of the Graves' ophthalmopathy quality of life questionnaire

Graves' ophthalmopathy (GO), associated with Graves' thyroid disease, is an incapacitating eye disease, causing visual problems, which can have an impact on daily functioning and well being, and psychological burden because of the progressive disfigurement of the eyes. Terwee *et al.* (1998) developed a disease-specific health-related quality of life questionnaire for patients with GO and called it GO-QOL. For the development of the GO-QOL questionnaire, items were selected from other questionnaires on the impact of visual impairments and from open-ended questionnaires completed by 24 patients with GO. In this way, 16 items were formulated.

For a complete UK version of GO-QOL, see www.clinimetrics.nl.

Terwee *et al.* (1998) performed PCA on a data set containing the data of 70 patients on these 16 items. The response categories were 'yes, seriously limited', 'yes, a little limited' and 'no, not at all limited' for items about impairments in daily functioning. For items on psychosocial consequences of the changed appearance, the response options were 'yes, very much so', 'yes, a little' and 'no, not at all'. For a complete UK version of the GO-QOL and the data set of Terwee *et al.* (1998) see www.clinimetrics.nl.

(a) Make a correlation matrix of the items. Are there items that you would delete before starting FA?

   (b) Perform PCA, following the steps described in Sections 4.4.2 and 4.4.3.

   (c) How many factors would you distinguish?

   (d) Perform PCA forcing a two-factor model and comment on the interpretation.

4. Cronbach's alpha: Graves' ophthalmopathy quality of life questionnaire

   (a) Calculate Cronbach's alpha for both subscales found in Assignment 3. What do these values mean?

   (b) Calculate Cronbach's alpha for the total of 16 items. How should this value be interpreted?

   (c) Try to shorten the subscales as much as possible, while keeping Cronbach's alpha above 0.80.

   (d) Can you give a reason why the authors did not reduce the scales?

5

Reliability

5.1 Introduction

An essential requirement of all measurements in clinical practice and research is that they are reliable. Reliability is defined as 'the degree to which the measurement is free from measurement error' (Mokkink *et al.*, 2010a). Its importance often remains unrecognized until repeated measurements are performed. To give a few examples of reliability issues: radiologists want to know whether their colleagues interpret X-rays or specific scans in the same way as they do, or whether they themselves would give the same rating if they had to assess the same X-ray twice. These are called the inter-rater and the intra-rater reliability, respectively. Repeated measurements of fasting blood glucose levels in patients with diabetes may differ due to day-to-day variation or to the instruments used to determine the blood glucose level. These sources of variation play a role in test–retest reliability. In a pilot study, we are interested in the extent of agreement between two physiotherapists who assess the range of movement in a shoulder, so that we can decide whether or not their ratings can be used interchangeably in the main study. The findings of such performance tests may differ for several reasons. For example, patients may perform the second test differently because of their experience with the first test, the physiotherapists may score the same performance differently or the instructions given by one physiotherapist may motivate the patients more than the instructions given by the other physiotherapist.

So, repeated measurements may display variation arising from several sources: measurement instrument; persons performing the measurement; patients undergoing the measurements; or circumstances under which the measurements are taken. Reliability is at stake in all these variations in measurements.

In addition to the general definition (i.e. that reliability is 'the degree to which the measurement is free from measurement error'), there is an extended definition. In full this is 'the extent to which scores for patients who have not changed are the same for repeated measurement under several conditions: e.g. using different sets of items from the same multi-item measurement instrument (internal consistency); over time (test–retest); by different persons on the same occasion (inter-rater); or by the same persons (i.e. raters or responders) on different occasions (intra-rater)' (Mokkink *et al.*, 2010a). Note that internal consistency, next to reliability and measurement error, is considered an aspect of reliability (see COSMIN taxonomy in Figure 1.1).

In other textbooks and articles on reliability a variety of terms are used. To list a few: reproducibility, repeatability, precision, variability, consistency, concordance, dependability, stability, and agreement. In this book, we will use the terms reliability and measurement error (see Figure 1.1).

At the beginning of this chapter we want to clear up the long-standing misconception that subjective measurements are less reliable than objective measurements, by referring to a recent overview published by Hahn *et al.* (2007), who summarized the reliability of a large number of clinical measurements. It appeared that among all kinds of measurements, such as tumour characteristics, classification of vital signs and quality of life measurements, there are instruments with high, moderate and poor reliability. As we will see in Section 5.4.1, the fact that measurement instruments often contain multiple items to assess subjective constructs increases their reliability.

We continue this chapter by presenting an example and explaining the concept of reliability. Subsequently, different parameters to assess reliability and measurement error will be presented, illustrated with data from the example. We will then discuss essential aspects of the design of a simple reliability study, and elaborate further on more complex designs. We will also explain why the internal consistency parameter Cronbach's alpha, that we already came across in Chapter 4, can be considered as a reliability parameter. After that, we will explain how measurement error and reliability can be assessed with item response theory (IRT) analysis. As reliability concerns the anticipation, assessment and control of sources of variation, last but not least, we will give some suggestions on how to anticipate measurement errors and how to improve reliability.

5.2 Example

This example is based on a reliability study carried out by De Winter *et al.* (2004) in 155 patients with shoulder complaints. Two experienced physiotherapists, whom we will call Mary and Peter, independently measured the range of movement of passive glenohumeral abduction of the shoulder joint with a Cybex Electronical Digit Inclinometer 320 (EDI). Both physiotherapists measured the shoulder of each patient once. Within 1 hour the second physiotherapist repeated the measurements. The sequence of the physiotherapists was randomly allocated. In this chapter, we use data from 50 patients and, for educational purposes, we deliberately introduce a systematic difference of about 5° between Mary and Peter. This data set can be found on the website: www.clinimetrics.nl, accompanied by instructions and syntaxes. Table 5.1 presents the values for some of the patients in a randomly selected sample of 50.

As is often done, the researchers started by calculating a Pearson's correlation coefficient (Pearson's r) to find out whether the scores of the two physiotherapists correlate with each other. They found a Pearson's r of 0.815 for this data set. They also performed a paired t-test to find out whether there are differences between Mary and Peter's scores. We see that, on average, Mary scores 5.94° higher than Peter (circled in Output 5.1). We will take up these results again in Sections 5.4.1 and 5.4.2.2.

5.3 The concept of reliability

A measurement is seldom perfect. This is true for all measurements, whether direct or indirect, whether based on a reflective or on a formative model. Measurements performed by a doctor (e.g. assessing a patient's blood pressure) often do not represent the 'true' score. 'True' in this context means the average score that would be obtained if the measurements were performed an infinite number of times. It refers to the consistency of the score, and not to its validity (Streiner and Norman, 2008). The observed score of a measurement can be represented by the following formula:

$Y = \eta + \varepsilon,$

Table 5.1 Mary and Peter's scores for range of movement for 50 patients

Patient code	Mary's score	Peter's score
1	88	90
2	57	45
3	82	68
4	59	53
5	75	80
6	70	45
7	68	54
8	63	58
9	78	68
10	69	61
11	60	69
.	.	.
.	.	.
.	.	.
48	40	19
49	66	78
50	68	70

Output 5.1 Output of the paired *t*-test comparing Mary and Peter's scores

		Paired samples statistics			
		Mean	*N*	SD	Std. error mean
Pair	Mary's score	68.300	50	17.860	2.526
	Peter's score	62.360		16.318	2.308

		Paired samples test							
		Paired differences							
				Std. error mean	95% CI of the difference				Sig.
		Mean	SD		Lower	Upper	*t*	df	(2-tailed)
Pair	Mary–Peter	(5.940)	10.501	1.485	2.956	8.924	4.000	49	.000

where Y represents the observed score, η (Greek letter eta) is the true score of the patient, and ε is the error term of the measurement. We have seen this formula before in Section 2.5.1 and know that it is the basic formula of the classical test theory (CTT). Each observed score can be subdivided into a true score (η) and an error term ε, and this applies to all measurements: not only indirect measurements (i.e. multi-item measurement instruments to estimate an unobservable construct (η)), but also direct measurements, such as blood pressure. However, η and ε can only be disentangled when there are repeated measurements. In that case, the formula becomes:

$$Y_i = \eta + \varepsilon_i, \tag{5.1}$$

where the subscript i indicates the repeated measurements, performed either by different raters, on different measurement occasions, under different circumstances, or with different items, as we saw in Chapter 2. We stated in Section 2.5.1 that the assumptions in the CTT are that the error terms are uncorrelated with the true score, and are also uncorrelated with each other. Hence, the variances of the observed scores can be written as

$$\sigma^2(Y_i) = \sigma^2(\eta) + \sigma^2(\varepsilon_i). \tag{5.2}$$

The term $\sigma^2(Y_i)$ denotes total variance, which can be subdivided into true variance $\sigma^2(\eta)$ and error variance $\sigma^2(\varepsilon_i)$. An additional assumption is that error variances $\sigma^2(\varepsilon_i)$ are constant for every repetition i. This implies that $\sigma^2(Y_i)$ is also constant. Denoting the observed variances and error variances as $\sigma^2(Y)$ and $\sigma^2(\varepsilon)$, respectively, we can rewrite Formula 5.2 as follows:

$$\sigma^2(Y) = \sigma^2(\eta) + \sigma^2(\varepsilon).$$

This formula holds for each repeated measurement i. In the remainder of this chapter the error variance $\sigma^2(\varepsilon)$ will be discussed several times. To make sure that it will not be confused with many other variance terms, from now on we will write σ^2_{error} to indicate the error variance. We will also replace $\sigma^2(\eta)$ with the notation σ^2_p because the constructs we are interested in are usually measured in persons or patients. If we now apply the COSMIN definition of the measurement property *reliability* (Mokkink *et al.*, 2010a) as the proportion of the total variance in the measurements (σ^2_y), which is due to 'true' differences between the patients (σ_p^2), the reliability parameter (Rel) can be represented by

$$\text{Rel} = \frac{\sigma_p^2}{\sigma_y^2} = \frac{\sigma_p^2}{\sigma_p^2 + \sigma_{\text{error}}^2}. \tag{5.3}$$

A reliability parameter relates the measurement error to the variability between patients, as shown in Formula 5.3. In other words, the reliability parameter expresses how well patients can be distinguished from each other despite the presence of measurement error. From this formula, we can also calculate the standard error of measurement (SEM) as a parameter of measurement error, which equals $\sqrt{\sigma_{\text{error}}^2}$.

As shown in Formula 5.3, reliability and measurement error are related concepts, but this does not mean that they represent the same concept. We can illustrate the distinction between reliability and measurement error through the example of the two physiotherapists (Mary and Peter) performing measurements of the range of shoulder movement in the same patients. Figure 5.1 shows scores for five patients, each dot representing a patient. For three different situations, the parameters of reliability (Rel) and measurement error (expressed as SEM) are presented. The measurement error is reflected by how far the dots are from the 45° line. The between-patient variation (expressed as SD) is reflected by the spread of values along the 45° line.

Reliability parameters range in value from 0 (totally unreliable) to 1 (perfect reliability). If measurement error is small in comparison with variability between patients, the reliability parameter approaches 1. In situation A in Figure 5.1, variation between patients is high and the measurement error is low. This means that discrimination between patients is scarcely affected by measurement error, and therefore the reliability parameter is high. In situation B, measurement error is as low as in situation A, but now variation between the five patients is much smaller, which results in a lower value of the reliability parameter. In this situation, the sample is more homogeneous. If patients have almost the same value it is hard to distinguish between them, and even a small measurement error hampers the distinction of these patients. In situation C, there is considerable measurement error (i.e. the dots are farther from the 45° line than in situations A and B),

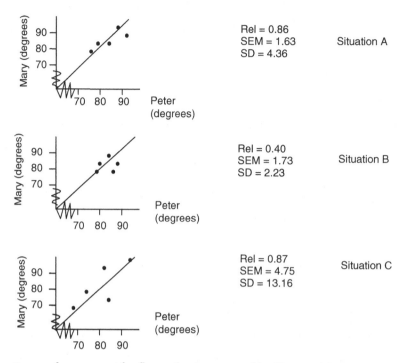

Figure 5.1   Range of movement for five patients, assessed by Mary and Peter.
Rel, reliability; SEM, standard error of measurement; SD, standard deviation.

but reliability is still high. This is due to the greater variation among the patients in situation C (i.e. a more heterogeneous sample), and thus measurement error is small in relation to variation between patients. In other words, in this situation measurement error does not obscure differences between patients.

This example not only shows the distinction between reliability and measurement error. It also emphasizes that reliability is a characteristic of an instrument used in a population, and not just of an instrument.

Now that we have explained the relationship between reliability and measurement error, we will present parameters to assess reliability and parameters to assess measurement error. Our example concerns inter-rater reliability, but all the parameters also apply to intra-rater and test–retest analysis. Parameters for continuous variables will be presented in Section 5.4, followed by parameters for categorical variables in Section 5.5.

5.4 Parameters for continuous variables

5.4.1 Parameters of reliability for continuous variables

We continue with our example, the range of shoulder movement among 50 patients, assessed by physiotherapists Mary and Peter. First, we plot Mary's scores against Peter's for each of the 50 patients (Figure 5.2). This plot immediately reveals the similarity of Mary's and Peter's scores. If reliability were perfect, we would expect all the dots to be on the 45° line. This plot also shows whether there are any outliers, which might indicate false notations or other errors. Should we delete outliers? No, because in reality such errors also occur. Moreover, outliers may give information about difficulties with measurement read-outs or interpretation of the scales.

5.4.1.1 Intraclass correlation coefficients for single measurements

In this data set, the first reliability parameter we will determine is the intraclass correlation coefficient (ICC) (Shrout and Fleiss, 1979; McGraw and Wong, 1996). There are several ICC formulas, all of which are variations on

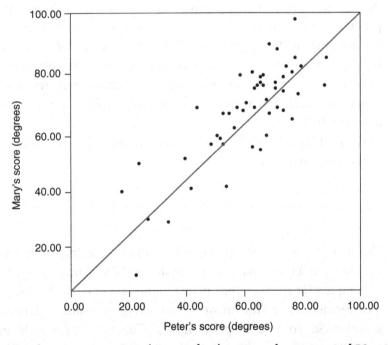

Figure 5.2 Mary's scores versus Peter's scores for the range of movement of 50 patients.

Table 5.2 Variance components in the range of movement example

Variance component	Meaning
σ_p^2	Variance due to systematic differences between 'true' scores of patients (patients to be distinguished)
σ_o^2	Variance due to systematic differences between observers (i.e. physiotherapists)
$\sigma_{\text{residual}}^2$	Residual variance (i.e. random error variance), partly due to the unique combination of patients (p) and observers (o)

the basic formula for a reliability parameter, as presented in Formula 5.3. All ICC formulas consist of a ratio of variances. Let us first focus on variance components. Variance components can be obtained through analysis of variance (ANOVA), in which the range of movement is the dependent variable and the patients and raters (in this example, physiotherapists) are considered random factors. The syntax can be found on the website (www.clinimetrics.nl). From this ANOVA, three variance components, namely σ_p^2, σ_o^2 and $\sigma_{\text{residual}}^2$ can be obtained (Table 5.2): σ_p^2 represents the variance of the patients (i.e. the systematic differences between the 'true' scores of the patients), σ_o^2 represents the variance due to systematic differences between the therapists, and $\sigma_{\text{residual}}^2$ represents the random error variance. The residual variance component ($\sigma_{\text{residual}}^2$) consists of the interaction of the two factors, patients and raters, in addition to some random error. As we cannot disentangle the interaction and random variance any further, we simply use the term 'residual variance'.

We start with an ICC formula, which contains all the variance components mentioned above:

$$ICC = \frac{\sigma_p^2}{\sigma_p^2 + \sigma_o^2 + \sigma_{\text{residual}}^2}.$$

The σ_o^2 component requires more attention. One important question is whether or not this variance due to systematic differences between the physiotherapists (or between time points in the case of test–retest) is part of the measurement error. The answer is not straightforward: it depends on the situation. Suppose we are performing a pilot study to assess the inter-rater variability of Mary and Peter. As they are the potential researchers for the main study, we are interested in how much their scores for the same patients will differ. Therefore, we compare their mean values, and for example discover that, on average, Mary scores 5.94° higher than Peter. We can adjust for this in the main study by subtracting 5.94° from Mary's scores. Then, only random errors remain, and σ_0^2 is not considered to be part of the measurement error. In this pilot study we are interested only in Mary and Peter, thus the physiotherapists are considered 'fixed'. However, if our aim is to assess how much physiotherapists in general differ in their scores, then we consider Mary and Peter to be representatives, i.e. a random sample of all possible physiotherapists. In that case, we want to generalize the results to all physiotherapists, and the physiotherapists are considered as a random factor. In this situation, σ_0^2 is part of the measurement error, because if we had taken physiotherapists other than Mary and Peter, systematic differences would also have occurred. In this case, we cannot adjust for the systematic differences, and therefore they are part of the measurement error.

So, if the raters are considered to be a random sample of all possible raters, then variance due to systematic differences between raters is 'usually' included in the error variance. We say 'usually', because it may be possible that we are not interested in absolute agreement between the raters, but only in consistency (i.e. ranking). To illustrate the difference, let us draw a parallel with education. When teachers mark students' tests to determine whether or not they have passed their exams, absolute agreement should be sought. The teachers should agree about whether the marks are below or above the cut-off point for passing the exam. However, if they mark the tests in order to identify the 10 best students, only consistency is relevant. In that case, we are only interested in whether the teachers rank students in the same order. In medicine, we are mainly interested in absolute agreement, because we want raters to draw the same conclusions about the severity of a disease or other characteristics. We are rarely interested in the ranking of patients. An example of the latter would be if we have to assign priorities to people on a waiting list for kidney transplantation, and the most severe patients should be highest on the list. Then, systematic differences are not of interest, because only the ranking is important.

As we have said before, there are several ICC formulas. For example, if we are interested in consistency, only the residual variance is considered as error variance. This ICC is called $ICC_{consistency}$. If we are interested in absolute

Output 5.2 Output of VARCOMP analysis of Mary and Peter's scores for the range of movement of 50 patients

Variance estimates

Component	Estimate
Var(p)	237.502
Var(o)	16.539
Var(residual)	55.131
Var(total)^a	309.172

Dependent variable: range of movement.
Method: ANOVA (Type III Sum of Squares).
^{a} Last row of this table is not provided by SPSS output.

agreement, variance due to systematic difference is part of the error variance, and we use the formula for ICC$_{\text{agreement}}$. In that case, the error variance consists of the residual variance plus variance due to systematic differences.

The formulas for ICC$_{\text{agreement}}$ and ICC$_{\text{consistency}}$ are as follows:

$$\text{ICC}_{\text{agreement}} = \frac{\sigma_p^2}{\sigma_p^2 + \sigma_o^2 + \sigma_{\text{residual}}^2}, \quad \sigma_{\text{error}}^2 = \sigma_o^2 + \sigma_{\text{residual}}^2, \tag{5.4}$$

$$\text{ICC}_{\text{consistency}} = \frac{\sigma_p^2}{\sigma_p^2 + \sigma_{\text{residual}}^2}, \quad \sigma_{\text{error}}^2 = \sigma_{\text{residual}}^2. \tag{5.5}$$

In ICC$_{\text{agreement}}$ the variance for the systematic differences between the raters (σ_o^2) is part of the error variance, and in ICC$_{\text{consistency}}$ σ_o^2 is not included in the error variance.

We now take a look at how these ICCs can be calculated in SPSS. We have already observed that ANOVA provides the values of the necessary variance components. In this ANOVA the range of movement is the dependent variable and the patients and raters (in this example the physiotherapists) are considered to be random factors. The syntax can be found on the website (www.clinimetrics.nl).

Output 5.2 shows the results of the SPSS VARCOMP analysis. The VARCOMP output does not show the value of the ICC, but it provides the elements from which ICC is built. The advantage is that this analysis gives insight into the magnitude of the separate sources of variation. Calculating $\text{ICC}_{\text{agreement}}$ and $\text{ICC}_{\text{consistency}}$ by hand gives $\text{ICC}_{\text{agreement}}$ of $237.502/(237.502 + 16.539 + 55.131) = 0.768$, and $\text{ICC}_{\text{consistency}}$ amounts to $237.502/(237.502 + 55.131) = 0.812$. As can be seen directly from Formulas 5.4 and 5.5, $\text{ICC}_{\text{agreement}}$ will always be smaller than $\text{ICC}_{\text{consistency}}$. The values of $\text{ICC}_{\text{agreement}}$ and $\text{ICC}_{\text{consistency}}$ will only coincide if there are no systematic differences between the raters. Using the VARCOMP analysis, the output readily shows the magnitude of the random error and systematic error in relation to variation of the patients. Expressed as proportions, the patients account for 0.768 ($237.502/309.172$) to the total variance, the systematic error for 0.053 ($16.539/309.172$), and the random error accounts for 0.178 ($55.131/309.172$). In this example, the systematic error is about 23% ($0.053/(0.053 + 0.178)$) of the total error variance.

Another way to calculate ICCs in SPSS is by using the option 'scale analysis' and subsequently 'reliability analysis'. Here we choose under ICC the option 'two-way analysis', and then we have to decide about agreement or consistency. In Output 5.3, we have to look at the single measures ICC to obtain the correct ICC value (circled in the output). The meaning of average measures ICC will be explained in Section 5.4.1.2.

Using this method to calculate ICC, we cannot obtain the values of the separate variance components on which the ICC formula is based. Output 5.4 shows the value of $\text{ICC}_{\text{consistency}}$. By comparing $\text{ICC}_{\text{agreement}}$ with $\text{ICC}_{\text{consistency}}$ we can deduce whether there is a systematic error. However, its magnitude is difficult to infer. By considering $\text{ICC}_{\text{consistency}}$, we only know the relative value of the error variance to the between-patient variance, but we do not know the actual values. For an overview of methods to calculate the ICC in SPSS, we refer to the website www.clinimetrics.nl.

5.4.1.2 Intraclass correlation coefficients for averaged measurements

Outputs 5.3 and 5.4 also show an ICC for average measures. First, we will explain how this ICC should be interpreted and then how it can be calculated.

In medicine, it is well known that a patient's blood pressure measurements vary a lot, either because it fluctuates, or because of the way in which it is measured by the clinician. It is common practice to measure a patient's blood pressure three times, and average the results of the three measurements.

Output 5.3 Output of reliability analysis to obtain ICC$_{agreement}$ for Mary and Peter's scores

| | Intraclass correlation[a] | 95% Confidence interval | | F test with true value 0 | | | |
		Lower bound	Upper bound	Value	df1	df2	Sig
Single measures	(0.768)	0.530	0.879	9.616	49	49	0.000
Average measures	0.869	0.682	0.937	9.616	49	49	0.000

Two-way random effects model where both people effects and measures (= *raters*) effects are random.

[a] Type A (= *agreement*) intraclass correlation coefficients using an absolute agreement definition.

Output 5.4 Output of reliability analysis to obtain ICC$_{consistency}$ for Mary and Peter's scores

| | Intraclass correlation[a] | 95% Confidence interval | | F test with true value 0 | | | |
		Lower bound	Upper bound	Value	df1	df2	Sig
Single measures	(0.812)	0.690	0.889	9.616	49	49	0.000
Average measures	0.896	0.817	0.941	9.616	49	49	0.000

Two-way random effects model where both people effects and measures (= *raters*) effects are random.

[a] Type C (= *consistency*) intraclass correlation coefficients using a consistency definition – the between measure (= *between-rater*) variance is excluded from the denominator variance.

This practice is based on the knowledge that repeating the measurements and averaging the results gives a more reliable result than a single measurement. The ICC for average measures applies to the situation where we are interested in the reliability of mean values of multiple measurements. In the example of shoulder movements, an ICC$_{consistency}$ of 0.896 (Output 5.4) holds for the situation that the range of movement is measured twice and averaged scores are used. Thus, when in clinical practice, a single measurement is used to assess the range of shoulder movement, as is current practice, the reliability of the obtained value is 0.812. When the range of shoulder movement is assessed by two different physiotherapists and their mean value is used in clinical practice, the reliability of that value would be 0.896.

In calculating this average measures ICC, we use a very important characteristic of the CTT. Recall our Formula 5.1 in Section 5.3:

$$Y_i = \eta + \varepsilon_i. \tag{5.1}$$

Suppose we have k measurements, then the formula for the sum of Ys (Y_+) is

$$Y_+ \equiv \sum_{i=1}^{k} Y_i = k\eta + \sum_{i=1}^{k} \varepsilon_i$$

and is accompanied by the following variance:

$$\sigma^2(Y_+) = k^2\sigma^2(\eta) + k\sigma^2(\varepsilon).$$

As in Section 5.3, we replace $\sigma^2(\varepsilon)$ by σ^2_{error} and $\sigma^2(\eta)$ by σ^2_p; then the reliability parameter can be written as

$$\text{Rel} = \frac{k^2\sigma^2_p}{k^2\sigma^2_p + k\sigma^2_{error}} = \frac{\sigma^2_p}{\sigma^2_p + \dfrac{\sigma^2_{residual}}{k}}.$$

This formula shows us that when we average several measurements, the error variance can be divided by the number of measurements over which the average is taken.

For our example of shoulder movements $\text{ICC}_{consistency}$ for scores averaged over two physiotherapists is

$$\text{ICC}_{consistency} = \frac{\sigma^2_p}{\sigma^2_p + \dfrac{\sigma^2_{error}}{2}} = \frac{\sigma^2_p}{\sigma^2_p + \dfrac{\sigma^2_{residual}}{2}} = \frac{237.502}{237.502 + \dfrac{55.131}{2}} = 0.896.$$

We have seen in Formula 5.4 that the component σ^2_o is part of the error variance in $\text{ICC}_{agreement}$:

$$\text{ICC}_{agreement} = \frac{\sigma^2_p}{\sigma^2_p + \dfrac{\sigma^2_{error}}{2}} = \frac{\sigma^2_p}{\sigma^2_p + \dfrac{\sigma^2_o + \sigma^2_{residual}}{2}} = \frac{237.502}{237.502 + \dfrac{16.539 + 55.131}{2}} = 0.869.$$

Hence, we always get a more reliable measure when we take the average of scores, because the measurement error becomes smaller.

5.4.1.3 Pearson's *r*

At the beginning of this chapter, we calculated Pearson's *r* to see whether Mary's and Peter's scores were correlated. If we compare the value of the Pearson's *r* with the $ICC_{agreement}$ (0.815 versus 0.768), we see that the Pearson's *r* is higher. Pearson's *r* is not a very stringent parameter to assess reliability, as is shown in Figure 5.3. If Mary's and Peter's scores are exactly on the same (line A), Pearson's *r*, $ICC_{agreement}$ and $ICC_{consistency}$ will all be 1. $ICC_{consistency}$ and Pearson's *r* will also be 1 if Mary's scores (*y*-axis) are 5° lower than Peter's scores (line B). This means that these two parameters do not take systematic errors into account. Pearson's *r* will even be 1 if Mary's scores are twice as low as Peter's scores (line C). In that case, neither ICCs will equal 1. Although the ranking of persons is the same, $ICC_{consistency}$ deviates from 1, because the variances of Peter's scores are larger than of Mary's scores. So, Pearson's *r* does not require a 45° line. However, if there are only random errors, the Pearson's *r* will give a good indication of the reliability. As could be expected, in our example Pearson's *r* is about equal to the $ICC_{consistency}$ (0.815 and 0.812, respectively). Therefore, because Pearson's *r* is less critical, we recommend the ICC as a reliability parameter for continuous variables.

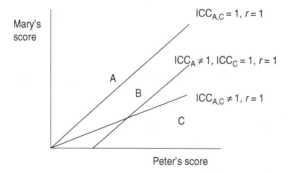

Figure 5.3 Values of Pearson's *r* and ICC for different relationships between Mary and Peter's scores.

5.4.2 Parameters of measurement error for continuous variables

5.4.2.1 Standard error of measurement

In Section 5.3, we introduced the SEM as a parameter of measurement error. The SEM is a measure of how far apart the outcomes of repeated measurements are; it is the SD around a single measurement. For example, if a patient's blood pressure is measured 50 consecutive times, and the SD of these values is calculated, then this SD represents the SEM. Three methods can be used to obtain the SEM value.

First, the SEM value can be derived from the error variance (σ^2_{error}) in the ICC formula. The general formula is

$$\text{SEM} = \sqrt{\sigma^2_{error}}.$$

As we have seen, σ^2_{error} may or may not include the systematic error (see Section 5.4.1.1). Therefore, as with the ICC, we have agreement and consistency versions of the SEM:

$$\text{SEM}_{agreement} = \sqrt{(\sigma^2_o + \sigma^2_{residual})},$$

$$\text{SEM}_{consistency} = \sqrt{\sigma^2_{residual}}.$$

In our example, using data from Output 5.2, the value of $\text{SEM}_{agreement} = \sqrt{(\sigma^2_o + \sigma^2_{residual})} = 8.466$, and $\text{SEM}_{consistency} = \sqrt{\sigma^2_{residual}} = 7.425$.

The second method that can be used to calculate the SEM is via the SD of the differences between the two raters ($\text{SD}_{difference}$). We seldom have so many repeated measurements of one patient that the SEM can be obtained from the SD of the patient. But often we do have two measurements of a sample of stable patients (e.g. because these patients are measured by two raters). We then take the difference of the values of the two raters, and calculate the mean and the SD of these differences ($\text{SD}_{difference}$). We can use this $\text{SD}_{difference}$ to estimate the SD around a single measurement to derive $\text{SEM}_{consistency}$ with the following formula:

$$\text{SEM}_{consistency} = \text{SD}_{difference}/\sqrt{2} = 10.501/\sqrt{2} = 7.425. \quad (5.6)$$

The $\sqrt{2}$ in the formula arises from the fact that we now use difference scores, and difference scores are based on two measurements. As each measurement is accompanied by the measurement error, we have twice the measurement error present in the variances. We know that, in general, SDs (σ)

are the square root of variances (σ^2), and therefore, the factor $\sqrt{2}$ appears in Formula 5.6. As $SD_{difference}$, by definition, does not include the systematic error, it is $SEM_{consistency}$ which is obtained here.

We have doubted whether or not to describe the third method that can be used to calculate the SEM, because we want to warn against its use. However, we decided to present the formula, and explain what the fallacies are.

The formula is the original ICC formula, rewritten as follows

$$SEM = \sigma_y \sqrt{(1 - ICC)} = SD_{pooled}\sqrt{(1 - ICC)}. \tag{5.7}$$

In this formula, σ_y represents the SD of the sample in which the ICC is determined. The corresponding term in Formula 5.5 for $ICC_{consistency}$ is σ_y^2, that contains the total variance, i.e. a summation of all terms in the denominator (see Formula 5.3). This formula is often misused. First, it is misused by researchers who want to know the SEM value, but who have not performed their own test–retest analysis, or intra-rater or inter-rater study. They take an ICC value from another study and then use Formula 5.7 to calculate an SEM. In this case, the population from which the ICC value is derived is often unknown or ignored. We saw earlier that the ICC is highly dependent on the heterogeneity of the population. Therefore, Formula 5.7 can only be used for populations with approximately the same heterogeneity (i.e. SD) as the population in which the ICC is calculated. If we were to apply the ICC found in our example to a more homogeneous population, we would obtain SEMs that are far too small and extremely misleading. Therefore, we discourage the use of this formula. Assignment 5.3 contains an example of consequences of the misuse of this formula. Secondly, some researchers insert Cronbach's alpha instead of the ICC for test–retest, inter-rater or intra-rater reliability. Although Cronbach's alpha is a reliability parameter, as we will explain in Section 5.12, it cannot replace the ICCs described above if one is interested in the SEM as the measurement error for test–retest, inter-rater or intra-rater situations (i.e. repeated measurements). The reason for this is that Cronbach's alpha is based on a single measurement. Thirdly, this formula applies only to $SEM_{consistency}$, because the SD to be inserted in this formula can be assessed only when there are no systematic differences.

To show that Formula 5.7 leads to the same result for $SEM_{consistency}$ as we have derived by the other methods, we take the SD_{pooled} (see Output 5.1 for the SD_1 of Mary's and SD_2 of Peter's scores) as

$$\sqrt{\frac{SD_1^2 + SD_2^2}{2}} = \sqrt{\frac{17.860^2 + 16.318^2}{2}} = 17.106$$

and $\text{ICC}_{\text{consistency}} = 0.812$. This leads to $\text{SEM} = \text{SD}_{\text{pooled}}\sqrt{(1 - \text{ICC}_{\text{consistency}})} = 17.106 \times \sqrt{(1 - 0.812)} = 7.417$.

By using this method, keep in mind that it only holds for the population in which the ICC was determined. We refer to Assignment 3 for an illustration of an incorrect use of this formula.

5.4.2.2 Limits of agreement (Bland and Altman method)

Another parameter of measurement error can be found in the limits of agreement, proposed by Bland and Altman (1986). In Figure 5.2, Mary's and Peter's scores are plotted. Without the straight 45° line drawn in Figure 5.2 it is very hard to see how much Mary's and Peter's scores deviate from each other and whether there are systematic differences (i.e. whether there are more dots on one side of the line). Bland and Altman designed a plot in which systematic errors can easily be seen (see Figure 5.4).

For each patient the mean of the scores assessed by Mary (M) and Peter (P) is plotted on the x-axis, against the difference between the scores on the y-axis. The output of the paired t-test analysis, as presented in Output

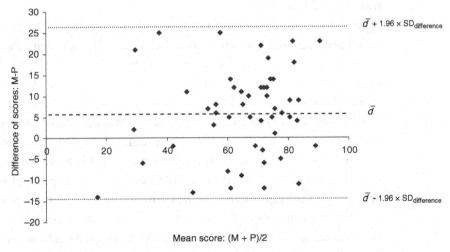

Figure 5.4   Bland and Altman plot for Mary and Peter's scores for the range of movement of 50 patients.

5.1 in Section 5.2, then provides all the relevant data to draw a Bland and Altman plot.

The dashed line $\bar{d}$ represents the mean systematic difference between Mary's and Peter's scores, which amounts to 5.940 (95% CI: 2.956 to 8.924) in our example (circled in Output 5.1 of the paired t-test). It appears that this mean difference is statistically significant. The two dotted lines above and below the line $\bar{d}$ represent the limits of agreement, and these are drawn at $\bar{d} \pm 1.96 \times \text{SD}_{\text{difference}}$. We can interpret $\bar{d}$ as the systematic error and $1.96 \times \text{SD}_{\text{difference}}$ as the random error. Assuming that the difference scores have a normal distribution, this means that about 95% of the dots will fall between the dotted lines. If Mary's and Peter's scores differ a lot, the SD of the differences will be large and the lines will be further away from the line $\bar{d}$. The limits of agreement here are −14.642 to 26.522. As these are expressed in the units of measurement, clinicians and researchers have a direct indication of the size of the measurement error.

We have seen in Section 5.4.2.1 that $\text{SEM}_{\text{consistency}} = \text{SD}_{\text{difference}}/\sqrt{2}$. So, the limits of agreement can also be written as $\bar{d} \pm 1.96 \times \sqrt{2} \times \text{SEM}_{\text{consistency}}$. However, if there are systematic differences the limits of agreement cannot be transformed into $\text{SEM}_{\text{agreement}}$. The reason for this is that in $\text{SEM}_{\text{agreement}}$ the systematic error is included in the error variance, while in the limits of agreement it is expressed in the $\bar{d}$ line. Therefore, only $\text{SEM}_{\text{consistency}}$ can be transformed in this way.

An important assumption of the Bland and Altman method is that the differences between the raters do not change with increasing mean values (Bland and Altman, 1999). In other words, the calculated value for the limits of agreement holds for the whole range of measurements. This assumption also underlies the calculation of SEM and ICC, but in the Bland and Altman plot we can readily observe whether the magnitudes of differences remains the same over the whole range of mean values. If the $\text{SD}_{\text{difference}}$ does change with increasing mean values, it is sometimes possible to transform the data in such a way that the transformed data satisfy the assumption of a constant $\text{SD}_{\text{difference}}$. An example of this can be found in the measurement of skin folds to assess the proportion of bodily fat mass. When skin folds become thicker, the measurement errors become larger. For an example of how such a transformation works, we refer to Euser $et\ al.$ (2008).

5.4.2.3 Coefficient of variation

The coefficient of variation (CV) is another parameter of measurement error that medical researchers might encounter. The CV is used primarily to indicate the reliability of an apparatus, when numerous measurements are performed on test objects in the phase of calibration and testing. It is not used to assess inter-rater or intra-rater reliability or test–retest reliability in the field of medicine. However, because researchers in the more physical disciplines will encounter CV values, it is worthwhile to explain what these represent.

The CV relates the SD of repeated measurements to the mean value, as is shown in the following formula:

$$CV = SD_{repeated\ measurements}/mean.$$

The CV is usually multiplied by 100% and expressed as a percentage. It is very appropriate to calculate this parameter if the measurement error grows in proportion to the mean value, because a stable percentage can then be obtained. This is often the case in physics. Note that the CV can only be calculated, or interpreted adequately, when we are using a ratio scale (i.e. there should be a zero point and all values should be positive).

5.5 Parameters for categorical variables

5.5.1 Parameters of reliability for categorical variables

5.5.1.1 Cohen's kappa for nominal variables

The example we use to illustrate parameters of reliability for categorical variables is the classification of precancerous states of cervical cancer. Screening for cervical cancer takes place by scraping cells from the cervix, and in case of abnormalities a biopsy (tissue sample) is taken to detect abnormal cells and changes in the architecture of the cervical tissue. Based on the biopsy, potentially precancerous lesions are classified into five stages: no abnormalities (no dysplasia: ND); three stages of dysplasia or cervical intraepithelial neoplasia, i.e. CIN1, CIN2, CIN3, corresponding to mild, moderate and severe dysplasia, respectively; and carcinoma in situ (CIS). This is a typical example of an ordinal scale. However, for our first example we dichotomize the classes as ND, CIN1 and CIN2 on the one hand, requiring no further action except careful observation, and CIN3 and CIS on the other hand, in which case excision of the lesion takes

Table 5.3 Classification of scores of pathologists A and B for 93 biopsies in two categories

Pathologist B	Pathologist A		
	CIN3 or CIS	No severe abnormalities	Total
CIN3 or CIS	15	10	25
No severe abnormalities	8	60	68
Total	23	70	93

place. The result is a dichotomous scale. De Vet *et al.* (1992) examined the inter-observer variation of the scoring of cervical biopsies by different pathologists. The scores of two pathologists (A and B) for the biopsy samples of 93 patients are presented in Table 5.3.

Cohen's kappa

The two pathologists (A and B) agree with each other in 75 of 93 cases, both observing severe abnormalities in 15 cases, and no severe abnormalities in 60 cases. This results in a fraction of 0.806 (75 of 93) of observed agreement (P_o). However, as is the case in an exam with multiple choice questions, a number of questions may be answered correctly by guessing. So, pathologist B would agree with pathologist A in some cases by chance, even if neither of them looked at the biopsies. Cohen's kappa is a measure that adjusts for the agreement that is expected by chance (Cohen, 1960). This chance agreement is also called expected agreement (P_e). Statisticians know that expected agreement could easily be calculated by assuming statistical independence of the measurements, which is obtained by multiplication of the marginals. The sum of the upper left and the lower right cells then becomes:

$$P_e = \frac{25}{93} \times \frac{23}{93} + \frac{68}{93} \times \frac{70}{93} = 0.617.$$

The following reasoning may help clinicians to understand the estimation of the expected number of biopsies on which both pathologists classify as CIN3 or CIS. Pathologist B classified 27% (25 of 93) of the samples as severe. If he did this without even looking at the biopsies, his scores would be totally independent of the score of pathologist A. In that case, pathologist B would probably also have rated as severe 27% of the 23 cases (i.e. 6.183 cases) that

Table 5.4 Classification of observed scores and expected numbers of chance (dis)agreements (between brackets)

Pathologist B	Pathologist A		
	CIN3 or CIS	No severe abnormalities	Total
CIN3 or CIS	15 (6.183)	10 (18.817)	25
No severe abnormalities	8 (16.817)	60 (51.183)	68
Total	23	70	93

were classified as severe by pathologist A. The same holds for the 70 samples that were rated non-severe by pathologist A; 73% (68 of 93) of these 70 (i.e. 51.183 cases) would be rated as non-severe by pathologist B. The number of chance agreements expected in all four cells are presented between brackets in Table 5.4.

Now we can calculate the fraction of the expected agreement (P_e), which amounts to a fraction of $(51.183 + 6.183)/93 = 0.617$. The formula for Cohen's kappa is as follows:

$$\kappa = \frac{P_o - P_e}{1 - P_e}.$$

In the numerator, the expected agreement is subtracted from the observed agreement. Therefore, the denominator should also be adjusted for the expected agreement. Thus, kappa relates the amount of agreement that is observed beyond chance agreement to the amount of agreement that can maximally be reached beyond chance agreement.

For this example, $P_o = 0.806$ and $P_e = 0.617$. Filling in the formula results in $\kappa = (0.806 - 0.617)/(1 - 0.617) = 0.493$.

5.5.1.2 Weighted kappa for ordinal variables

Weighted kappa
In the example concerning cervical dysplasia, the pathologists actually assigned the 93 samples to five categories of cervical precancerous stages.

We can also calculate a kappa value for a 5×5 table, using the same methods as we did before. The observed agreement $P_o = (1 + 13 + 18 + 15 + 2)/93 = 49/93 = 0.527$. The expected agreement by chance can again

Table 5.5 Classifications of scores of pathologists A and B for 93 biopsies in five categories

Pathologist B	Pathologist A					
	CIS	CIN3	CIN2	CIN1	ND	Total
CIS	1 (0.022)	0	0	0	0	1
CIN3	1	13 (5.419)	9	1	0	24
CIN2	0	7	18 (13.892)	9	0	34
CIN1	0	1	11	15 (8.731)	2	29
ND	0	0	0	3	2 (0.215)	5
Total	2	21	38	28	4	93

be derived from the marginals of each cell. So, for the middle cell with an observed number of 18, the expected number is $(34 \times 38)/93 = 13.892$. And $P_e = (0.022 + 5.419 + 13.892 + 8.731 + 0.215)/93 = 28.279/93 = 0.304$. So, this amounts to a value of kappa (κ) = $(P_o - P_e)/(1 - P_e) = (0.527 - 0.304)/(1 - 0.304) = 0.320$. This is called an unweighted kappa value.

However, it is also possible to calculate a weighted Cohen's kappa (Cohen, 1968). The rationale for a weighted kappa is that misclassifications between adjacent categories are less serious than those between more distant categories, and that the latter should be penalized more heavily. The formula for the weighted kappa is

$$\kappa = 1 - \frac{\sum w_{ij} \times P_{o_{ij}}}{\sum w_{ij} \times P_{e_{ij}}},$$

where summation is taken over all cells (i, j) in Table 5.5 with row index i (scores of pathologist B) and column index j (scores of pathologist A), w_{ij} is the weight assigned to cell (i, j) and $P_{o_{ij}}$ and $P_{e_{ij}}$ are the observed and expected proportions of cell (i, j), respectively.

Sometimes linear weights are used, but quadratic weights are usually applied. The linear and quadratic weights are presented in Table 5.6.

It is laborious to calculate weighted kappa values manually. Therefore, we recommend a website http://faculty.vassar.edu/lowry/kappa.html that can be used to calculate weighted kappas. You only have to enter the numbers in the cross-table, and the program calculates the values for the unweighted

Table 5.6 Linear and quadratic weights used in the calculation of weighted kappa values

	Same category	Adjacent category	2 categories apart	3 categories apart	4 categories apart
Linear weights	0	1	2	3	4
Quadratic weights	0	1	4	9	16

kappa, and for the weighted kappa, using linear and quadratic weights. The 95% confidence intervals are also presented, together with a large number of other details. For the example above the kappa values are

unweighted kappa = 0.320 (95% CI = 0.170–0.471), and
weighted kappa with quadratic weights = 0.660 (95% CI = 0.330–0.989).

Cohen's kappa is a reliability parameter for categorical variables. Like all reliability parameters, the value of kappa depends on the heterogeneity of the sample. In the case of cross-tables, the heterogeneity of the sample is represented by the distribution of the marginals. An equal distribution over the classes represents a heterogeneous sample. A skewed distribution points to a more homogeneous sample (i.e. almost all patients or objects are the same). In a homogeneous sample it is more difficult to distinguish the patients or objects from each other, often resulting in low kappa values. A weighted kappa, using quadratic weights, equals $ICC_{agreement}$ (Fleiss and Cohen, 1973). Note, that by calculating weighted kappa, we are ignoring the fact that the scale is still ordinal (i.e. the distance between the classes is unknown), while by assigning weights we pretend that these distances are equal.

5.5.2 No parameters of measurement error for categorical variables

For ordinal and nominal levels of measurement, there is only classification and ordering and no units of measurement. Therefore, there are no parameters of measurement error that quantify the measurement error in units of measurement. It can be examined, however, which percentage of the measurements are classified in the same categories. We call this the percentage of agreement.

Table 5.7 presents an overview of parameters of reliability and measurement error for continuous and categorical variables.

Table 5.7 Overview of parameters of reliability and measurement error for continuous and categorical variables

	Continuous scale	Ordinal scale	Nominal scale
Reliability	ICC	ICC or weighted kappa	unweighted kappa
Measurement error/ agreement	SEM or limits of agreement	% agreement	% agreement

5.6 Interpretation of the parameters

5.6.1 Parameters of reliability

5.6.1.1 Intraclass correlation coefficient

Calculating parameters for reliability is not the end of the story; we want to know which values are satisfactory. The ICC values range between 0 and 1. The ICC value approaches 1 when the error variance is negligible compared with the patient variance. The value approaches 0 when the error variance is extremely large compared with the patient variance, and this value is obtained in very homogeneous samples. Note that ICC = 0 when all patients have the same score (i.e. patient variance is 0). Typically, an ICC value of 0.70 is considered acceptable (Nunnally and Bernstein, 1994), but values greater than 0.80 or even greater than 0.90 are, of course, much better. We have seen that the ICC is sample-dependent: patients in a heterogeneous population are much easier to distinguish than patients who are very similar with regard to the characteristic to be measured. This is not a disadvantage of an ICC in particular: it is typical of every reliability parameter. However, it stresses the importance that the ICC should be determined in the population for which the instrument will be used. In addition, by the same token, if one is going to use a measurement instrument and wants to know its reliability, one should look for an ICC for that instrument determined in a comparable population.

5.6.1.2 Kappa

Kappa values range between −1 and 1. Kappa equals 1 when all scores are in the upper left cell or lower right cell of the 2 × 2 table (or, more generally, all scores are in cells along the diagonal of a bigger table). A kappa value of 0

Interpretation of kappa values

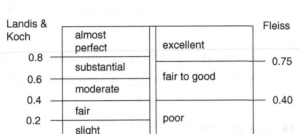

Figure 5.5   Classifications for interpretation of Cohen's kappa values.

means that there is no more agreement than can be expected by chance. If the kappa value is negative but still close to 0, this points to less agreement than would be expected by chance. However, a kappa value close to –1 is usually caused by reversed scaling by one of the two raters. In our example concerning cervical dysplasia the unweighted kappa value was 0.493. Is this kappa value acceptable? Figure 5.5 presents two slightly different methods that can be used to interpret kappa values (Landis and Koch, 1977; Fleiss, 1981). A value of about 0.5 is considered to be 'moderate' or 'fair to good', depending on which method of classification is used. Of course, when the kappa value is 0.77, researchers prefer to use the classification of Fleiss (1981), because that classifies this value as excellent. Although the differences between the methods may be confusing, they illustrate clearly the ambiguity and arbitrariness of these classifications.

As explained in Section 5.5.1, kappa values are influenced by the distribution of the marginals. Kappa values can also be influenced by the number of classes and by systematic differences between the raters, so a kappa value on its own is not very informative. Therefore, it is strongly recommended that the content of the cross-tables is presented, in addition to the kappa value. This content provides information about:

- The marginal distribution: a more skewed distribution (i.e. a more homogeneous population) leads to a higher fraction of chance agreement, leaving less room for real agreement. Although, theoretically, the kappa value can still approach 1, in practice the values are usually lower.
- Systematic differences: by comparing the marginal distributions of the raters, one can see whether there are systematic differences between

the raters. In Tables 5.3 (2 × 2 table) and 5.5 (5 × 5 table) it can be seen that pathologists A and B had similar distributions over the various categories.

Many clinicians gain a clearer view of the amount of misclassification by looking at the numbers in a 2 × 2 table than by knowing the kappa value.

5.6.2 Parameters of measurement error

5.6.2.1 Standard error of measurement

Parameters of measurement error are expressed in the unit of measurement. Therefore, it is impossible to give general guidelines regarding what values are acceptable. Fortunately, such guidelines may also be less necessary than for reliability coefficients. If clinicians are familiar with the measurements in question, they have an immediate feeling as to whether the measurement error is small or not. For example, clinicians know what a 5 mmHg measurement error in blood pressure means, or an error of 1 mmol/l in fasting glucose levels, and physiotherapists are familiar with the meaning of a difference of 5° in range of movement measurements. This is the advantage of the parameters of measurement error: they are easily interpreted by clinicians and researchers.

However, if we are using multi-item measurements, it is not intuitively clear what a certain value means. For example, the Roland–Morris Disability Questionnaire (RDQ) (Roland and Morris, 1983) that assesses the disability of patients with low back pain, is scored on a 0–24-point scale. On this scale it is more difficult to decide whether a SEM of 3 points is acceptable. To enhance the interpretation of the size of the measurement error, the limits of agreement are often calculated, and then related to the range of the scale.

5.6.2.2 Bland and Altman method

A SEM value of 3 points leads to limits of agreement of $\bar{d} \pm 1.96 \times \sqrt{2} \times 3$ (see the Bland and Altman method in Section 5.4.2.2). When there are no systematic errors between the two raters, the value of $\bar{d}$ is 0 and the limits of agreement are ±8.3. Relating the limits of agreement to the range of the scale may give an impression of the magnitude of the measurement error. By definition, 95% of the differences between repeated measurements fall between the limits of agreement. If we observe, for example, a change of 5 points on the RDQ, there is a reasonable chance that this is due to measurement error. However, if we observe a change of 10 points, which is outside the limits of agreement, it is improbable that this is due to measurement error, and it possibly indicates a real change. Therefore, limits of agreement give information about the smallest detectable change (i.e. change beyond measurement error). This will be further discussed in Chapter 8, Section 8.5.3.

As we will see in Chapter 8, which focuses on interpretation, efforts are made to define values for minimal important change or other measures of clinical relevance for measurement instruments. If such measures are available, it is clear that measurement errors are acceptable if the smallest detectable change is smaller than the values for minimally important change.

5.7 Which parameter to use in which situation?

Reliability parameters assess how well patients can be distinguished from each other, and parameters of measurement error assess the magnitude of the measurement error. In clinical practice, a clinician tries to improve the health status of individual patients, and is thus interested in the evaluation of health status. In research, much attention is also paid to evaluative questions, such as 'does the health status of patients change?', 'does a treatment work?' or 'is there a relevant improvement or deterioration in health?'. All these questions require a quantification of the measurement error, in order to determine whether the changes are real, and not likely to be due to measurement error. Parameters of measurement error are relevant for the measurements of changes in health status. In diagnostic and prognostic research, the aim is to distinguish between different (stages of) diseases or between different courses or outcomes of the disease. For these discriminative purposes, reliability parameters are primarily indicated (De Vet *et al.*, 2006).

Although parameters of measurement error are often relevant for measurements in the field of medicine, only reliability parameters are presented in many situations. In two systematic reviews of evaluative measurement instruments we assessed whether reliability parameters or parameters of measurement error were presented (Bot *et al.*, 2004b; De Boer *et al.*, 2004). All 16 studies focusing on shoulder disability questionnaires presented parameters of reliability, but only six studies also reported a parameter of measurement error. For 31 measurement instruments used to assess quality of life in visually impaired patients, a parameter of reliability was reported for 16 instruments, but a parameter of measurement error was reported for only seven instruments. As we have seen in Section 5.4.2.1, in theory, the SEM can be derived from the ICC formula, but this is only possible if all the components of the ICC formula are presented. Usually only the bare ICC value is provided, often with no mention at all as to which ICC formula has been used. We strongly recommend and promote the use of parameters of measurement error, or the provision of details about the variance components underlying the ICC.

5.8 Design of simple reliability studies

Now that we have discussed many questions concerning reliability that can be answered by calculating the right measurement error and reliability parameters, it is time to take a closer look at the design of a reliability study. There is more to this than just repeating measurements and calculating an adequate parameter.

The crucial question that must be kept in mind when designing a reliability study is 'For which situation do we want to know the reliability?', because the design of the study should mimic that situation. We list a number of relevant issues that should be taken into consideration.

- Which sample or population? The study sample should reflect the population that we are interested in, because we have seen that reliability is highly dependent on the distribution of the characteristic under study in the population. If we want to know the reliability of measurements of patients, it is of no use to test the reliability of measurements of healthy subjects. The reliability study should be performed in a sample of those patients in which we want to apply the measurement instrument in the future.
- Which part of the measurement process are we interested in? For example, when assessing the inter-rater reliability of an electroencephalograph (EEG), we should specify whether we are only interested in the reliability of the readings and interpretation of the EEGs, or whether we are interested in the reliability of the whole procedure, including the positioning

and fixation of the electrodes on the skull. And for performance tests, are we interested in the inter-observer reliability of only the judgement of the quality of performance, or are we interested in the variation among physiotherapists performing the whole test with the patient independently, i.e. the physiotherapists each give their own instructions and the patient performs the test twice? Note that in the latter situation both the patient variation in performance and the influence of the physiotherapists' instructions are included.

- Which time interval? In the design of a test–retest reliability study we have to decide on the appropriate time interval between the measurements. If the characteristic under study is stable, a longer time interval can be allowed, but if it changes rapidly the length of time between two tests should be as short as justified. There are no standard rules for this. The choice is based on common sense, finding a good balance, in general terms, between the stability of the characteristics and the independence of the repeated tests (i.e. absence of interferences). In performance tests, interference can occur, due to pain, tiredness or muscle pain resulting from the first test. Interference can also occur in questionnaires if patients can remember their previous answers. If the questionnaire contains a long list of questions about everyday business, a shorter time interval can be used than when there are only a few rather specific questions, because then patients will find it easier to remember their previous answers. To give an indication, we often use a time interval of 2 weeks between questionnaires but there is no standard rule, given above-mentioned considerations.

- Which situation? Situation or circumstances can be interpreted in several ways, as illustrated in the following examples. In an inter-rater reliability study, do we want to assess the situation as it is in routine care, or are we interested in a perfect situation? If we want to assess the reliability of the performance of radiologists in everyday practice, it is of no use to select the best radiologists in the country, or to train the radiologists beforehand. If practically and ethically feasible, the radiologists should not even know that they are participating in the study, or whether the X-rays they assess are from the study sample. But when we are testing a new measurement instrument, for example a special positron emission tomography (PET) scan, on its intra-rater and inter-rater reliability, it is more appropriate to select the best trained specialists to interpret the scans in order to get an estimation of the maximum possible reliability.

- For a proper interpretation, we should be aware of the assumptions made. Assessing the inter-rater reliability of X-ray interpretation, we know that the X-rays are exactly the same and the variation in outcomes is due to the raters. However, when assessing the reliability of blood pressure measurements in patients performed by one rater within 10 min, we either assume that the blood pressure is stable and attribute the variation to the rater, or we assume that variation in outcome may be attributed to both the rater and to the variation in blood pressure. When these blood pressure measurements are performed on different days, we probably assume that it will vary between measurements and we attribute the variation in outcome to both biological variation in blood pressure and variation in measurement by the rater. Note that if we assume that the rater is stable in his or her measurements, we might draw a conclusion about the biological variation of blood pressure. Therefore, the underlying assumptions determine the interpretation.

In conclusion, the key point is that the situation for the reliability study resembles the situation in which the measurement instrument is going to be used. Another important issue in the study design is to decide on how many patients and how many repeated measurements are needed.

5.9 Sample size for reliability studies

How many patients are needed for reliability studies? If researchers ask us this question, we usually say 50. About 50 patients are required to reasonably fill a 2 × 2 table to determine the kappa value, and to provide a reasonable number of dots in a Bland and Altman plot to estimate the limits of agreement. This sample size of 50 is often the starting point for negotiations. Of course, researchers will argue that it is very difficult for logistic reasons to have so many patients examined by more than one clinician. However, if it concerns photographs, slides or other samples that can easily be circulated among the raters, a sample of 50 is usually quite feasible.

Sample size estimations for reliability parameters are not a matter of statistical significance, because the issue is whether the reliability parameter approaches 1, and not its statistical difference from 0. An adequate sample size is important to obtain an acceptable confidence interval (CI) around

Table 5.8 Required sample size for ICC 0.7 and 0.8 for two to six repeated measurements

ICC = 0.7			ICC = 0.8		
m repeated measurements	95% CI ± 0.1 n	95% CI ± 0.2 n	*m* repeated measurements	95% CI ± 0.1 n	95% CI ± 0.2 n
2	100	25	2	50	13
3	67	17	3	35	9
4	56	14	4	30	8
5	50	13	5	28	7
6	47	12	6	26	7

CI, confidence interval.

the estimated reliability parameter. Guidelines for the calculation of sample sizes for reliability studies are difficult to find in the literature. For ICC values, we can calculate how many patients (or objects of study) and how many measurements (or raters) per patient are necessary to reach a pre-specified CI. Giraudeau and Mary (2001) provide a formula for the calculation of the sample size n:

$$n = \frac{8z_{1-\alpha/2}^2(1-ICC)^2[1+(m-1)ICC]^2}{m(m-1)w^2}.$$

In this formula, m stands for the number of measurements per patient and w stands for the total width of the $100(1-\alpha)$% CI for ICC, i.e. $w = 0.2$ for a CI ± 0.1. In Table 5.8 sample sizes for situations that occur frequently are presented.

Table 5.8 shows that lower ICC values require a larger sample size to reach the same CI. Moreover, by performing more measurements per patient, the sample size can be reduced. Logistical aspects may play a role in determining about the most efficient design. Note that the sample size required to obtain a CI of 0.1 is four times larger than for a CI of 0.2. This can easily be seen in the formula, where w^2 appears in the denominator. Thus, to obtain a CI of 0.15 the numbers needed for a CI of 0.1 should be divided by $(1.5)^2 = 2.25$.

Sample size calculations for kappa values are difficult to perform, because in addition to the expected kappa value, we need information about the distribution of the marginals. To obtain the same width of confidence for kappa values as for ICCs, a larger sample size is needed. This has to do with the ordinal or nominal nature of kappa values. As is the case for ICC, if the kappa value is lower a larger sample size is needed to reach the same CI.

Quite often small samples of patients are used to determine reliability coefficients. We recommend that a 95% CI is presented with the parameters of reliability. Most statistical software programs provide these for kappa and ICC values, but nevertheless they are seldom presented. For the limits of agreement, a 95% CI of the higher or lower limit of agreement can be calculated as the limit of agreement $\pm$ 1.96 $\times$ $\sqrt{3}$ $\times$ $SD_{difference}/\sqrt{n}$ (Bland and Altman, 1999). The 95% CIs of SEM values, and in particular for $SEM_{agreement}$, are more difficult to obtain.

These considerations of sample size concern the number of patients and repeated measurements in relation to the efficiency of the design to reach the same CI (i.e. the precision of the estimation). However, in addition to efficiency there is the issue of external validity, which concerns the generalizability of the results to other situations. In the example concerning the range of shoulder movements, De Winter *et al.* (2004) took a sample of 155 patients who were assessed by two physiotherapists. If their intention was to generalize their results to all physiotherapists, the involvement of only two physiotherapists would seem to be inadequate and assessments by more than two physiotherapists would have been a better choice. Using designs in which various physiotherapists assess a sample of the patients would have been an option, but for these more complex designs, it is advisable to consult a statistician.

5.10 Design of reliability studies for more complex situations

Until now, we have looked at reliability studies that focus on one source of variation at a time (e.g. the variance among raters or the variance between different time-points). However, many situations involve more than one source of variation. For example, we might be interested in variation among raters who assess patients on different days and at different time-points during the day. Sometimes we want to know the contribution of each of these several sources of variation (raters, days, time) separately. In particular, this is the case if our aim is to improve the reliability of measurements. In this section, we will deal with more complex questions of reliability. A reliability study of blood pressure measurements will serve as an example. We

Table 5.9 Measurement scheme of 350 boys: systolic blood pressure is measured three times by four different clinicians

	Clinician 1			Clinician 2			Clinician 3			Clinician 4		
	M1	M2	M3	M1	M2	M3	M1	M2	M3	M1	M2	M3
1												
2												
3												
•												
•												
349												
350												

M, moment.

composed a set of variance components inspired by the study carried out by Rosner *et al.* (1987), who assessed blood pressure in children. They assessed the blood pressure at four different visits (each 1 week apart), and at each visit three measurements were performed.

In our example, we use the data of 350 boys, aged 8–12 years, and assume that instead of four different visits, there were four different clinicians that performed the measurements. Each clinician performed three measurements: M_1, M_2, and M_3. Table 5.9 presents the measurement scheme corresponding to the design of this example, and Table 5.10 shows the variance components that can be distinguished.

The total variance of one measurement in Table 5.9 can be written as

$$\sigma_y^2 = \sigma_p^2 + \sigma_o^2 + \sigma_m^2 + \sigma_{po}^2 + \sigma_{pm}^2 + \sigma_{om}^2 + \sigma_{\text{residual}}^2.$$

The variance of the patients (σ_p^2) is of key interest, because we want to distinguish between the blood pressure levels of these boys, beyond all sources of measurement error. The variance components σ_o^2 and σ_m^2 represent systematic differences between clinicians and between measurements, respectively, over all patients. The variance components σ_{po}^2 and σ_{pm}^2, pointing to interaction, are more difficult to interpret. For example, interaction between boys and clinicians occurs if some boys become more relaxed because the clinician is friendlier, resulting in lower blood pressure values. This variance is expressed as σ_{po}^2. If all boys react in this way, it would become visible as

Table 5.10 Variance components corresponding to the measurement scheme above

Source of variability	Meaning of variance component	Variance notation
Patients (p)	Variance due to systematic differences between 'true' score of patients (patients to be distinguished)	σ_p^2
Observers (o)	Variance due to systematic differences between the observers (clinicians in this example)	σ_o^2
Measurements (m)	Variance due to systematic differences between the measurements (the three measurements by the same clinician in this example)	σ_m^2
$p \times o$	Variance due to the interaction of patients and observers (in this example boys and clinicians)	σ_{po}^2
$p \times m$	Variance due to the interaction of patients and measurements (in this example boys and measurements by the same clinician)	σ_{pm}^2
$o \times m$	Variance due to the interaction of observers and measurements (in this example clinicians and measurements by the same clinician)	σ_{om}^2
$p \times o \times m$	Residual variance, partly due to the unique combination of p, o and m	$\sigma_{\text{residual}}^2$

a systematic difference between the clinicians, and would be expressed as σ_o^2. Interaction between clinicians and measurements occurs if, for example, some clinicians concentrate less when performing the second or third measurement. The residual variance component consists of the interaction of the three factors (patients, observers and moments), in addition to some random error.

In our example, we assumed that we have a crossed design, meaning that the four clinicians performed the three repeated measurements for all boys. However, for logistical reasons, crossed designs are not often used. For example, a doctor will often measure his/her own patients, which means that patients are 'nested' within the factor 'doctor'. Factors can be nested or overlap in many ways. For a more detailed explanation of nested designs, we refer to Shavelson and Webb (1991), and strongly advise that a statistician should be consulted if you are considering using one of these complex designs.

Now that we have repeated measurements by different clinicians, we can answer many questions. For example:

(1) What is the reliability of the measurements, if we compare for all boys, one measurement by one clinician with another measurement by another clinician?

(2) What is the reliability of the measurements if we compare for all boys the measurements performed by the same clinician (i.e. intra-rater reliability)?

(3) What is the reliability of the measurements if we compare for all boys the measurements performed by different clinicians (i.e. inter-rater reliability)?

(4) Which strategy is to be recommended for increasing the reliability of the measurement: using the average of more measurements of the boys by one clinician, or using the average of one measurement by different clinicians?

The answers to these questions are relevant, not only for clinical practice, but also for logistical reasons when designing a research project. These questions can all be answered by generalizability and decision studies.

5.11 Generalizability and decision studies

5.11.1 Generalizability studies

Generalizability and decision (G and D) studies first need to be explained in the context of reliability. For example, in question 3 above (Section 5.10) we investigate the inter-rater reliability. If this reliability is low, we might expect different answers from different clinicians, but if the reliability is high, almost similar values for blood pressure will be found by different clinicians. In other words, we can generalize the values found by one clinician to other clinicians. Therefore, these reliability studies are called generalizability (G) studies. Question 4 above asks to choose the most reliable strategy and involves a decision (D) to be taken. To answer this question we have to see which strategy has the highest reliability. In G and D studies we need formulas for a G coefficient, which is analogous to ICC, except that it contains more than one source of variation.

The total variance σ_y^2 at each blood pressure measurement in the example above can be subdivided as follows:

$$\sigma_y^2 = \sigma_p^2 + \sigma_o^2 + \sigma_m^2 + \sigma_{po}^2 + \sigma_{pm}^2 + \sigma_{om}^2 + \sigma_{residual}^2.$$

In the same manner as in Section 5.3, the reliability parameter can be written as

$$\text{Rel} = G = \frac{\sigma_p^2}{\sigma_p^2 + \sigma_o^2 + \sigma_m^2 + \sigma_{po}^2 + \sigma_{pm}^2 + \sigma_{om}^2 + \sigma_{residual}^2}.$$

To understand these G coefficients properly we have to go back to the COSMIN definition of the measurement property reliability: the proportion of the total variance in the measurements, which is due to 'true' differences between the patients (Mokkink *et al.*, 2010a):

$$\text{Rel} = \frac{\sigma_p^2}{\sigma_p^2 + \sigma_{error}^2}.$$

The true variance of the patients we want to distinguish appears in the numerator, and the total variance is represented by $\sigma_p^2 + \sigma_{error}^2$ in the denominator. But as we address each of the four questions in turn, the subdivision into σ_p^2 and σ_{error}^2 will be done in different ways. While doing this we must not forget that the total variance is the sum of the patient variance and error variance, and thus: patient variance = total variance – error variance. We will see how this works out for questions 1, 2 and 3.

The results of three-way ANOVA to estimate the variance components of patients, clinicians, measurements and their interactions are reported in Table 5.11.

Question 1

What is the reliability of the measurements if we compare for all the boys, one measurement by one clinician with another measurement by another clinician?

This question refers to generalization across clinicians and across measurements and, therefore, all the variance components involving clinicians and measurements are included in the error variance. In practical terms, all the variances that have *o* or *m* as subscripts are considered to be error variances. Analogous to ICC, the G coefficients have an agreement and a

Table 5.11 Values of various variance components

Variance component	Value
σ_p^2	70
σ_o^2	6
σ_m^2	2
σ_{po}^2	30
σ_{pm}^2	12
σ_{om}^2	3
$\sigma_{residual}^2$	15

consistency version. Using the data from Table 5.11, we can calculate the G coefficients for agreement corresponding to question 1 as follows:

$$G_{agreement} = \frac{\sigma_p^2}{\sigma_p^2 + \sigma_o^2 + \sigma_m^2 + \sigma_{po}^2 + \sigma_{pm}^2 + \sigma_{om}^2 + \sigma_{residual}^2}$$

$$= \frac{70}{70+6+2+30+12+3+15} = 0.507.$$

In the consistency version of the G coefficient, the variance due to the systematic differences between clinicians σ_o^2, the variance due to the systematic differences between the measurements σ_m^2, and the interaction term between clinicians and measurements σ_{om}^2, are omitted from the error variance:

$$G_{consistency} = \frac{\sigma_p^2}{\sigma_p^2 + \sigma_{po}^2 + \sigma_{pm}^2 + \sigma_{residual}^2} = \frac{70}{70+30+12+15} = 0.551.$$

In the presence of systematic errors, $G_{consistency}$ will be larger than $G_{agreement}$. The considerations for choosing between the agreement or consistency version of the G coefficient are exactly the same as explained for the ICC in Section 5.4.1. However, because the G coefficient is easier to explain for the consistency version, we will use only the consistency version from now on.

Question 2

What is the reliability of the measurements if we compare for all boys the measurements performed by the same clinician (i.e. intra-rater reliability)?

This question refers to generalization across the measurements and not across the clinicians. Therefore, the variance components that involve the multiple measurements, i.e. that include m in the subscript, are included in the error variance. So, the error variance consists of $\sigma^2_{error} = \sigma^2_{pm} + \sigma^2_{residual}$. As the total variance remains the same, this implies that the variance components not part of the error variance automatically become part of the patient variance, and the patient variance is now $\sigma^2_p + \sigma^2_{po}$. For this situation the formula for $G_{consistency}$ is as follows:

$$G_{consistency} = \frac{\sigma^2_p + \sigma^2_{po}}{\sigma^2_p + \sigma^2_{po} + \sigma^2_{pm} + \sigma^2_{residual}} = \frac{70+30}{70+30+12+15} = 0.787.$$

There is another way to explain why σ^2_{po} appears in the numerator. If we didn't know that there were different clinicians involved, the variance due to the different clinicians would have been incorporated in the observed differences between the boys.

Question 3

What is the reliability of the measurements if we compare for all boys the measurements performed by different clinicians (i.e. inter-rater reliability)?

This question refers to generalization across the clinicians, and not across measurements, if only one measurement is taken by each clinician. Therefore, the variance components that involve multiple observers, i.e. that include o in the subscript, are included in the error variance. So, the error variance consists of $\sigma^2_{error} = \sigma^2_{po} + \sigma^2_{residual}$. By the same reasoning as above, σ^2_{pm} will appear in the numerator as part of the patient variance. For this situation the formula for $G_{consistency}$ is as follows:

$$G_{consistency} = \frac{\sigma^2_p + \sigma^2_{pm}}{\sigma^2_p + \sigma^2_{pm} + \sigma^2_{po} + \sigma^2_{residual}} = \frac{70+12}{70+12+30+15} = 0.646.$$

Notice that generalizability across different clinicians is lower than across different measurements ($0.65 < 0.79$). This means that the value of the blood pressure measured at one moment by one clinician can be generalized better to another measurement by the same clinician than to a measurement taken by another clinician. In other words, there is more variation between the different clinicians than between the measurements taken by one clinician. This leads to the fourth question.

5.11.2 Decision studies

For question 4, we switch from G studies to D studies. That is because question 4 concerns a strategy, i.e. a decision about the most efficient use of repeated measurements in order to achieve the highest reliability.

Question 4

Which strategy is to be recommended for increasing the reliability of the measurement: using the average of more measurements of the boys by one clinician, or using the average of one measurement by different clinicians?

This question requires generalization across clinicians and measurements. Therefore, all variance components with o and m in the subscript in the $G_{consistency}$ formula appear in the error variance.

In the situation in which more measurements of the boys are made by one clinician, we average the three values of the repeated measurements per clinician. In that case, as we have seen in Section 5.4.1.2, all variances with m in the subscript are divided by the factor 3. This also applies to the residual variance because, as can be seen in Table 5.10, the residual variance includes interaction between factors p, o and m. If the value of three repeated measurements are averaged, the formula for the G coefficient is

$$G_{consistency} = \frac{\sigma_p^2}{\sigma_p^2 + \sigma_{po}^2 + \dfrac{\sigma_{pm}^2}{3} + \dfrac{\sigma_{residual}^2}{3}} = \frac{70}{70 + 30 + \dfrac{12}{3} + \dfrac{15}{3}} = 0.642.$$

In the situation in which the boys have one single measurement by four different clinicians, we average the values of the repeated measurements of the four clinicians. In this case, all variances with o in the subscript are divided by a factor 4. The G coefficient formula then becomes

$$G_{consistency} = \frac{\sigma_p^2}{\sigma_p^2 + \dfrac{\sigma_{po}^2}{4} + \sigma_{pm}^2 + \dfrac{\sigma_{residual}^2}{4}} = \frac{70}{70 + \dfrac{30}{4} + 12 + \dfrac{15}{4}} = 0.751.$$

Thus, the idea is that error variance can be reduced by performing repeated measurements and assessing the reliability of the averaged values: each variance component that contains the factor over which the average is taken is divided by the number of measurements being averaged. Averaging over different clinicians is the more advantageous strategy, because the G coefficient is larger (0.751 versus 0.642). This is not simply because there are more clinicians than there are measurements. You might check that averaging over three clinicians leads to a G coefficient of 0.722, which is still larger than the 0.642 obtained when averaging over three measurements made by one clinician.

Deciding how to achieve the most efficient measurement design is referred to as a D study. Note that this is not really a study in which new data are collected, it just implies drawing additional conclusions from the data of the G study. We can take decisions about all the sources of variability that have been included in the G study. For example, using the variances found in our G study on blood pressure measurements, we can calculate the G coefficient for a situation in which we use 10 repeated measurements per patient or in which we use the measurements made by two or five clinicians.

It is evident that maximum gain in reliability is achieved if we can average over the largest sources of variation. In the example above, the variation among clinicians is greater than the variation among multiple measurements by the same clinician (see Table 5.11). Therefore, averaging over clinicians turned out to be more advantageous. However, apart from the G coefficient, practical consequences must also be taken into account. For logistical reasons, we might choose multiple measurements per clinician, because the involvement of different clinicians costs more time and effort. One has to weigh these costs against the gain in reliability.

For didactical reasons, we have used the formulas to come to this conclusion. However, it is clear which strategy would be best: dividing the largest variance components will result in the greatest increase in reliability. Therefore, to improve the reliability we have to identify the source of variation that contributes most to the error. If we are able to reduce this source, the gain in reliability will be highest. We have presented the proportional contribution of the various components to the total variance in Table 5.12.

Using the variance components in this table, we can calculate the G coefficients, and after considering the practical consequences, we can decide on the most efficient measurement strategy. If we were to calculate the G coefficients for agreement, the variance components of the systematic differences would also need to appear in Table 5.12. As we have said before

Table 5.12 Values of various variance components

Variance notation	Value	Proportion of total variance
σ_p^2	70	0.551
σ_{po}^2	30	0.236
σ_{pm}^2	12	0.095
$\sigma_{residual}^2$	15	0.118
Total variance:		
$\sigma_p^2 + \sigma_{po}^2 + \sigma_{pm}^2 + \sigma_{residual}^2$	127	1.000

the $G_{agreement}$ formulas are more complex, and we recommend consulting a statistician when these are to be used.

5.12 Cronbach's alpha as a reliability parameter

In the beginning of this chapter, we promised to demonstrate that Cronbach's alpha is a reliability parameter. For this reason, instead of the term 'internal consistency', the terms 'internal reliability' and 'structural reliability' are also used in the literature. The repetition is not measurement by different observers, on different occasions or at different time-points, the repetition is rather measurement by different items in the multi-item measurement instrument, which all aim to measure the same construct. Therefore, Cronbach's alpha can be based on a single measurement. We recall here Formula 5.1, in which we presented the basic formula of the CTT for repeated measurements:

$$Y_i = \eta + \varepsilon_i. \tag{5.1}$$

In Section 5.4.1.2, we saw that when we take the average value of multiple measurements, the error variance can be divided by the number of measurements over which the average is taken. This principle can be applied to Cronbach's alpha: in a multi-item instrument, if we consider one scale based on a reflective model, the construct is measured repeatedly by each item, but then to calculate the score of the scale we take the sum or the average of all items. Let us return to the somatization scale (Terluin *et al.*, 2006) as an example. The somatization scale consists of 16 symptoms, measuring among other things: headache, shortness of breath and tingling in the fingers. The questions refer to whether the patient suffered from these symptoms during the previous week and the response options are 'no', 'sometimes', 'regularly', 'often' and 'very often or constantly'. All 16 symptoms are indicative of somatization, and the scale has been shown to be unidimensional. Each item is scored 0 ('no'), 1 ('sometimes') or 2 (all other categories), which results in a score from 0 to 32, a higher score indicating a higher tendency to somatize.

The items are summed (or averaged) to obtain a score for the construct, and by using 16 items to get the best estimation of the construct, the error term is divided by 16 (the number of items). We calculate the G coefficient for consistency as follows:

$$G_{consistency} = \frac{\sigma_p^2}{\sigma_p^2 + \dfrac{\sigma_{error}^2}{16}}.$$

This G coefficient is Cronbach's alpha. Based on the notion that Cronbach's alpha is one of the many ICC versions, there are a number of interesting characteristics of Cronbach's alpha:

- As we already noticed in Chapter 4, Cronbach's alpha depends on the number of items. The explanation becomes apparent in the formula above. If we had measured somatization with 32 items instead of 16, the error variance would be divided by 32. This increases the reliability, and thus also Cronbach's alpha.
- Cronbach's alpha, like all other reliability parameters, depends on the variation in the population. This means that in heterogeneous populations a higher value of Cronbach's alpha will be found than in homogeneous populations. So, be aware that Cronbach's alpha is sample-dependent and, just like validity and test–retest reliability, a characteristic of an instrument used in a population, and not a characteristic of a measurement instrument.

Together with the output of reliability analysis for $ICC_{agreement}$ and $ICC_{consistency}$ (Section 5.4.1), comes Cronbach's alpha. Notice that the value for Cronbach's alpha equals the average ICC measures for consistency. By running these analyses yourselves you will see that both the outputs of $ICC_{agreement}$ and $ICC_{consistency}$ mention a value for Cronbach's alpha of 0.896. By now you should be able to understand why that is the case.

5.13 Reliability parameters and measurement error obtained by item response theory analysis

As we have already seen in Chapters 2 and 4, IRT can be used to investigate various characteristics at item level. In the CTT the SEM is calculated, and assumed to be stable, over the total scale. Recall that in constructing the Bland and Altman plot we explicitly made this assumption. In the IRT, the item characteristic curves i.e. the discrimination (slope) and the difficulty parameter, can be estimated per item. The next step is that the ability (θ) of the patients in the sample is estimated from the discrimination and difficulty parameters of the items. This estimation of a patient's ability is accompanied by a standard error (SE), which concerns the internal consistency, indicating how good the items can distinguish patients from each other. Like Cronbach's alpha, the SE is based on a single measurement, and not on test–retest analysis.

In IRT, reliability is determined by the discriminating ability of the items. In Figure 5.6 (similar to Figure 2.6), item 2 has a higher discriminating value than item 1. We say that high discriminating items provide more information about a patient's ability. A measurement instrument with a large number of highly discriminating items, like item 2, will give more precise information about the location of persons on the ability (θ) axis than a measurement instrument containing items like item 1. Therefore, it will be better able to

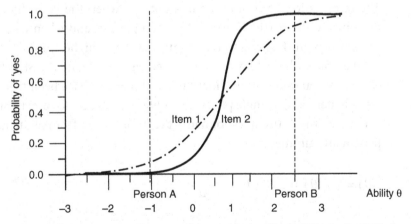

Figure 5.6   Item characteristic curves for two items with the same difficulty but differing in discrimination.

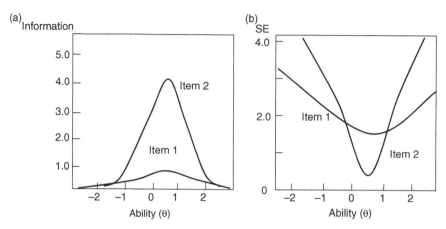

Figure 5.7　Information curves (a) and standard error curves (b) for two items.

distinguish patients from each other. To illustrate this principle, the information curves of items 1 and 2 in Figure 5.6 are shown in Figure 5.7(a,b).

Figure 5.7(a) shows the information curves of these two items, and Figure 5.7(b) shows the SEs of these items. The less discriminating item 1 has a flatter and more widely spread information curve. Item 2 is better able to discriminate between the ability of the patients than item 1 and contains more information. The formula is as follows:

$$I_i(\theta) = a_i^2 P_i(\theta)[1 - P_i(\theta)].$$

The information level of an item is optimal when the item difficulty corresponds to the particular trait score of a patient, and when item discrimination is high. If the amount of information is highest, the SE (which is comparable with the SEM) is lowest (see Figure 5.7(b)). The SE is the reciprocal of the amount of information. Until now, we have been talking about a single item and a single patient. To obtain a total SE for a patient that has completed the entire questionnaire, the information from all items for this patient are summed:

$$I(\theta) = \sum_i I_i(\theta) \text{ and } SE(\theta) = \frac{1}{\sqrt{I(\theta)}}.$$

As a last step, the SE of each patient can be averaged over the population to obtain a summary index of reliability for the population. However, the advantage of having information about the varying reliability over the scale is then lost.

5.14 Reliability and computer adaptive testing

As described in Chapter 2, the essential characteristic of computer adaptive testing (CAT) is that the test or questionnaire is tailored to the 'ability' of the individual. This means that for each respondent, items are chosen that correspond to his/her ability. Without any previous information, one would usually start with items with a difficulty parameter between −0.5 and +0.5. If a patient gives a confirmative answer to the first item, the next item will be more difficult, but if the answer is negative, the next item will be easier. With a few questions, the computer tries to locate the patient at a certain range of positions on the scale. Knowing that an item gives the most information about a respondent if he/she has a probability of 0.5 of giving a confirmative answer, items in this range will be used to estimate a patient's position on the x-axis. Thinking about this strategy in terms of reliability, it is obvious that with a small number of items one tries to obtain the maximum amount of information. As we learned in Section 5.13, this implies a small measurement error, and thus high reliability. It is this very principle that makes the CAT tests shorter. An important question is: when does one stop administering new items to a respondent? The most commonly applied stopping rule is to keep administering items until the SE is below a certain a priori defined value. In general, fewer items are needed for CAT tests than for the corresponding 'regular' tests. Moreover, with fewer items there is an equal or even lower level of measurement error. This is shown in Figure 5.8, which is based on the PROMIS item bank for measuring physical functioning (Rose *et al.*, 2008).

Figure 5.8 shows the measurement precision, expressed as SE for a CAT questionnaire consisting of 10 questions compared with other instruments that assess physical functioning. With fewer items, there are smaller SEs. Only the 53-item questionnaire resulted in smaller SEs. The SE values of 5.0, 3.3 and 2.3 as shown in Figure 5.8, correspond to reliability parameters of 0.80, 0.90 and 0.95, respectively, if we assume that SD = 10. In Figure 5.8 the SE is presented on the y-axis, but sometimes the number of items needed to obtain a certain SE value is represented on the y-axis.

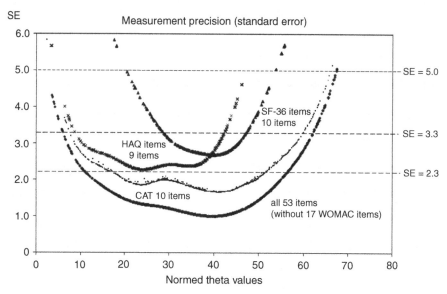

Figure 5.8   Standard errors for various questionnaires to assess physical functioning, including a 10-item Computer Adaptive Testing (CAT) questionnaire. Rose *et al.* (2008), with permission.

5.15 Reliability at group level and individual level

In the literature on reliability, it is often stated that ICC values of 0.70 are acceptable if an instrument is used in measurements of groups of patients. However, for application in individual patients, ICC values as high as 0.90 and preferably 0.95 are required (Nunnally and Bernstein, 1994). In this section, we explain why higher values for reliability are required for the measurement of individual patients.

The first reason is that measurement of individual patients is usually followed by a specific decision for this particular patient, while the consequences of research findings for clinical practice are only indirect. Therefore, for use in clinical practice one has to have high confidence in the obtained value. Note that with an ICC value of 0.90, using the formula $\text{SEM} = \text{SD} \sqrt{(1 - \text{ICC})}$ presented in Section 5.4.2.1, SEM values are 1/3 SD. In section 5.4.1.2, we described how measurement errors could be reduced by taking the average of multiple measurements. The error term can be divided by a factor $\sqrt{k}$, when k is the number of repeated measurements. When the measurement error decreases, the value of ICC will increase.

This is illustrated by the following formulas, assuming a situation with a single score per patient, and a situation in which the scores of k measurements are averaged, respectively:

When using a single measurement

$$ICC_{consistency} = \frac{\sigma_p^2}{\sigma_p^2 + \sigma_{error}^2} \, .$$

When using the mean value of k measurements

$$ICC_{consistency} = \frac{\sigma_p^2}{\sigma_p^2 + \dfrac{\sigma_{error}^2}{k}} \, .$$

Repeating the number of measurements and averaging the results is an adequate way in which to increase the ICC value to an acceptable level.

The second reason why higher values for reliability parameters are required for individual patients, compared with groups of patients has to do with the statistical principles of calculating group mean and SE. If measurements of patients are averaged to obtain a group mean, this is accompanied by SE of the mean, which, as we all learned in our basic courses in statistics, equals SD/$\sqrt{n}$. This SD consists of deviations of the scores of individual group members from the value of the group mean, plus measurement error.

The basic formula of the classical test theory (Formula 5.1) is slightly rewritten as

$$Y_i = \theta_i + \varepsilon_i$$

in which θ_i now represents the score of each patient i in the group. The variance of Y_i is:

$$\text{Var } Y_i = \sigma_\theta^2 + \sigma_e^2$$

and the variance of the mean value of Y ($\bar{Y}$) is

$$\text{Var } \bar{Y} = (\sigma_\theta^2 + \sigma_e^2)/n.$$

As the Var $\bar{Y}$ equals $SE_{\bar{Y}}^2$, it follows that:

$$SE_{\bar{Y}} = \sqrt{\frac{\sigma_\theta^2 + \sigma_e^2}{n}} = \sqrt{\frac{\sigma_\theta^2 + SEM^2}{n}} \, .$$

In this formula, it can be seen that by using the SE of the mean, the standard error of measurement is divided by $\sqrt{n}$. Therefore, when we are examining groups of patients, the measurement error is reduced by a factor $\sqrt{n}$, when the group consists of n patients. However, we can not distinguish the measurement error variance from the between-patient variance.

Therefore, the reason why ICC values of 0.70 suffice for application in groups of patients (Nunnally and Bernstein, 1994) is that one anticipates that averaging the scores reduces the measurement error. In fact, in both clinical practice and research very reliable instruments are required. In clinical practice, this has to be achieved by using a measurement instrument with a small measurement error, or by averaging the scores of repeated measurements. In research, increasing the sample size will help. Note that, as a consequence, more reliable measurement instruments are required for use in clinical practice.

5.16 Improving the reliability of measurements

In Section 5.1, we stated that reliability concerns the anticipation, assessment and control of sources of variation, and that the ultimate aim of reliability studies is to improve the reliability of measurements. Throughout this chapter, we have already encountered a number of strategies that can be used for this purpose, but here we will summarize these strategies to give an overview.

- *Restriction.* Restriction means that we avoid a specific source of variation. For example, when we know that the amount of fatigue that patients experience increases during the day, we can exclude this variation by measuring every patient at the same hour of the day.
- *Training and standardization.* The reliability of measurements can be improved by intensive training of the raters or by standardization of the procedure. For example, physiotherapists can be trained to carry out performance tests. They should be trained to use exactly the same text to instruct the patients, they should try to do that with a similar amount of enthusiasm, and there should be agreement on whether, and to what extent, they should encourage the patients during the performance of the tests.

- *Averaging of repeated measurements.* In the previous section we have explained how averaging repeated measurements reduces the measurement error. This only affects the random error, not the systematic error. If it is possible to make repeated measurements of the largest sources of variation, the increase in reliability is highest. We have described how this works, using the G coefficient.

5.17 Summary

Reliability and measurement error are two different, but related, concepts. Important parameters for assessing reliability are Cohen's kappa for measurements on a nominal scale (unweighted kappa) or ordinal scale (weighted kappa) and the ICC for measurements with continuous outcomes. There are various ICC formulas. We have differentiated between $ICC_{consistency}$ and $ICC_{agreement}$. In $ICC_{consistency}$ systematic errors are not included in the error variance, and this applies when the source of variation is fixed (e.g. we are only interested in the raters involved in this specific reliability study). If our aim is to generalize and consider the source of variation as a random factor, we can choose between $ICC_{consistency}$ and $ICC_{agreement}$. In that case, we use $ICC_{agreement}$ when interested in the absolute agreement between the repeated measurements, and $ICC_{consistency}$ when we are only interested in the ranking. For the assessment of measurement error, we have mentioned the SEM and limits of agreement (Bland and Altman method).

The interpretation of all these parameters is facilitated by a detailed presentation of the results. This holds for the Bland and Altman plot, for a full presentation of the tables underlying the kappa values, and a presentation of the variance components incorporated in the ICC formula.

Parameters of measurement error are of great value for clinicians. They are expressed in the units of measurement, which often facilitates interpretation for clinicians. Moreover, they are most relevant when monitoring the health status of patients, and when deciding whether changes exceed the measurement errors. Unfortunately, in medicine, too often only parameters of reliability are used. The SEM can only be derived if the error variance is reported in addition to an ICC value, or when the SD of the population in which the ICC is determined is known.

When designing a reliability study, the aim of the study should be kept in mind. Important questions are: To which raters do you want to generalize? For which part of the measurement process do you want to know the reliability? What is the target population? The latter is of major importance, because the heterogeneity of the study population has substantial influence on the parameters of reliability.

In the case of multi-item measurement instruments, the number of items that are included can be used to increase the reliability of the instrument. We have shown that Cronbach's alpha is a reliability parameter. CAT also makes use of the principle that the SE can be reduced by repeated measurements, and that by tailoring the measurements to the ability of the patients, the internal reliability of measurements can be substantially improved. A high internal reliability or internal consistency does not imply that the test–retest reliability is also high, because these are different sources of variation. Therefore, internal consistency cannot replace test–retest reliability.

In G and D studies, it becomes clear that knowledge about the different sources of variation is vital to improve the reliability of measurements. Anticipating large sources of variation reduces measurement errors. Strategies to avoid measurement errors are, for example, restriction to one rater, or standardization of the time-points of measurement. Measurement error can be reduced, for example, through better calibration of measurement instruments, or more intensive training for raters. Consensus among raters with regard to the scoring criteria may also help to increase reliability. If these strategies cannot be applied, multiple measurements can be made and the values averaged to reduce measurement error. We can only improve the quality of measurements by paying attention to reliability and measurement errors.

Assignments

1. Calculation and interpretation of intraclass correlation coefficient

In the example concerning range of movement (ROM) in patients with shoulder complaints we used data on 50 patients, and we purposefully introduced a systematic error. For the current assignment, we use the complete data set for 155 patients (De Winter *et al.*, 2004), which can be found on the website www.clinimetrics.nl.

(a) Use this data set to calculate the means and SDs of Mary's and Peter's scores, the mean difference and the SD of the difference, and both the ICC for agreement and the ICC for consistency (and 95% CI).

(b) Which parameter do you prefer: $ICC_{consistency}$ or $ICC_{agreement}$?

(c) Can you explain why there is such a difference between the ICCs for the affected side and the non-affected side?

2. Calculation of measurement error

(a) Calculate $SEM_{agreement}$ and $SEM_{consistency}$ for the affected shoulder and the non-affected shoulder.

(b) Now that you have seen that SEMs for the affected shoulder and non-affected shoulder are roughly the same, what is your explanation for assignment 1(c)?

(c) Draw a Bland and Altman plot for the affected side.

(d) Calculate the limits of agreement.

3. Calculation of standard error of measurement by rewriting the intraclass correlation coefficient formula

In Section 5.4.2.1, we warned against the use of the formula $SEM = \sigma_y \sqrt{(1 - ICC)}$. Suppose researchers measured the ROM of shoulders in the general population, and the SD of the scores in this population was 8.00. In the literature, the researchers find an ICC value of 0.83 for the ROM of shoulders. They decide to calculate the SEM for these measurements as $SEM = SD_{pooled}\sqrt{(1 - ICC_{consistency})} = 8.00 \times \sqrt{(1 - 0.83)} = 3.30$.

Comment on this calculation.

4. Calculation of kappa

EEG recordings have been introduced as a potentially valuable method with which to monitor the central nervous function in comatose patients. In these patients, it is relevant to detect refractory convulsive status epilepticus, because patients experiencing such seizures may easily recover from the coma if they receive medication. Ronner et al. (2009) designed an inter-observer study with nine clinicians to evaluate EEG recordings, and these clinicians had to decide for each EEG whether or not there was any evidence

Table 5.13 Results of two clinicians

	Clinician 1		
Clinician 2	EEG+	EEG⁻	Total
EEG+	17	0	17
EEG⁻	5	8	13
Total	22	8	30

EEG+ denotes evidence of seizure and EEG⁻ denotes no evidence of seizure on the encephalo-electrogram.

of an electrographic seizure. The results of two clinicians are presented in Table 5.13.

(a) Calculate Cohen's kappa value for these two observers. You may try to do it manually to practise using the formulas presented in this chapter.

(b) In order to obtain a 95% CI for the kappa value you have to use a computer program (see Section 5.5.1.2). Check your calculated kappa value, and calculate the 95% CI.

(c) How do you interpret this kappa value?

5. Calculation of weighted kappa

In Section 5.5.1.2, we presented the formula that should be used to calculate weighted kappa values, and the weights that are often used. For Table 5.5 in this section we provided the result of the weighted kappa obtained by a computer program. Are you able to reproduce this value, filling in the formula?

6. Design of a generalizability study

Researchers developed the Pain Assessment Checklist for Seniors with Limited Ability to Communicate (PACSLAC), an observation scale for the assessment of pain in elderly people with dementia. Nursing home doctors decide to introduce this scale in their nursing homes, but they want to know how the scale should be used to obtain a reliable outcome.

(a) What sources of variation can you think of?

(b) Draw a measurement scheme for a G study, with four different factors.

7. Exercise on generalizability and decision studies

(a) In Table 5.12 we presented the variance components for the G and D study focusing on blood pressure measurements in boys. We saw that different clinicians were a larger source of variation than multiple measurements made by the same clinician. To increase reliability, we can either have measurements made by different clinicians or multiple measurement made by one clinician. When do we achieve the highest reliability: when one measurement is made by two different clinicians, or when five measurements are made during one visit by the same clinician? We first assume that there are no systematic errors, and use $G_{consistency}$ for the calculations.

(b) We had ignored systematic errors, but if there are any, which ones do you expect to be larger: those between clinicians or those between multiple measurements made by the same clinician? Does that change the decision about the most reliable measurement strategy?

6

Validity

6.1 Introduction

Validity is defined by the COSMIN panel as 'the degree to which an instrument truly measures the construct(s) it purports to measure' (Mokkink *et al.*, 2010a). This definition seems to be quite simple, but there has been much discussion in the past about how validity should be assessed and how its results should be interpreted. Psychologists, in particular, have struggled with this problem, because, as we saw in Chapters 2 and 3, they often have to deal with 'unobservable' constructs. This makes it difficult for them to judge whether they are measuring the right thing. In general, three different types of validity can be distinguished: content validity, criterion validity and construct validity. Content validity focuses on whether the content of the instrument corresponds with the construct that one intends to measure, with regard to relevance and comprehensiveness. Criterion validity, applicable in situations in which there is a gold standard for the construct to be measured, refers to how well the scores of the measurement instrument agree with the scores on the gold standard. Construct validity, applicable in situations in which there is no gold standard, refers to whether the instrument provides the expected scores, based on existing knowledge about the construct. Within these three main types of validity, there are numerous subtypes, as we will see later in this chapter.

We will start with a concise overview of the literature about the concept of validity, and point out a number of important implications for our current thoughts about validation. Then we will focus on several types of validity, and discuss their roles and applications in the validation process. The examples we use are derived from different medical disciplines.

6.2 The concept of validity

The discussion about validity started in the mid fifties in psychological literature. Before that time, validation was mostly a matter of predicting outcome. However, it became clear that this method of validation did not add much to the knowledge about the constructs and to the formation of theories. Therefore, Cronbach and Meehl (1955) proposed to start from theories about the construct, and then formulate hypotheses. These hypotheses concern relationships of the construct under study with other constructs or hypotheses about values of the construct, dependent on characteristics of patient groups. Thus, validation consists of testing hypotheses. If these hypotheses are not rejected then the instrument is apparently suitable to measure that construct. Thus, the issue is not simply whether an instrument truly measures a construct, but whether scores of the instrument are consistent with a theoretical model of the construct (Cronbach and Meehl, 1955).

In a recent overview, Strauss and Smith (2009) nicely summarized these ideas about the concept of validation. For those who are interested in philosophical issues, this paper offers much 'food for thought'. Although the discussions took place in the field of psychology, they have influenced current thoughts about validation in all fields of medicine. We have extracted a number of important implications from this overview, as listed and discussed below. These concern the following issues:

- knowledge about the construct to be measured
- complexity of the construct
- dependency on the situation
- validation of scores, not measurement instruments
- formulation of specific hypotheses
- validation as a continuous process.

Knowledge about the construct
We emphasized the theoretical foundations of constructs and the presentation of conceptual models in Chapter 2. Now we see why this is of crucial importance for validation, i.e. we can only assess whether a measurement instrument measures what it purports to measure if researchers have clearly described the construct they intend to measure. Subsequently, we have to formulate hypotheses about what scores we expect to find on the measurement

instruments, based on our knowledge of the construct. Therefore, detailed knowledge of the construct and a conceptual model to hypothesize relationships with other constructs are indispensable for a sound validation process.

Complexity of the construct

A simple (unidimensional) construct is often easier to validate than a complex (multidimensional) construct. For example, if we want to evaluate an instrument to measure fatigue, it is much easier to formulate hypotheses about specific aspects of fatigue (e.g. only physical fatigue, or only mental fatigue) than about fatigue in general. As described in Section 3.3, when measuring overall fatigue we are not sure which aspects are included and how respondents weight these, which makes it difficult to predict relationships with related constructs. It might be much easier to predict relationships with related constructs for physical fatigue or mental fatigue. Note that when using a multidimensional instrument, each scale or each part of the instrument that measures a specific dimension should be validated, by formulating hypotheses for each dimension separately.

Dependency on the situation

A measurement instrument should be validated again if it is applied in a new situation or for another purpose. Suppose we have a measurement instrument to assess mobility, which was developed for adults with mobility problems. If we want to use this instrument in an elderly population, we have to validate it for use in this new target population, because this is a new situation. The Food and Drug Administration (FDA) Guidance Committee has described in detail what they consider to be new situations (FDA Guidance, 2009, pp. 20–1). For example, the application of an instrument in another target population, another language, or another form of administration (e.g. interview versus self-report) is considered to be a new situation. A well-known type of validation is cross-cultural validation, i.e. validation when an instrument is applied in countries with a different culture and language. For example, the Short-Form 36 (SF-36) has been translated and cross-culturally validated for a large number of languages (Wagner *et al.*, 1998).

It is also common practice to use instruments for broader applications than those for which they were originally developed. As an example, the

Roland–Morris Disability Questionnaire was originally developed for patients with non-specific low back pain, but later applied to patients with radiating low back pain (sciatica) (Patrick *et al.*, 1995). A new validation study was therefore performed in the new target population.

Validation of scores, not measurement instruments

Validation focuses on the scores produced by a measurement instrument, and not on the instrument itself. This is a consequence of the previous point, i.e. that a measurement instrument might function differently in other situations. As Nunnally (1978) stated: 'strictly speaking, one validates not a measurement instrument, but rather some use to which the measurement instrument is put'. So, we can never state that a measurement instrument is valid, only that it provides valid scores in the specific situation in which it has been tested. Therefore, the phrase that you often read in scientific papers, that 'valid instruments were used', should always be doubted, unless there is an indication as to which population and context this statement applies.

Formulation of specific hypotheses

Tests of validation require the formulation of hypotheses, and these hypotheses should be as specific as possible. Existing knowledge about the construct should drive the hypotheses. When researchers decide to develop a new instrument in a field in which other instruments are available, they should state on which points they expect their instrument to be better than the already existing instruments. The validation process should be based on hypotheses regarding these specific claims about why the new instrument is better. For example, if we want to develop an instrument mainly to measure physical functioning, and not focus so much on pain as other instruments do, there should be hypotheses stating that the correlation with pain is less for the new instrument than for the existing instruments.

Validation as a continuous process

A precise theory and extensive knowledge of the construct under study enables a strong validation test. This represents the ideal situation. However, when a construct is newly developed, at first there are only vague thoughts, or less detailed theories and construct definitions. In that case, the hypotheses are much weaker, and consequently, this also applies to the evidence they generate about the validity of the measurement instrument. When knowledge in a certain field is evolving, the initial theory will be rather weak but during the process of validation, theories about the construct and validation of measurements will probably become stronger. The same applies to the extension of empirical evidence concerning the construct. This is an iterative process in which testing of partially developed theories provides information that leads to refinement and elaboration of the theory, which in turn provides a stronger basis for subsequent construct and theory, and strengthen the validation of the measurement instrument. For these reasons, and also because measurements are often applied in different situations, validation is a continuous process.

This overview shows that validation of a measurement instrument cannot be disentangled from the validity of underlying theories about the construct, and from scores on the measurement instrument. Recently, the discussion about validity has been revived by Borsboom *et al.* (2004) who state that a test is valid for measuring a construct if and only if (a) the construct exists, and (b) variations in the construct causally produce variations in measurement outcomes. They emphasize that the crucial ingredient of validity involves the causal role of the construct in determining what value the measurement outcomes will take. This implies that validity testing should be focused on the process that convey this role, and tables of correlations between test scores and other measures provide only circumstantial evidence for validity. However, examples of such validation processes have been scarce until now.

In the validation process different types of validation can be applied, and the evidence from these different types of validation should be integrated to come to a conclusion about the degree of validity of the instrument in a specific population and context. We will now discuss various types of validation, and present some specific examples.

6.3 Content validity (including face validity)

Content validity is defined by the COSMIN panel as 'the degree to which the content of a measurement instrument is an adequate reflection of the construct to be measured' (Mokkink *et al.*, 2010a). For example, if the construct we want to measure is body weight, a weighing scale is sufficient. To measure the construct of obesity, defined as a body mass index

(BMI = weight/height^2) > 30 kg/m^2, a weighing scale and a measuring rod are needed. Now, suppose that we are interested in the construct of undernutrition in the elderly, with undernutrition defined as a form of malnutrition resulting from an insufficient supply of food, or from inability to digest, assimilate and use the necessary nutrients. In that case, a weighing scale and a measuring rod will not be sufficient, because the concept of undernutrition is broader than just weight and height.

6.3.1 Face validity

A first aspect of content validity is face validity. The COSMIN panel defined face validity as 'the degree to which a measurement instrument, indeed, looks as though it is an adequate reflection of the construct to be measured' (Mokkink *et al.*, 2010a). It concerns an overall view, which is often a first impression, without going into too much detail. It is a subjective assessment and, therefore, there are no standards with regard to how it should be assessed, and it cannot be quantified. As a result, the value of face validation is often underestimated. Note that, in particular, 'lack of face validity' is a very strong argument for not using an instrument, or to end further validation. For example, when selecting a questionnaire to assess physical activity in an elderly population, just reading the questions may give a first impression: questionnaires containing a large number of items about activities that are no longer performed by elderly people are not considered to be suitable. Other questionnaires may be examined in more detail to assess which ones contain items corresponding to the type of activities that the elderly do perform.

6.3.2 Content validity

When an instrument has passed the test of face validation, we have to consider its content in more detail. The purpose of a content validation study is to assess whether the measurement instrument adequately represents the construct under study. We again emphasize the importance of a good description of the construct to be measured. For multi-item questionnaires, this implies that the items should be both relevant and comprehensive for the construct to be measured. Relevance can be assessed with the following three questions: Do all items refer to relevant aspects of the construct to be measured? Are all items relevant for the study population, for example, with respect to age, gender, disease characteristics, languages, countries, settings? Are all items relevant for the purpose of the application of the measurement instrument? Possible purposes (Section 3.2.3) are discrimination (i.e. to distinguish between persons at one point in time), evaluation (i.e. to assess change over time) or prediction (i.e. to predict future outcomes). All these questions assess whether the items are relevant for measuring the construct. Comprehensiveness is the other side of the coin, i.e. is the construct completely covered by the items.

The process of content validation consists of the following steps:

(1) consider information about construct and situation
(2) consider information about content of the measurement instrument
(3) select an expert panel
(4) assess whether content of the measurement instrument corresponds with the construct (is relevant and comprehensive)
(5) use a strategy or framework to assess the correspondence between the instrument and construct

1: Consider information about construct and situation

To assess the content validity of an instrument, the construct to be measured should be clearly specified. As described in Chapter 3 (Section 3.2), this entails an elaboration of the theoretical background and/or conceptual model, and a description of the situation of use in terms of the target population, and purpose of the measurement. A nice example of elaboration of a construct is provided by Gerritsen *et al.* (2004), who compared various conceptual models of quality of life in nursing home residents.

Information about the construct should be considered by both the developer of a measurement instrument (who should provide this information), and by the user of a measurement instrument (who should collect this information about the construct).

2: Consider information about content of the measurement instrument

In order to be able to assess whether a specific measurement instrument covers the content of the construct, developers should have provided full details about the measurement instrument, including procedures. If the new measurement instrument concerns, for example, a MRI procedure, or a new laboratory test, the materials, methods and procedures, and scoring must be described in such a way that researchers in that specific field can repeat it. If the measurement instrument is a questionnaire, a full copy of the questionnaire (i.e. all items and response options, including the instructions) must be available, either in the article, appendix, on a website or on request from the authors. Furthermore, details of the development process may be relevant, such as a list of the literature that was used or other instruments that were used as a basis, and which experts were consulted. All this information should be taken into consideration in the assessment of content validity.

3: Select an expert panel

The content validity of a measurement instrument is assessed by researchers who are going to use it. Note, however, that developers of a measurement instrument are often biased with regard to their own instrument. Therefore, content validity should preferably be assessed by an independent panel. For all measurement instruments, it is important that content validity should be assessed by experts in the relevant field of medicine. For example, experts who are familiar with the field of radiology are required to judge the adequacy of various MRI techniques. For patient-reported outcomes (PROs), patients and, particularly representatives of the target population, are the experts. They are the most appropriate assessors of the relevance of the items in the questionnaire, and they can also indicate whether important items or aspects are missing. In Chapter 3 (Section 3.4.1.3) we gave an example of how patients from the target population were involved in the development of an instrument to assess health-related quality of life (HRQL) in patients with urine incontinence.

4: Assess whether the content of the measurement instrument corresponds with the construct

Like face validation, content validation is also only based on judgement, and no statistical testing is involved. The researchers who developed the measurement instrument should have considered relevance and comprehensiveness during the development process. However, users of the instrument should always check whether the instrument is sufficiently relevant and comprehensive for what they want to measure. Assessment of content validity by the users is particularly important if the measurement instrument is applied in other situations, i.e. another population or purpose than for which it was originally developed. For example, we want to measure physical functioning in stroke patients, and we find a questionnaire that was developed to assess physical functioning in an elderly population. To assess the content validity of this questionnaire, we have to judge whether all the activities mentioned in this questionnaire are relevant for the stroke population, and also to ensure that no important activities for stroke patients are missed (i.e. is the instrument comprehensive?). Another example, an accelerometer attached to a belt around the hip to measure physical activity may adequately detect activities such as walking and running, but may poorly detect activities such as cycling, and totally fail to detect activities involving only the upper extremities. Therefore, an accelerometer lacks comprehensiveness to measure total physical activity.

5: Use a strategy or framework to assess the correspondence between the instrument and construct

Although content validation is based on qualitative assessment, some form of quantification can be applied. At least the assessment of the content can be much more structured than is usually the case. As an example, we present the content of a number of questionnaires concerning physical functioning. Table 6.1 gives an overview of the items in the domain of 'physical functioning' in a number of well-known questionnaires. Cieza and Stucki (2005) classified the items according to the internal classification of functioning (ICF). In this example, the ICF is used as a framework, to compare the content of various questionnaires. If we need a questionnaire to measure physical functioning in depressive adolescents, the Nottingham Health Profile (NHP) may be the most suitable choice, because adolescents have the potential to be very physically active. However, for post-stroke patients the Quality of Life-Index (QL-I) may be more appropriate, because items concerning self-care and simple activities of daily living (I-ADL) are particularly relevant for severely disabled patients.

This type of content analysis is very useful if one wishes to select one measurement instrument that best fits the construct in the context of interest out of a large selection of measurement instruments. To use it for content validation, one should have an idea about what kinds of activities are important.

Table 6.1 General health status measurement instruments – frequencies showing how often the activities-and-participation categories were addressed in different instruments. Adapted from Cieza and Stucki (2005), with permission

Content comparison

ICF category[a]	QL-I	WHO DASII	NHP	SF-36
d450 Walking			1	
d4500 Walking short distances				1
d4501 Walking long distances		1		2
d455 Moving around			2	
d4551 Climbing			2	
d510 Washing oneself	1	1		1
d530 Toileting	1			
d540 Dressing	1	1	1	1
d550 Eating	1	1		
d6309 Preparing meals, unspecified			1	
d640 Doing housework	1	1	1	2
d6509 Caring for household objects		1		

[a] The numbers correspond to various disability (d) categories in the ICF classification. ICF, International Classification of Functioning; QL-I, Quality of Life-Index; WHO DASII, World Health Organization Disability Assessment Schedule; NHP, Nottingham Health Profile.

6.4 Criterion validity

Criterion validity is defined by the COSMIN panel as 'the degree to which the scores of a measurement instrument are an adequate reflection of a gold standard' (Mokkink *et al.*, 2010a). This implies that criterion validity can only be assessed when a gold standard (i.e. a criterion) is available.

Criterion validity can be subdivided into concurrent validity and predictive validity. When assessing concurrent validity we consider both the score for the measurement and the score for the gold standard at the same time, whereas when assessing predictive validity we consider whether the measurement instrument predicts the gold standard in the future. It is not surprising that the latter validation is often used for instruments to be used in predictive applications, while concurrent validity is usually assessed for instruments to be used for evaluative and diagnostic purposes. In case of concurrent validity and predictive validity, there is usually only one hypothesis that is not clearly stated but rather implicit. This hypothesis is that the measurement instrument under study is as good as the gold standard. In practice, the essential question is whether the instrument under study is sufficiently valid for its clinical purpose. It is not possible to provide uniform criteria to determine whether an instrument is sufficiently valid for application in a given situation, because this depends on the weighing of a number of consequences of applying the measurement instrument instead of the gold standard. These consequences include not only the costs and burden of the gold standard versus those of the measurement instrument, but also the consequences of false positive and false negative classifications resulting from the measurement instrument.

The general design of criterion-related validation consists of the following steps:

(1) identify a suitable criterion and method of measurement
(2) identify an appropriate sample of the target population in which the measurement instrument will ultimately be used
(3) define a priori the required level of agreement between measurement instrument and criterion
(4) obtain the scores for the measurement instrument and the gold standard, independently from each other
(5) determine the strength of the relationship between the instrument scores and criterion scores.

1: Identify a suitable criterion and method of measurement

The gold standard is considered to represent the true state of the construct of interest. In medicine, this will usually be a disease status or a measure of the severity of a disease, if the instrument is used to measure at ordinal level or interval level. In theory, the gold standard is a perfectly valid assessment. However, a perfect gold standard seldom exists in practice. It is usually a measurement instrument for the construct under study, which is regarded as ideal by experts in the field, i.e. a measurement instrument that has been accepted as a gold standard by experts. For example, the gold standard used to identify cancer is usually based on histological findings in the tissues, extracted by biopsy or surgery.

PROs, which often focus on subjective perceptions and opinions, almost always lack a gold standard. An exception is a situation in which we want to develop a shorter questionnaire for a construct, when a long version already exists. In that case, one might consider the long version as the gold standard.

To be able to assess the adequateness of the gold standard, it is important that researchers provide information about the validity and reliability of the measurement instrument, that is used as gold standard. For example, a histological diagnosis can only be considered to be a gold standard for cancer, if the reliability of assessment has been shown to be high.

2: Identify an appropriate sample of the target population in which the measurement instrument will ultimately be used

As discussed previously in Section 6.2, for all types of validation the instrument should be validated for the target population and situation in which it will be used. For example, if we are interested in the validity of the scores of a measurement instrument in routine clinical care, it is important that in the validation study the measurements are performed in the same way as in routine clinical care (i.e. without involvement of experts or any special attention being paid to the quality of measurements, as is usually the case in a research setting).

3: Define a priori the required level of agreement between measurement instrument and criterion

In criterion validation, there is usually one implicit hypothesis that the measurement instrument should be as good as the gold standard. Therefore, most studies on criterion validity lack a hypothesis specifying the extent of agreement. Quite often, the conclusion is that the agreement is not optimal, but sufficient for its purpose. However, it is better to decide a priori which level of agreement one considers acceptable. This makes it possible to draw firm conclusions afterwards, and certainly prevents one from drawing positive conclusions on the basis of non-convincing data (e.g. being satisfied with a correlation of 0.3 for scores on instruments that measure similar constructs).

When formulating hypotheses, the unreliability of measurements must be taken into account. Suppose that the comparison test is not a perfect gold standard, and has a reliability (Rel [Y]) of 0.95 and the measurement instrument under study has a reliability (Rel [X]) of 0.70. In that case, the observed correlation of the measurement instrument with the gold standard cannot be expected to be more than $\sqrt{(\text{Rel }[Y] \times \text{Rel }[X])} = \sqrt{(0.95 \times 0.70)} = 0.82$ (Lord and Novick, 1968).

It is difficult to provide criteria for the level of agreement between the scores of the measurement instrument and the gold standard that is considered acceptable, because this totally depends on the situation. Correlations above 0.7 are sometimes reported to be acceptable, analogous to ICCs of 0.70 and higher, which are considered as good reliability. Acceptable values for sensitivity, specificity and predictive values also depend on the situation, and on the clinical consequences of positive and negative misclassifications.

4: Obtain the scores for the measurement instrument and the gold standard, independently from each other

Independent application of the measurement instrument and the gold standard is a well-known requirement for diagnostic studies, but this is also necessary for the validation of measurement instruments. Moreover, the measurement instrument should not be part of the gold standard, or influence it in any way. This could happen if the gold standard is based on expert opinion, as sometimes occurs in diagnostic studies. In that case, the measurement instrument under study should not be part of the information on which the expert opinion is based. In the situation in which a short version of a questionnaire is validated against the original long version, the scores for each instrument should be collected independently from each other. The assignments at the end of this chapter include an example of such a criterion validation study.

5: Determine the strength of the relationship between the instrument scores and criterion scores

To assess criterion validity, the scores from the measurement instrument to be validated are compared with the scores obtained from the gold standard. Table 6.2 gives an overview of the statistical parameters used at various measurement levels of gold standard and measurement instruments. If both the gold standard and the measurement instrument under

Table 6.2 Overview of statistical parameters for various levels of measurement for the gold standard and measurement instrument under study

Level of measurement		Same units	Statistical parameter
Gold standard	Measurement instrument		
Dichotomous	Dichotomous	Yes	Sensitivity and specificity
	Ordinal	NA	ROC
	Continuous	NA	ROC
Ordinal	Ordinal	Yes	Weighted kappa
		No	Spearman's r[a] or other measures of association
	Continuous	NA	ROCs[b]/Spearman's r
Continuous	Continuous	Yes	Bland and Altman limits of agreement or ICC[c]
		No	Spearman's r or Pearson's r

[a] r = correlation coefficient; [b] ROCs: for an ordinal gold standard a set of ROCs may be used, dichotomizing the instrument by the various cut-off points; [c] ICC, intraclass correlation coefficient; NA, not applicable.

study have a dichotomous outcome, which is often the case with diagnostic measurement instruments, the criterion validity of the instrument, also referred to as the diagnostic accuracy, is expressed in sensitivity and specificity. If the measurement instrument has an ordinal or continuous scale, receiver operating characteristic curves (ROCs) are adequate. If the gold standard is a continuous variable, criterion validity can be assessed by calculating correlation coefficients. If the measurement instrument and the gold standard are expressed in the same units, Bland and Altman plots and ICCs can be used. Analyses with the gold standard as an ordinal variable do not often occur. The gold standard's ordinal scale is usually either considered as a continuous variable, or classes are combined to make it a dichotomous instrument.

In a number of examples, using different measurement levels, we will show the assessment of concurrent (Section 6.4.1) and predictive validity (Section 6.4.2). Note that Table 6.2 applies to both concurrent and predictive validity.

6.4.1 Concurrent validity

Example of concurrent validity (dichotomous outcome)

Lehman *et al.* (2007) determined the diagnostic accuracy of MRI for the detection of breast cancer in the contralateral breast of a woman who had just been diagnosed with cancer in the other breast. This means that MRI was tested in a situation in which no abnormalities were found by mammography and clinical examination of the contralateral breast. MRI is the measurement instrument under study, scored according to the standard procedure. The gold standard, based on the clinical course, was considered to be positive for cancer if there was histological evidence of invasive carcinoma or ductal carcinoma in situ within 1 year after the MRI, and negative for cancer if the study records, including the 1-year follow-up, contained no diagnosis of cancer. The primary aim of the study was to determine the number of cases with contralateral cancer that could be detected by MRI in women with recently diagnosed unilateral cancer. However, we use these data to validate the MRI scores in a situation in which no abnormalities were found by mammography and clinical examination of the contralateral breast. Table 6.3 shows the 2 × 2 table of the MRI results and the presence of breast cancer according to the gold standard.

According to the gold standard, 3.4% (33 of 969) of the women had breast cancer. Sensitivity and specificity are often used as parameters, in case of a dichotomous gold standard. Note that the gold standard, being perfectly valid, has a sensitivity of 100% (i.e. it identifies all individuals with the target condition and does not produce any false-negative results) and a specificity of 100% (i.e. it correctly classifies all individuals without the target condition and does not produce any false-positive results). Validating the MRI scores against this gold standard, the sensitivity of the MRI was 90.9% (TP/[TP + FN] = 30/33) and its specificity was 87.8% (TN/[FP + TN] = 822/936). However, when one has to decide whether the instrument under study is sufficiently valid for its clinical purpose, other diagnostic parameters, such as predictive values, are more informative. The positive predictive value is defined as the proportion of patients with a positive test result (MRI+) who have cancer according to the gold standard. The positive predictive value was 20.8% (TP/[TP + FP] = 30/144) in this example, and the negative predictive value (i.e. the proportion of negative test results without cancer) was 99.6% (TN/[FN + TN] = 822/825). This means that when no abnormalities

Table 6.3 Cross-tabulation of the MRI results and gold standard

MRI results	Gold standard Breast cancer	Gold standard No breast cancer	
MRI+	30 (TP)	114 (FP)	144
MRI–	3 (FN)	822 (TN)	825
	33	936	969

TP, true positive; FP, false positive; FN, false negative; TN, true negative.
Adapted from Lehman *et al.* (2007), with permission.

are observed on the scan, it is almost certain there is no cancer in the contralateral breast. However, if abnormalities are observed on the MRI, the probability that this is breast cancer is 20.8%, and 79.2% of the positive MRI scans are false positive results. This implies that when the MRI scan is made of the contralateral breast of all patients who have been diagnosed with breast cancer, a large number of results will be false positive.

In the same study, doctors were also asked to score the MRI results on a five-point malignancy scale, with a score of 1 indicating 'definitively not malignant' and a score of 5 indicating 'definitely malignant'. Figure 6.1 shows the ROC curve, in which each dot represents the sensitivity and 1-specificity when points 1–5 are taken as cut-off points. After fitting a curve through these points, it is possible to calculate the area under the curve (AUC), which amounted to 0.94 in this study. An AUC has a maximum value of 1.0, which is reached if the curve lies in the upper left-hand corner; a value of 0.5, represented by the diagonal, means that the measurement instrument can not distinguish between subjects with and without the target condition. Although the researchers did not specify beforehand which values of the assessed diagnostic parameters they would consider acceptable, they concluded that a measurement instrument with an AUC of 0.94 could be considered to be highly valid for its purpose.

This is an example of concurrent validity (as opposed to predictive validity), because the cancer is assumed to be present at the time when the MRI was made. It is only the procedure of verification that takes time, and for that reason the researchers decided to look at the available evidence for the presence of histologically confirmed breast cancer during a period of 1

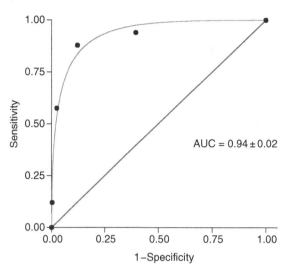

year. Note that in diagnostic research, clinical course is often used as a gold standard for the verification of negative test results.

Example of concurrent validity (continuous outcome)

Hustvedt *et al.* (2008) assessed the validity of an ambulant activity monitor (ActiReg®) for the measurement of total energy expenditure (TEE) in obese adults. A doubly labelled water (DLW) method was considered to be the gold standard for the assessment of TEE. ActiReg® is an instrument that uses combined recordings of body position and motion to calculate energy expenditure (EE). To calculate the TEE, a value for the resting metabolic rate (RMR) should be added to the EE. So, TEE = EE + RMR. RMR was measured by indirect calorimetry. As TEE is a continuous variable, and expressed in megajoules (MJ: 1 MJ = 1000 kilojoules) per day by both the activity monitor and the gold standard (DLW), it is possible to assess the agreement between the two methods with the Bland and Altman method. To do this, the difference between the calculated TEE based on ActiReg® (TEE_{AR}) and TEE measured by the DLW technique (TEE_{DLW}) is plotted against the mean of these values.

TEE was measured with the DLW method for a period of 14 days in 50 obese men and women (BMI $\geq$ 30 kg/m^2). Recordings were obtained from the activity monitor for 7 days during the same period. Because EE may

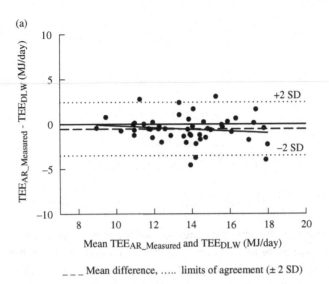

Figure 6.2   Bland and Altman plot of total energy expenditure measured with the doubly labelled water method and the activity monitor. Hustvedt *et al.* (2008), with permission.

disproportionately increase in obese subjects during weight-bearing activities, a new set of physical activity ratios were established to calculate EE on the basis of the activity monitor. Figure 6.2 shows the Bland and Altman plot for the TEE, as measured with the activity monitor and the DLW method.

The mean TEE, according to the DLW, was 13.94 (standard deviation [SD] 2.47) MJ/day, and the mean TEE based on data from the activity monitor and the RMR was 13.39 (SD 2.26). This resulted in a mean difference, and thus consistent underestimation of 0.55 MJ/day (95% CI 0.13–0.98 ($P < 0.012$)) of the activity monitor results (i.e. 3.9%). The Bland and Altman plot shows this slight underestimation, and that the limits of agreement are –3.47 to 2.37 MJ/day. The researchers conclude that, despite the slight underestimation, the activity monitor can be used to measure TEE in obese subjects, if an increase in their EE during weight-bearing activities is taken into account.

6.4.2 Predictive validity

An example of a study on predictive validity can be found in the field of heart surgery. The European System for Cardiac Operative Risk Evaluation (EuroSCORE) was developed to predict 'in-hospital' mortality in patients

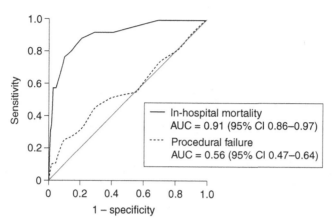

Figure 6.3   ROC curves showing the sensitivity and 1-specificity of prediction of in-hospital mortality and procedure-related failure for the EuroSCORE risk algorithm. Reproduced from Romagnoli *et al.* (2009), with permission from BMJ Publishing Group Ltd.

undergoing open heart surgery, and has been validated to predict 'in-hospital' mortality of 1173 patients undergoing percutaneous myocardial revascularization (Romagnoli *et al.*, 2009). The EuroSCORE is based on weighted, patient-related, cardiac-related and procedure-related risk factors, expressing the probability of 'in-hospital' mortality. It is a continuous variable with a range from 0 to 100%. The EuroSCORE appeared to be an independent predictor of mortality, in addition to other predictors of outcome. The performance of the EuroSCORE was presented in a ROC graph, in which the AUC was 0.91 (95% CI: 0.86–0.97) (see Figure 6.3). The researchers conclude that the EuroSCORE is a good predictor of 'in-hospital' mortality after percutaneous myocardial revascularization. The figure also shows that the EuroSCORE was not able to predict procedure-related failure during surgery.

The predictive validity of a measurement instrument should be assessed in a different sample from the one in which it has been developed. Risk scores or prognostic instruments are often constructed in regression analyses in a large data set, and are constructed in such a way that they fit the data best. Therefore, they may be rather optimistic. Although there are methods that can be used to adjust for optimism, it is better to determine the predictive validity in another, but similar sample of the target population.

In this example, the predictive validity is expressed as the area under a ROC curve. However, for clinical use it is important to decide about a cut-off point for the measurement instrument above which patients are considered a high-risk group. Ideally, this should be done before the validation study commences. Romagnoli *et al.* (2009) suggested a cut-off point of 6, which is the same cut-off point used in open heart surgery. This cut-off also appeared to be suitable for the new target population.

6.5 Construct validity

In situations in which a gold standard is lacking, construct validation should be used to provide evidence of validity. Construct validity was defined by the COSMIN panel, as the degree to which the scores of a measurement instrument are consistent with hypotheses, e.g. with regard to internal relationships, relationships with scores of other instruments or differences between relevant groups (Mokkink *et al.*, 2010a). It is based on the assumption that the measurement instrument validly measures the construct to be measured. Construct validation is often considered to be less powerful than criterion validation. However, with strong theories and specific and challenging hypotheses, it is possible to acquire substantial evidence that the measurement instrument is measuring what it purports to measure. There are three aspects of construct validity: structural validity, hypotheses testing and cross-cultural validity. We will start with structural validity, because we first have to determine whether a construct exists of one or more dimensions, as this has to be taken into account in further hypothesis testing.

6.5.1 Structural validity

Structural validity is defined as 'the degree to which the scores of a measurement instrument are an adequate reflection of the dimensionality of the construct to be measured' (Mokkink *et al.*, 2010a). This can be assessed by factor analysis. In Chapter 4, we explained the difference between exploratory and confirmatory factor analysis – the first method being applied if there are no clear ideas about the number and types of dimensions, and the latter if a priori hypotheses about dimensions of the construct are available, based on theory or previous analyses. Therefore, for validation purposes, confirmatory factor analysis is more appropriate. Nevertheless, exploratory factor analysis is often performed when confirmatory factor analysis (i.e. confirmation of the existence of predefined dimensions) would have been more adequate (De Vet *et al.*, 2005). In a confirmatory analysis, fit-parameters are used to test whether the data fit the hypothesized factor structure. In addition, it is possible to test whether the proposed model is better than alternative models. An example will illustrate how this works.

Example of confirmatory factor analysis

The example concerns the validation of the Center of Epidemiological Studies Depression Scale (CES-D) in patients with systemic sclerosis (SSc). SSc or scleroderma is a chronic, multisystem disorder of connective tissue characterized by thickening and fibrosis of the skin, and by involvement of internal organs. Patients with SSc report high levels of pain, fatigue and disability. The CES-D is a widely used 20-item self-report measure that was originally developed for assessing depressive symptoms in the general population, consisting of four factors: depressive affect symptoms (seven items), somatic/vegetative symptoms (seven items), (lack of) positive affect symptoms (four items) and interpersonal symptoms (two items). The frequency of occurrence of symptoms is rated on a 0–3 Likert scale ranging from 'rarely or none of the time' to 'most of the time', resulting in a scale from 0 to 60. Thombs *et al.* (2008) used confirmatory factor analysis to examine the validity of the CES-D in 470 patients with SSc by hypothesizing that the four-factor model (see Figure 6.4) has an adequate fit in these patients, and performs well in comparison with other possible factor solutions.

They tested various models as depicted in Table 6.4, a one- and two-factor model, two three-factor models, and two four-factor models. To assess the fit of the models to the data, chi-square tests for fit are highly sensitive to sample size and can lead to rejection of well-fitting models. Therefore, to evaluate model fit: the comparative fit index (CFI), the root mean square error of approximation (RMSEA) and the standardized root mean square residual (SRMR) were used. Guidelines proposed by Hu and Bentler (1999) suggest that models with CFI close to 0.95 or higher, RMSEA close to 0.06 or lower, and SRMR close to 0.08 or lower are representative of good-fitting models. From Table 6.4, showing the fit indices, it appears that the four-factor model

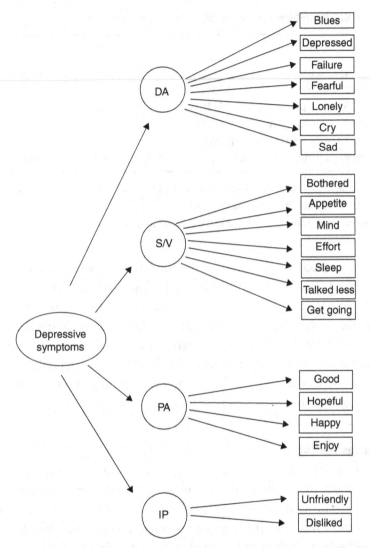

Figure 6.4   Second-order factor model with the domains depressed affect (DA), somatic/ vegetative affect (S/V), positive affect (PA) and interpersonal (IP). Thombs *et al.* (2008), with permission.

(model 4A) has adequate fit indices, also in comparison with the others, implying that the CES-D consists of four different domains. In addition, it was tested whether a model containing a second-order factor, which we labelled as 'depressive symptoms', would also fit. A second-order factor is

Table 6.4 Fit indices for confirmatory factor analysis models

Model fit indices	CFI	RMSEA	SRMR
Model 1: 1 factor	0.70	0.19	0.14
Model 2: 2 factor (DA + S/V + IP, PA)	0.95	0.08	0.06
Model 3A: 3 factor (DA + S/V, PA, IP)	0.96	0.07	0.06
Model 3B: 3 factor (DA + PA, S/V, IP)	0.73	0.19	0.13
Model 4A: 4 factor (DA, S/V, IP, PA)	0.97	0.06	0.05
Model 4B: 4 factor, second-order (DA, S/V, IP, PA)	0.97	0.06	0.06

CFI, comparative fit index; RMSEA, root mean square error of approximation; SRMR, standardized root mean square residual.
Adapted from Thombs *et al.* (2008), with permission.

a factor based on the scores of the four underlying factors as depicted in Figure 6.4. This model 4B also showed adequate fit indices.

This confirmatory factor analysis shows that the a priori hypothesized four-factor structure has an adequate fit. This analysis of structural validity gives evidence that CES-D adequately reflects the dimensionality of the construct depression in SSc patients. The four-factor model holds (model 4A) and the scores of the four factors can be combined in one overall score for depression (model 4B).

6.5.2 Hypotheses testing

The basic principle of construct validation is that hypotheses are formulated about the relationships of scores on the instrument under study with scores on other instruments measuring similar or dissimilar constructs, or differences in the instrument scores between subgroups of patients. These hypotheses have then to be tested. Although evidence for construct validity is typically assembled through a series of studies, the process generally consists of the following steps:

(1) describe the construct to be measured in as much detail as possible, preferably with the conceptual model on which it is based
(2) formulate hypotheses about expected relationships with measurement instruments assessing related constructs or unrelated constructs, or with respect to expected differences between subgroups of patients

(3) describe the measurement instruments with which the measurement instrument under study is compared, in terms of the constructs they measure, and present data about their measurement properties. In addition, describe the characteristics of the subgroups to be discriminated

(4) gather empirical data that will permit the hypotheses to be tested

(5) assess whether the results are consistent with the hypotheses

(6) discuss the extent to which the observed findings could be explained by rival theories or alternative explanations (and eliminate these if possible)

1: Describe the construct

A detailed description of the construct to be measured (see Chapter 3, Section 3.2), preferably embedded in a conceptual model, is the starting point for construct validation. This is indispensable in order to assess whether a chosen measurement instrument validly measures the construct of interest.

2: Formulate hypotheses

Based on this conceptual model or theories about the construct, hypotheses can be formulated with regard to expected relationships with instruments measuring related constructs. Researchers often think, in the first place, about positive correlations with similar constructs (convergent validity). However, part of the definition of the construct may contain statements about what the construct of interest is *not*. For example, if the researchers want a measurement instrument to measure physical functioning, and not pain, then the hypothesis could be formulated that the measurement instrument should have no correlation, or only a slight correlation with measurement instruments that measure pain (discriminant validity). Another type of hypotheses concerns expected differences between subgroups of patients. If a measurement instrument is intended to measure depression, it should be able to differentiate between patients with mild, moderate and severe depression (known group or discriminative validity). For this purpose, mean scores on the measurement instrument for the subgroups are usually compared.

The hypotheses should be formulated in advance, i.e. before data collection commences. The specific expectations with regard to certain relationships can be based either on an underlying conceptual model, or on data in the literature. It is important to report the hypotheses together with their justification in the publication, to enable the readers to judge the plausibility of the hypotheses.

The hypotheses should be as specific as possible, i.e. not only the direction of the correlation or difference should be given, but also the magnitude. For instance, a statement that the new instrument to measure 'physical functioning in the elderly' should correlate with other measures of physical functioning is too vague. Looking at the content of the measurement instruments in Table 6.1, one could hypothesize that the new instrument has a 0.1 higher correlation with the QL-I Spitzer scale than with the NHP, because the QL-I Spitzer contains more activities that elderly people tend to perform.

3: Describe the comparable measurement instruments or subgroups to be discriminated

It is important to present details about the other measurement instruments, to which the new measurement instrument is related, in terms of the construct(s) they measure and their measurement properties. To assess their similarity or dissimilarity, one must have insight into the content of these comparable measurement instruments. In addition, there should be a description of what is known about the validity and other measurement properties of these instruments in the specific situation under study. This part of the validation study is often taken too easily. There should at least be references to papers describing the content and measurement properties of these instruments in the same target population.

When hypotheses are formulated about differences between known groups, details about the demographic, clinical and other relevant characteristics of these groups should be presented.

4: Gather empirical data

This is a straightforward step. However, attention must be paid to the population and situation in which these data are collected. Validation is dependent on these issues, so the study sample and situation should be representative of the target population and conditions in which the measurement instrument will be used.

5: Assess whether the results are consistent with the hypotheses

This step should also be straightforward if the previous steps have been performed correctly, in which case it is just a matter of counting how many hypotheses were confirmed and how many were rejected. However, if the hypotheses were vaguely formulated, this step becomes problematic. Can one say that a correlation coefficient of 0.35 is moderate, and can one conclude that subgroups have a different mean value, if this difference did not reach statistical significance in a small study? So, defining explicitly beforehand the correlations and magnitude of differences one considers acceptable, will prevent the need for these post-hoc, data-dependent decisions.

6: Explain the observed findings

In the discussion section of a publication describing a validation study, one often finds many explanations why the hypotheses were not confirmed. Quite often, the construct and the hypotheses are debatable. There seldom is a firm conclusion about the lack of validity for this situation, which is the only acceptable explanation if the construct and hypotheses were well thought out. As we will see in the examples, weak theories and hypotheses leave much room for discussion and alternative explanations. Only validation studies with explicitly defined constructs, and hypotheses based on theory or literature findings, make it possible to draw firm conclusions about the (lack of) construct validity of the scores of a measurement instrument.

Example of discriminative validation

In Chapter 3 (Section 3.6.2) we introduced a stool chart as an instrument to characterize faecal output (Whelan *et al.*, 2004). This stool chart combines the consistency and weight of the faeces into a score, and together with the frequency of faecal output, this is expressed in a faecal score. The stool chart consisted of a visual representation of faecal output, using three weight categories (< 100 g, 100–200 g, > 200 g) and four consistency categories (hard and formed, soft and formed, loose and unformed, liquid). To validate the stool chart, the researchers used data from 36 patients who they measured over several days, resulting in data on 171 patient-days. They hypothesized that both the frequency and weights of the faeces were higher, and the consistency was less formed, resulting in a higher faecal score for the following subgroups: patients with a positive *Clostridium difficile* toxin compared

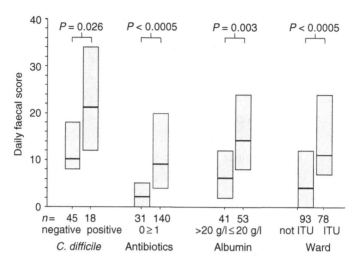

Figure 6.5 Daily faecal scores showing comparison between different patient groups (the bold line indicates the median faecal score and the box the interquartile range). Reprinted by permission from Macmillan Publishers Ltd: Whelan *et al.* (2004).

with patients with a negative assay; patients receiving antibiotics compared with patients not receiving antibiotics; patients with severe hypoalbuminaemia (≤20 g/l) compared with patients with no severe hypoalbuminaemia (>20 g/l); and patients on an intensive therapy unit (ITU) compared with patients not on an ITU (Whelan *et al.*, 2004). The researchers did not specify the magnitude of the differences. Figure 6.5 shows the distribution of the faecal scores for the various groups. As the differences between the subgroups were statistically significant, the authors concluded that the daily faecal score using the stool chart showed good construct validity.

Example of convergent, discriminant and discriminative validation
Another example concerns the validation of a number of health status questionnaires that are used to assess children with acute otitis media (AOM), which is a common childhood infection. Repetitive episodes of pain, fever and general illness during acute ear infections, as well as worries about potential hearing loss and disturbed language development, may all compromise the quality of life of the child and its family. Brouwer *et al.* (2007) validated a number of generic questionnaires and disease-specific questionnaires that have been used to assess functional health

status in children with AOM. They analysed data of 383 children, aged 1–7 years. The generic questionnaires were the RAND SF-36, the Functional Status Questionnaire (FSQ) Generic, measuring age appropriate functioning and emotional behaviour, and the FSQ Specific, measuring general impact of illness on functioning and behaviour. The disease-specific questionnaires for otitis media were the Otitis Media-6 (OM-6), assessing physical functioning, hearing loss, speech impairment, emotional distress, activity limitations and caregivers concern, a numerical rating scale (NRS) to assess health-related quality of life (HRQL) of the child (reported by the caregiver), an NRS to assess the HRQL of the caregiver, and a Family Functioning Questionnaire (FFQ).

They formulated, among other things, the following hypotheses with regard to correlations between various measurement instruments (convergent and discriminant validity):

- The correlation between the FSQ Generic and the NRS caregiver was predicted to be weak ($r = 0.1$–0.3), as they were expected to assess two different constructs.
- Moderate to strong correlations ($r > 0.40$) were expected between the RAND SF-36 and the NRS caregiver.
- Moderate to strong correlations were also expected between the OM-6 and the FSQ specific, the NRS child (reported by the caregiver), the NRS caregiver and the FFQ, because they all assessed OM-related HRQL or functional health status.

Table 6.5 shows the correlations between the various questionnaires. The correlations that were expected on the basis of the hypotheses are printed in bold. It can be seen that the NRS child does not perform as hypothesized, and the NRS caregiver shows a lower correlation than was expected with the FSQ Specific and the OM-6.

The researchers also formulated a number of hypotheses about the differences between known groups: discriminative validity. They hypothesized that the children with four or more episodes of OM per year ($n = 242$) would have lower scores on all the measurement instruments than the children with only two or three episodes per year ($n = 141$). However, they did not specify the magnitude of the differences. We see that there was a statistical significant difference between the two groups in the scores

Table 6.5 Construct validity: correlations[a] between the questionnaires

	RAND	FSQ Generic	FSQ Specific	OM-6	NRS child	FFQ	NRS caregiver
RAND	1.00	**0.52**[b]	**0.49**	**0.34**	**0.33**	**0.43**	**0.49**
FSQ Generic		1.00	**0.80**	**0.37**	0.25	**0.43**	0.24
FSQ Specific			1.00	**0.49**	0.26	**0.52**	0.24
OM-6				1.00	0.23	**0.74**	0.28
NRS child					1.00	0.22	**0.47**
FFQ						1.00	0.39
NRS caregiver							1.00

[a] Spearman correlation coefficients were calculated.
[b] Appropriately a priori predicted correlations are bold-printed.
Brouwer *et al.* (2007), with permission.

of all measurement instruments but the NRS child and the NRS caregiver (Table 6.6).

The researchers concluded that the global ratings of HRQL (NRS child and NRS caregiver) did not perform as well as was expected. These were hypothesized to correlate moderately with the ratings of the other disease-specific questionnaires, but the correlations were weak. Moreover, the NRS scores could not distinguish between the children with moderate AOM (2–4 episodes) and serious (≥ 4 episodes) AOM in the previous year. The results of the convergent and discriminative validation support each other. The researchers concluded that most of the generic and disease-specific questionnaires showed adequate construct validity. Only the NRS child and the NRS caregiver showed poor convergent validity, and low to moderate discriminative validity.

Note that these researchers validated a number of measurement instruments at the same time, which often happens when there are many existing instruments to measure the same construct. They do not state, however, which measurement instruments they considered to be acceptable to measure the construct under study, and which they use as standard to validate the others against. When validating a measurement instrument using convergent validity, it is always necessary to choose as standard an existing instrument with known validity.

Table 6.6 Known groups (discriminative validity): scores of children with 2–3 versus 4 or more episodes of AOM in the previous year[a]

	2–3 AOM episodes	≥ 4 AOM episodes	P value[b]
Generic			
RAND SF-36	21.1	19.6	0.004
FSQ Generic	76.5	72.2	0.002
FSQ Specific	83.9	78.4	0.001
Disease-specific			
OM-6	18.9	17.0	<0.001
NRS child	5.2	5.4	0.48
FFQ	84.9	78.5	<0.001
NRS caregiver	6.6	6.2	0.22

[a] Two to three episodes indicate moderate acute otitis media (AOM), and > 4 episodes indicate serious AOM.
[b] Calculated by Mann–Whitney test.
Brouwer *et al.* (2007), with permission.

Example of hypotheses testing of the COOP/WONCA scales

The Dartmouth COOP/WONCA charts are intended to measure HRQL of patients. Hoopman *et al.* (2008) validated these COOP/WONCA charts in a Turkish and a Moroccan minority population in the Netherlands. They hypothesized that the items in the COOP/WONCA charts correlated more strongly with conceptually similar scales of the SF-36 than with conceptually less similar scales. The SF-36 has been found to be a reliable and valid instrument for use in such ethnic minority groups. Seven COOP/WONCA charts that had corresponding SF-36 scales were selected (SF-Vitality, and SF-Role Emotional were excluded). Pearson's correlation coefficients were calculated. They hypothesized that each COOP/WONCA chart should correlate more strongly (at least 0.10) with the corresponding SF-36 scale than with the non-corresponding SF-36 scales.

Based on Table 6.7, the researchers concluded that the construct validity of the COOP/WONCA charts in relation to the SF-36 was good for the Turkish group, because 74% (31 of 42) of the correlations were as expected, and fairly good for the Moroccan group, because 67% (28 of 42) of the correlations were as expected.

Table 6.7 Pearson's correlations of the COOP/WONCA charts and SF-36 subscales

	COOP-PF	COOP-DA	COOP-PA	COOP-SA	COOP-FE	COOP-OH	COOP-CH
Turkish (n = 87)							
SF-36-PF	**0.46**	0.56	0.51[a]	0.37[a]	0.24[a]	0.43	0.27[a]
SF-36-RP	0.35[a]	**0.44**	0.44[a]	0.48[a]	0.28[a]	0.48	0.09[a]
SF-36-BP	0.37	0.60	**0.66**	0.46[a]	0.37[a]	0.43	0.13[a]
SF-36-SF	0.31[a]	0.56	0.42[a]	**0.64**	0.37[a]	0.40[a]	0.06[a]
SF-36-MH	0.19[a]	0.61	0.40[a]	0.52[a]	**0.51**	0.43	0.07[a]
SF-36-GH	0.27[a]	0.37	0.37[a]	0.37[a]	0.47	**0.52**	0.23[a]
SF-36-CH	0.06[a]	0.14[a]	0.16[a]	0.05[a]	0.09[a]	0.33[a]	**0.53**
Moroccans (n = 73)							
SF-36-PF	**0.44**	0.57	0.50[a]	0.50	0.50[a]	0.61	0.31[a]
SF-36-RP	0.37	**0.34**	0.50[a]	0.39[a]	0.31[a]	0.52	0.22[a]
SF-36-BP	0.34[a]	0.39	**0.83**	0.46	0.48[a]	0.67	0.37[a]
SF-36-SF	0.18[a]	0.34	0.41[a]	**0.49**	0.48[a]	0.48[a]	0.37[a]
SF-36-MH	0.22[a]	0.33	0.38[a]	0.36[a]	**0.71**	0.50	0.34[a]
SF-36-GH	0.34	0.37	0.53[a]	0.48	0.37[a]	**0.58**	0.28[a]
SF-36-CH	0.20[a]	0.32	0.30[a]	0.18[a]	0.33[a]	0.31[a]	**0.51**

COOP dimensions: PF, Physical Fitness; DA, Daily Activities; PA, Pain; SA, Social Activities; FE, Feelings; OH, Overall Health; CH, Change of Health. SF-36 dimensions (scales): PF, Physical Functioning; RP; Physical Role Functioning; BP, Bodily Pain; SF, Social Functioning; MH, Mental Health; GH, General Health Perceptions; CH, Change of Health.
[a] The COOP/WONCA chart correlated higher (at least 0.10) with the corresponding SF-36 scale (printed in bold) than with the non-corresponding SF-36 scales, as hypothesized.
Hoopman *et al.* (2008), with permission.

This study is an example in which the magnitudes of differences in correlations were quantified in the hypotheses. Quite often though, hypotheses are vaguely formulated such as 'we expect the instrument to be correlated with available measurement instruments for the same constructs'. These hypotheses lack sufficient detail. It is more challenging to hypothesize whether one expects a moderate or strong correlation, or, for example, correlations between 0.3 and 0.6 or between 0.6 and 0.8. Other possibilities are hypotheses that state the researchers expect a stronger correlation with comparable instrument A than with comparable instrument B, but quantification of the expected correlations and expected differences is highly preferred. Statistical significance of the correlation is not useful, for two reasons: first, because low correlations can become statistical significant in large populations, and secondly, the issue is not whether the correlation deviates from zero, but whether there is some predefined degree of correlation.

For discriminating validity, hypotheses containing a statement about the magnitude of the difference are recommended, and including a requirement of statistical significance in the hypotheses can be misleading, as small differences can easily reach statistical significance in large studies. It is informative to provide box plots, showing minimum and maximum values, together with the median value and interquartiles, for differences between groups, as in the stool chart example. This facilitates the interpretation of the discriminating potential of a measurement instrument better than mean and SD.

This study is also a nice example of a multitrait-multimethod (MTMM) approach. The MTMM approach was described by Campbell and Fiske (1959), as a validation method, which combines convergent and discriminant validity. Hoopman et al. (2008) hypothesized that COOP/WONCA chart items correlated more strongly with conceptually similar scales of the SF-36 than with conceptually less similar scales. The two methods used in their example to measure specific domains of the HRQL were the SF-36 and COOP/WONCA instruments. They showed that subscales assessing similar domains measured by different methods (COOP/WONCA and SF-36) correlated with each other, but less with dissimilar domains (Table 6.6). Thus, they used a combination of convergent and discriminant validation. MTMM can be analysed more specifically using structural equation modelling (Eid et al., 2008).

6.5.3 Cross-cultural validity

Cross-cultural validity is defined as 'the degree to which the performance of the items on a translated or culturally adapted PRO instrument are an adequate reflection of the performance of items in the original version of the instrument' (Mokkink et al., 2010a). This is often assessed after the translation of a questionnaire. Apart from differences induced by the translations, there may also be differences in cultural issues. Some items in a questionnaire may be irrelevant in other cultures. For example, the ability to ride a bicycle is very important in the Netherlands, which almost everybody does for short distance transportation, while in the USA, cycling is considered as a type of sport, and only a minority of the population possesses a bicycle.

Cross-cultural validation starts with an accurate translation process. After the translation, or cultural adaptation, the real cross-cultural validation takes place. In cross-cultural validation, special attention is paid to the equivalence of scores in the original and the new target population. For this purpose, data from two similar populations are needed: one population completes the original version of the questionnaire, and the other population completes the new cross-culturally adapted version. Other terms for equivalence of scores of measurement instruments are measurement invariance, or differential item functioning (DIF). Measurement invariance means that patients or target populations with the same true score on the construct, for example with the same severity of a disease, have the same score on the measurement instrument. Measurement invariance can be assessed both at scale level and at item level. Measurement invariance at item level is also known as DIF. This means that there are items for which patients from both populations with the same severity of disease do not have the same scores on the original and cross-culturally adapted version. In that case, an item apparently measures different things in the two populations.

We will first present the steps to be taken in a proper translation of a questionnaire, followed by assessments of measurement invariance.

6.5.3.1 The translation process

Essential steps have been pointed out in several guidelines (Beaton *et al.*, 2000). The translation process consists of six steps, as presented in Figure 6.6.

Step 1: Forward translation

Two bilingual translators independently translate the questionnaire (i.e. instructions, item content and response options are all translated from the original language into the target language). The translators should have the target language as the mother tongue. They make a written report of the translation containing challenging phrases and uncertainties, and considerations for their decisions. One translator should have expertise on the construct under study, the second one being a language expert, but naive about

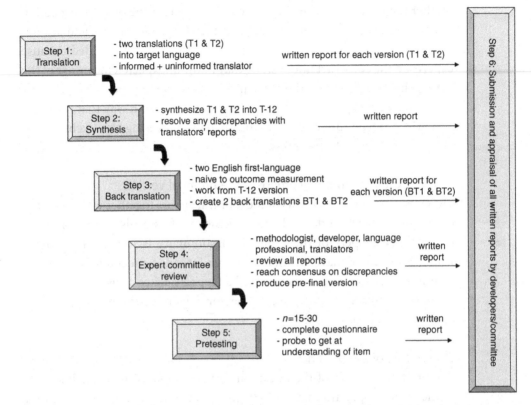

Figure 6.6   Graphic representation of the recommended stages of cross-cultural adaptation.
Beaton *et al.* (2000), with permission.

the topic. These types of expertise are required to obtain equivalence from both a topic-specific and language-specific perspective.

Step 2: Synthesis of the forward translation
The two translators and a recording observer (this may be the researcher) combine the results of both translations (T1 and T2 into T12), which results in one synthesized version of the translation, and a written report carefully documenting how they have resolved discrepancies.

Step 3: Back translation
The common translation version (T12) is then translated back into the original language by two other translators with the original language as the

mother tongue (BT1 and BT2). These are blinded for the original version of the questionnaire. These translators are both language experts and are not experts on the constructs to be measured. This is recommended because experts on the construct under study may know unexpected meanings of the items. They have background information about what aspects are relevant, while language experts translate the questions in such a way that respondents will probably understand them, thereby increasing the likelihood of detecting imperfect translations.

Step 4: Expert committee composes the pre-final version
The expert committee consists of the four translators together with researchers, methodologists and health and language professionals. If possible, contact with developers of the original questionnaire is important to check whether the items have maintained their intended meaning. The expert committee reviews all translations and all reports, takes decisions on all discrepancies and composes a pre-final version. Again, a written report is made of all considerations and decisions.

Step 5: Test of the pre-final version
The pre-final version of the questionnaire is completed by a small sample of the target population ($n = 15$–30) for pilot-testing. It is then tested for comprehensibility, as described in Section 3.7.1. Special attention should be paid to whether respondents interpret the items and responses as intended by the developers.

Step 6: Appraisal of the adaptation process by the developers
In the end, it is recommended to send all translations and written reports to the original developers of the instrument/questionnaire. They will perform a process audit, but they do not adapt the items. After their approval, the translated questionnaire is ready for cross-cultural validation.

6.5.3.2 Cross-cultural validation
The validity of the new, cross-culturally adapted instrument should be checked by assessing its construct validity. The researchers might check whether the translated instrument shows the expected correlations with related constructs, and is able to discriminate between relevant subgroups.

In this way, the performance of (sub)scales of the measurement instrument can be assessed. This hypotheses-testing becomes stronger if data on the same hypotheses in the original population are available. If so, the hypotheses can be formulated quite specifically, so that the same magnitude of correlations and/or differences is to be expected in the new population.

One can expect similar scores if the instrument is used in a similar target population. For example, the West Ontario and McMaster University osteoarthritis index (WOMAC) is an instrument developed to assess pain and physical functioning in patients with osteoarthritis. Patients in Canada and the Netherlands who have hip replacement surgery are expected to have about the same WOMAC scores 2 weeks after surgery, assuming that health status of the patients is comparable 2 weeks post-surgery and that healthcare provided for these patients is similar in Canada and the Netherlands. However, we can never be sure about this. When different mean and standard variations are found between populations, it is difficult to decide whether this is due to differences in the translated measurement instruments or differences in the populations. So, this method is sample dependent. Fortunately, there are more powerful ways in which to determine equivalence of an instrument's scores, based on the assessment of measurement invariance.

6.5.3.3 Assessment of measurement invariance

Measurement invariance means that a measurement instrument, a scale or an item functions in exactly the same way in different populations. In that case, it does not show DIF. There are several methods that can be used to assess measurement invariance (Teresi, 2006). We will present the following most commonly used methods in this section: factor analysis, logistic regression analysis and item response theory (IRT) techniques.

Factor analysis

Factor analysis is a method often used to assess differences between the original and translated version of a measurement instrument. The principle of assessing measurement invariance with factor analysis is that if one or more items do not load on the original factor after translation, this indicates that these items have a different meaning, either due to the translation, or due to cultural differences. In other words, if all items have kept the same meaning after translation, we expect the instrument to retain the same factor structure in the new population. As already discussed in Section 6.5.1, confirmatory factor analysis is strongly preferred over exploratory factor analysis for validation purposes. In assessing measurement invariance, the factor structure of data gathered in both the original and new populations are compared on three points (Gregorich, 2006):

(1) Are the same factors identified in both populations, and are these factors associated with the same items across the two populations?
(2) Do the factors have the same meanings across the two populations (i.e. do the items show the same factor loadings in both populations)?
(3) Do the items have the same mean values (intercepts) in both populations?

Examining the factor structure (question 1) is what is normally done in a confirmatory factor analysis (CFA), as shown in Section 6.5.1. In multiple group factor analysis, the equivalence of the factor loadings (question 2) in the two populations can be tested, as well as the equivalence of the intercepts reflecting the item mean scores (question 3). The method of assessing equivalence via factor analysis is not sample-dependent, because the factor loadings can be considered as regression coefficients, which are hardly dependent on sample means.

Logistic regression analysis

Logistic regression analysis is an appropriate method for assessing measurement invariance at item level (Petersen *et al.*, 2003). Again, data from two populations are needed, one completing the original version of the questionnaire, and the other completing the cross-culturally adapted version. An item displays DIF when patients from the two populations with the same 'true value' on the construct do not have the same probability of endorsing that item. According to the classical test theory, the overall scale score is used as an indication for this 'true value'. Uniform and non-uniform DIF can be distinguished. Uniform DIF means that in one population an item is endorsed less (or more) often at *all* values of the construct, compared with the other population. Non-uniform DIF means that in one population an item is endorsed less (or more) often at *some* values of the construct, but more (or less) often at *other* values of the construct compared with the other population.

In this regression analysis, the item response is the dependent variable, and the overall scale score, the dichotomous variable 'original questionnaire versus translated version', and an interaction term for 'questionnaire version', are the independent variables. When the item response is dichotomous, common logistic regression can be used. However, often the item response is an ordinal variable, in which case ordinal logistic regression analysis should be applied. It is possible to detect uniform and non-uniform DIF with this method. The interaction represents possible non-uniform DIF (i.e. indicating that the magnitude or direction of cultural or language differences in item scores differs between several ranges of the overall scale score). In the absence of non-uniform DIF, uniform DIF is tested by modelling the item responses (i.e. the dependent variable) as a function of the 'questionnaire version' and the scale score, with the variable 'questionnaire version' representing possible uniform DIF. Uniform DIF (testing the direction and magnitude of cultural/language differences in item scores) is considered to be present if the odds ratio (OR) of the variable 'questionnaire version' is statistically significantly different from 1. However, there are also other criteria: uniform DIF is sometimes considered to be present if the OR of the variable 'questionnaire version' is outside the interval of 0.53–1.89 (ln(OR) numerically larger than 0.64) (Zieky, 1993). And sometimes an increase (difference) in Nagelkerke's R^2 of more than 0.03 is used as a criterion to indicate noticeable DIF (combined uniform and non-uniform DIF) (Rose *et al.*, 2008). An example may clarify this theoretical presentation of assessing DIF by means of regression analysis.

Example

Hoopman *et al.* (2006) translated and validated the SF-36 for use among Turkish and Moroccan ethnic minority patients with cancer in the Netherlands. They compared the data from the Turkish sample ($n = 90$) and the Moroccan sample ($n = 79$) with those from a previous study of 376 Dutch patients with cancer (Aaronson *et al.*, 1998). They first tested for non-uniform DIF by modelling the item response as a logit linear (= logistic) function of the translation (Dutch versus Turkish, or Dutch versus Moroccan), the scale score and the interaction between translation and scale score. Non-uniform DIF was considered to be present if the interaction term was statistically significant at a P value of less than 0.001, and uniform DIF was considered to be present if the OR of the variable 'questionnaire version' was outside the interval of 0.53–1.89 (Zieky, 1993).

Table 6.8 shows the results of the tests for DIF expressed in OR of the variable 'questionnaire version' for the Mental Health domain. The item 'Down

Table 6.8 Results of the tests for uniform and non-uniform DIF by applying ordinal logistic regression analysis: OR, (and 95% CI) and P values of the Dutch sample versus the Turkish or Moroccan sample (corrected for age, gender and stage of disease)

	Turkish		Moroccan	
	Odds ratio	P value	Odds ratio	P value
Items in the mental health scale				
Nervous	0.68 (0.41–1.11)	0.12	1.24 (0.71–2.17)	0.44
Down in the dumps	**0.28 (0.16–0.50)**	<0.001	1.60 (0.86–2.99)	0.14
Calm and peaceful	0.96 (0.94–0.98)	<0.001*	1.19 (0.68–2.09)	0.54
Blue/sad	0.60 (0.36–1.01)	0.06	**1.98 (1.10–3.56)**	0.02
Happy	**2.76 (1.64–4.63)**	<0.001	0.67 (0.38–1.16)	0.15

Uniform DIF for language was considered to be present if the OR was outside the interval of 0.53–1.89, and this is presented in bold print. Non-uniform DIF was considered to be present if the interaction of languages with the total score was found to be statistically significant ($P < 0.001$), and is presented in the table with an asterisk. Hoopman *et al.* (2006), with permission.

in the dumps' had an OR of 0.28 (0.16–0.50) in the Turkish study sample. An OR of 0.28 means that the Turkish sample has a lower score for this item at the same level of mental health. The item 'blue/sad' had an OR of 1.98 (1.10–3.56) in the Moroccan study sample, meaning that the Moroccan sample scored higher on the item blue/sad than the Dutch sample at the same level of mental health. In the case of uniform DIF, this applies to all levels of mental health. Non-uniform DIF is indicated by an asterisk. We see that the item 'calm and peaceful' showed non-uniform DIF, which indicates that comparing the score for this item in the Dutch and Turkish samples, the differences found vary in magnitude and direction at various levels of mental health. We found a negative regression coefficient for the interaction, which means that at the higher scores on the 'Mental Health' scale the difference between the Turkish and Dutch samples will be smaller.

Item response theory techniques
IRT techniques are a powerful method with which to detect DIF, by comparing the item characteristic curves of the items in the original version and the

translated version. Where regression analysis uses the observed score, IRT can use the latent score (i.e. the estimated score on the latent trait). In IRT terminology, an item displays DIF when persons from the original and new population who have an equal score on the latent trait have a different probability of endorsing a specific item when completing the original and translated questionnaires. In other words, the item characteristic curve of the translated item differs from the item characteristic curve of the original item. Uniform DIF occurs if an item appears to be easier or more difficult in one of the populations at all levels of the trait (i.e. item difficulties have changed). Non-uniform DIF occurs if one item is easier for the new population, compared with the original population, at one level of the trait, and more difficult at another level of the trait (i.e. the item characteristic curves of the item before and after translation cross each other). In non-uniform DIF, item discrimination has changed. Figure 2.6 (Section 2.5.2) represented this situation if we presume that the two items depicted there are the same items scored by people from a different population. In IRT, interpretation problems due to different sample mean and standard deviations can easily be dealt with by calibrating both samples on the same trait level, or by using multiple group IRT (Embretson and Reise, 2000). The following example presents testing of the equivalence of WOMAC items after translation from English into Dutch.

Example

Roorda *et al.* (2004) translated and performed a cross-cultural validation of the original Canadian WOMAC with a Dutch version, using DIF analysis in patients with hip osteoarthritis who were waiting for hip replacement surgery. One of the subscales of the WOMAC is a physical functioning scale (17 items). We will use data from this scale in our example. Using a Rasch rating scale model, a mean item difficulty is calculated per polytomous item. The calibrated item difficulties, resulting from separate analysis of the Canadian and Dutch sample, were plotted against each other, with the Dutch items on the y-axis and the English items from the Canadian version on the x-axis (Figure 6.7). An identity line was drawn through the origin of the plot with a slope of 1. The dotted lines represent the 95% CI to guide interpretation. Items that fall outside the dotted lines demonstrate DIF.

For an adequate interpretation, we must remember that the position of items on the scales is determined by the 'probability of a positive response'

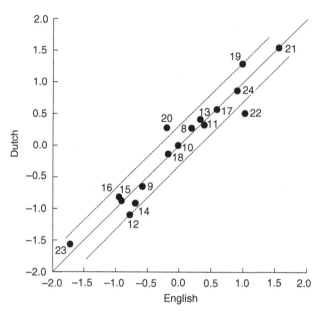

Figure 6.7   Calibration of physical functioning items for the Dutch WOMAC (*y*-axis) and the Canadian WOMAC (*x*-axis). Reproduced from Roorda *et al.* (2004), with permission from BMJ Publishing Group Ltd.

(see Section 2.5.2, Figure 2.5). The WOMAC items refer to difficulties when performing a number of activities. Items with a high probability of causing difficulties are located on the left-hand side of the scale. These items refer to heavy activities, which are difficult to perform, and people who are able to perform them have a higher level of physical functioning. Items on the right-hand side of the scale refer to activities that are less difficult to perform, and the probability of causing difficulties is lower. Patients experiencing problems with these light activities have a low level of physical functioning. By the same token, items that are very difficult to perform are found at the lower end of the *y*-axis, and items less difficult are found at the higher end of the *y*-axis. Patients with a lower level of physical functioning are located at the higher end of the *y*-axis. We observe that item 20 (getting in/out of the bath) was easier for the Dutch population, and item 22 (getting on/off the toilet) was easier for the Canadian population. There are several explanations for these DIF findings. They may be due to a poor translation, but there are also other explanations. They may be due to differences in the activities described in the items. With respect to item 22, the toilets in Canada may be higher than the toilets in the Netherlands, thus causing less difficulty. They also may be due to cultural or other differences in the population (e.g. the Dutch may have longer legs, which makes it more difficult for them to get on and off the toilet). However, we must be aware that these DIF tests are very sensitive, and in particular, DIFs found in large study samples may be statistically significant, but clinically of little relevance.

6.5.3.4 Dealing with measurement invariance

When some of the translated items turn out to show substantial DIF, we first take a look at these items to see whether there is a plausible explanation. That is often not the case. When there is DIF, we have the choice to adapt the translation of these items and test them again in a cross-cultural validation. Most often though these items are deleted. When DIF is identified by multiple group factor analysis or IRT, it is possible to adapt the model and calculate adjusted scores (see Embretson and Reise, 2000 for more details). When DIF is identified by logistic regression analysis, this possibility does not exist.

6.6 Validation in context

At the end of this chapter we will address sample sizes and missing values. However, we will also discuss design issues regarding validating measurement instruments along with clinical studies, and about the validity and its relation to the purpose of the measurement instrument, accumulation of evidence from validation studies, and to reliability and responsiveness.

6.6.1 Sample sizes

With regard to the sample size for validation studies, for criterion and construct validation studies in which correlation coefficients are calculated, we recommend a minimum of 50 patients, but larger samples (e.g. over 100 patients) are preferred. Criterion validation studies with dichotomized outcomes require larger samples if there is an uneven distribution over the two categories, to avoid small numbers in one of the columns of the 2×2 table. For known group validation, we recommend a minimum of 50 patients per subgroup.

For factor analysis, we already provided a rule of thumb in Chapter 4 (Section 4.4.5), i.e. a minimum of 4–10 cases per item, but with 100 patients as an absolute minimum. For IRT techniques, many more patients are needed, and several hundreds of patients are required to construct stable models.

6.6.2 Missing values

With regard to missing values, as in all research, these should be reported and, as far as possible, the reasons for missing values should be investigated. In effectiveness studies there may be selective drop-out or loss to follow-up related to (lack of) effectiveness, thereby inducing bias. In diagnostic studies, uninterpretable results or the fact that not all tests are indicated for all patients may cause missing values, and may lead to bias. In validation research, the relationship between missing values and the outcome of the study (e.g. correspondence between the scores of two instruments measuring the same construct) may be less clear-cut, and therefore there is probably less potential for bias. However, although missing values are less problematic in validation studies than in diagnostic or effectiveness studies, more than 15% of missing values might cause problems with regard to the generalizability of the results to the missing part of the population, especially if the reasons for missing values, and therefore the potential of selection bias, are unknown.

Note that missing values may occur when a measurement instrument is used in another population than for which it was originally developed. This may point to items that are not relevant for the new population.

6.6.3 Validation along clinical studies

As we already saw in Section 6.2, when a new construct is being developed it is very difficult to disentangle the theoretical development of the construct and validation of the measurement instrument. So, if the hypotheses cannot be confirmed by the validation studies, the researchers do not know whether there is a critical flaw in the ideas about the construct, in the instrument used to measure it, or both. Although this situation is well known in the development of new psychological constructs (Strauss and Smith, 2009), it occurs in every field of research in which new theories about diseases are being developed. This interference of construct and measurement instrument validation also occurs when validation takes place during a clinical study, in which case there are two objectives of the study. On the one hand, the instrument is used to answer a clinical question, and on the other hand, it is used to draw conclusions about the validity of the measurement instrument. This can cause problems in the interpretation of the results. For example, see the Alzheimer disease (AD) study in Section 3.4.1.4 where Scheltens *et al.* (1992) found that there was white matter involvement in late-onset AD, but not in pre-senile onset AD. Suppose that in a subsequent study the researchers are interested in finding out whether there is white matter involvement in an intermediate-onset AD group (clinical objective), but at the same time they want to know whether tiny hyperintensities can be observed on the MRI (instrument validation objective). Hence, there are two objectives in this study. MRI scans are therefore made of a large number of patients with intermediate AD onset. If the researchers observe tiny hyperintensities, they will conclude that there is white matter involvement in intermediate AD onset, and these hyperintensities can be observed on MRI. However, if they do not observe any hyperintensities, they can not draw conclusions about either of the two objectives: perhaps there are no hyperintensities in intermediate-onset AD, perhaps they can not be observed on MRI or perhaps both of these conclusions are true. This implies that the question whether MRI is able to detect tiny hyperintensities can only be assessed in situations where it is known, either by using another instrument or by theory, that the tiny hyperintensities are truly present.

6.6.4 Link with new clinical knowledge

In the above example, the purpose of the measurements was to learn more about the constructs to be measured, i.e. pathophysiology of AD. As the aim of medical research is generally to learn more about the pathophysiology and biological mechanisms of diseases, many measurement instruments are used to improve, extend and broaden our clinical knowledge, and the development or refinement of measurement instruments often keeps abreast of the clinical development. So, not only in the past, but also now and in the future, development of the construct and measurement instrument will go hand in hand. However, strong validation studies of the measurement instrument can only be performed after the construct has been fully developed.

Stronger validation is also possible when a measurement instrument that has shown an acceptable degree of validity in one situation is validated for another application. The findings of previous validation studies can then be used as a basis for hypotheses to assess whether the measurement instrument performs equally well in the new situation. These new situations might call for modifications to the measurement instrument (e.g. another language, another mode of administration, other response options, the addition of extra items, other target populations or other purposes of measurement).

6.6.5 Accumulation of evidence from validation studies

This chapter has shown that there are various types of validation that can be used to obtain evidence that a measurement instrument truly measures the construct it purports to measure. Face validity or content validity should always be assessed. Depending on the availability of a gold standard either criterion validation or construct validation can be applied. In case of criterion validation, usually one comparison is made. In case of construct validation, various forms can be applied: structural validation if it concerns a multidimensional instrument, and in addition as many hypotheses as considered relevant can be formulated. Every test of validity and every hypothesis adds to the body of evidence with regard to the validity of the instrument in a specific context.

6.6.6 Validity and reliability

Reliability was defined in Chapter 5 as the extent to which scores for patients who have not changed are the same for repeated measurements under several conditions. Figure 6.8 gives a very simple representation of the essentials of validity and reliability. The four boxes in this figure reflect various combinations of validity and reliability. The dots represent multiple measurements of one patient, and the cross within the circle represents the true score:

- the dots in cell A correspond to valid and quite reliable scores
- the dots in cell B correspond to mostly invalid, and definitely unreliable scores

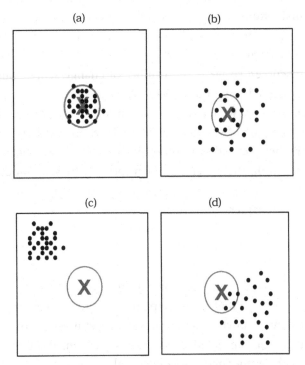

Figure 6.8   Various combinations of validity and reliability.

- the dots in cell C correspond to invalid, but quite reliable scores and
- the dots in cell D correspond to invalid and unreliable scores

In cell B we see that when a measurement does not provide a reliable score, a single measurement of this patient is probably not valid, because many scores fall outside the circle representing the 'true' value. However, we have learned in Chapter 5 (Section 5.4.1.2) that by averaging the scores of multiple measurements we might come to a more reliable score, and the mean score of multiple measurements of this patient in cell B would be valid. In Section 5.15, we applied the same reasoning to single scores of patients and the average score of the group of patients. In cell D averaging the scores of multiple measurements would lead to an invalid result.

We can now say that with regard to the single score, a score that is not reliable has a low probability of being valid. However, we can overcome this by performing multiple measurements, which will reduce the measurement error and produce a valid mean score (either within or over patients).

6.6.7 Validity and responsiveness

In this chapter, we have dealt with the validity of the scores of measurement instruments in various fields and applications. However, one issue that has not been discussed so far is the validity of change scores, but we will deal with this so-called longitudinal validity or responsiveness in the next chapter. Nevertheless, we want to emphasize in this chapter that we consider responsiveness as a part of validity. As you will see in Chapter 7, there are many similarities between validity and responsiveness. However, apart from discussing these similarities, there is much more to be said about responsiveness and the ways in which it can be assessed. Therefore, responsiveness deserves a separate chapter.

6.7 Summary

In this chapter, we have explained how various types of validation can be used to provide evidence that measurement instruments truly measure the constructs that they purport to measure. A good definition of the construct to be measured is indispensable for a correct validation, and this definition should preferably be embedded in a conceptual model.

Content validation is the start of the validation process; first, a global assessment is performed, referred to as face validation, followed by a more detailed assessment. Content validity can be clearly described for multi-item instruments, in which case content validation consists of assessment of the relevance and comprehensiveness of all items. However, other measurement instruments also have a phase of content or face validation, in order to assess whether they are suitable to measure the construct. For example, one should consider whether relevant tissues could be made visible on MRI.

The next step is criterion validation, which is a powerful step when an appropriate gold standard is available. Correspondence of the measurement instrument with the gold standard should be determined, followed by a conclusion, preferably on the basis of an a priori set level, as to whether this correspondence is acceptable for the purpose of the measurement.

If there is no gold standard, construct validation must provide the evidence. The definition of the construct and underlying conceptual model is a good starting point for the generation of hypotheses about the construct.

Confirmation of well-considered and specific hypotheses provides more evidence than weakly formulated hypotheses. When a large number of challenging hypotheses are tested, construct validation becomes a powerful tool in the validation process. Specific types of construct validation are structural validation and cross-cultural validation. Structural validation, which can be applied to multi-item instruments, is a strong tool if the structure of the instrument can be specified a priori, based on evidence from previous research or on a well-considered development process. Confirmatory factor analysis is highly preferred over exploratory factor analysis, because it makes it possible to draw firm conclusions about whether the items act as expected. If a questionnaire is translated or adapted to another culture, cross-cultural validation should be applied. Confirmatory factor analysis can be used for this purpose. In addition, DIF analysis by logistic regression analysis, and IRT techniques, if applicable, are also very suitable to determine whether the items have the same meaning after translation.

The validation of a measurement instrument is an ongoing process, which usually consists of a combination of various types of validation, accumulating evidence when hypotheses that are more specific are confirmed.

Assignments

1. Validation is a continuous process

Give two reasons why validation is a continuous process.

2. Drawing conclusions about construct validity

Suppose, in a validation study of the SF-36 as a measurement instrument for assessing general health status, one of the hypotheses is that the overall scores on both the physical component scale (PCS) and the mental component scale (MCS) show a high correlation ($r = 0.6 - 0.8$) with a global rating of the health status on a numerical rating scale of 0–10 points. The results show that correlation with the PCS is 0.75, but correlation with the MCS is only 0.49. Which of the following conclusions can be drawn from the above information?

    (a) The MCS scale has insufficient validity in this population.

    (b) The respondents apparently base their global assessment of general health status more on physical aspects than on mental aspects.

    (c) The SF-36 is focused more on the physical aspects than on the mental aspects of general health status.

3. Formulation of conclusions about validity

Below you will find the formulation of a number of conclusions that are often found in the abstracts of papers reporting on validation studies. Which ones do you think are adequate? Explain why the others are inadequate.

    (a) Instrument X is valid.

    (b) Instrument X is shown to be valid in this study.

    (c) Instrument X is shown to have satisfactory construct validity in this study, because 80% of the hypotheses were confirmed.

    (d) Instrument X is shown to be valid in population P.

    (e) Instrument X is shown to be valid for discriminating between subgroup A and subgroup B in population P.

    (f) Instrument X is shown to have good criterion validity in our population P.

    (g) Instrument X is shown to cover all relevant aspects of the construct.

4. Validation of a Short-Form version of the WOMAC versus the Long-Form version

Baron *et al.* (2007) validated a Short-Form (SF) version of the Western Ontario and McMaster Universities Osteoarthritis Index (WOMAC) physical functioning subscale in patients with hip and knee osteoarthritis. The Long-Form (LF) version of this physical functioning scale consisted of 17 items, and had previously been shortened to a version consisting of eight items.

A total of 1036 outpatients with osteoarthritis of the hip or knee participated in this validation study. They had to rate their pain during movement, give a global assessment of disease activity, and rate their impairment in physical functioning on a numerical rating scale, with a score ranging from 0 to 10 (a high score indicating a high level of symptoms). In order to validate the SF version against the LF version, half of the patients completed the LF version of the WOMAC physical functioning scale and the other half completed the SF version. In this way, the authors were able to compare the SF and LF versions between the two groups, by comparing the mean and SDs of both versions (Approach 1). In addition, they extracted the scores for the SF version from the half of the population that completed the LF version, and compared the scores of the SF and LF version within the same population, using the Bland and Altman plot (Approach 2). For both approaches the scores of the SF version (range 0–32) and the LF version (range 0–68) were transformed to a 0–100 scale to make them comparable.

(a) What are the advantages and disadvantages of these two approaches?
(b) Explain why they compared mean and SDs in Approach 1 and used a Bland and Altman plot in Approach 2.
(c) Construct validity was assessed by examining the correlation of the WOMAC LF and SF with the measures of pain during movement, impairment in physical functioning and global assessment of the disease activity. They expected these variables to correlate less with the LF version than with the SF version (no arguments given). How could you make these hypotheses more specific?

5. Interpretation of data on measurement invariance (differential item functioning)

A cancer-specific quality of life questionnaire was originally developed by the European Organization for Research and Treatment of Cancer (the EORTC QLQ 30) in English. It has been translated into Danish (DA), Dutch (NL), French (FR), German (DE), Italian (IT), Norwegian (NO), Spanish (ES) and Swedish (SV). Scott *et al.* (2009) tested for DIF in various translations. They used ordinal logistic regression analysis to test for DIF on the items of nine subscales and for the eight different languages. None of the items showed non-uniform DIF. Uniform DIF was considered to be present if the odds ratio (OR) of the translation term was outside the interval of 0.53–1.89 (ln(OR) numerically larger than 0.64). They performed separate analyses for baseline data, on-treatment data and off-treatment data. Table 6.9 shows the results. Uniform DIF is represented by '+' if the new population completing the translated version had higher scores, given a similar 'true' value based on the overall score, and by a '−' if this new population had lower scores.

Table 6.9 Summary of uniform DIF results

Scale	Item	DA	NL	FR	DE	IT	NO	ES	SV
QL	Q29	×oo	ooo	ooo	ooo	oo×	ooo	oo×	oo×
	Q30	×oo	ooo	ooo	ooo	oo×	ooo	oo×	oo×
PF	Q1	×××	oo×	o−×	oo×	o××	o××	oo×	−××
	Q2	×××	oo×	oo×	oo×	o××	o××	oo×	o××
	Q3	×××	+o×	oo×	oo×	o××	+××	oo×	o××
	Q4	×××	−−×	oo×	oo×	+××	+××	−−×	+××
	Q5	×××	oo×	oo×	oo×	o××	o××	oo×	o××
RF	Q6	×oo	oo+	oo+	oo+	oo×	ooo	o+×	oo×
	Q7	×oo	oo−	oo−	−o−	oo×	ooo	o−×	oo×
EF	Q21	ooo	ooo	ooo	ooo	oo×	ooo	o+×	oo×
	Q22	ooo	ooo	ooo	+++	oo×	− o	oo×	oo×
	Q23	ooo	−oo	ooo	o−o	oo×	ooo	−×	oo×
	Q24	ooo	oo−	ooo	ooo	oo×	+oo	oo×	++×
CF	Q20	ooo	+o+	ooo	ooo	oo×	ooo	oo×	+o×
	Q25	ooo	−o−	ooo	ooo	oo×	ooo	oo×	−o×
SF	Q26	+++	ooo	ooo	+++	o+×	ooo	oo×	oo×
	Q27	−−−	ooo	ooo	−−−	o−×	ooo	−o×	oo×
FA	Q10	ooo	ooo	ooo	ooo	oo×	ooo	−−×	oo×
	Q12	ooo	ooo	ooo	ooo	++×	oo+	++×	oo×
	Q18	ooo	ooo	ooo	ooo	o−×	−−−	oo×	oo×
NV	Q14	ooo	ooo	ooo	ooo	−o×	ooo	oo×	oo×
	Q15	ooo	ooo	ooo	ooo	+o×	ooo	oo×	oo×
PA	Q9	ooo	ooo	−o−	−−−	oo×	−o−	oo×	oo×
	Q19	ooo	ooo	+o+	+++	oo×	oo+	oo×	oo×

Translations: Danish (DA), Dutch (NL), French (FR), German (DE), Italian (IT), Norwegian (NO), Spanish (ES), Swedish (SV). The three symbols in each cell refer to (from left to right): DIF analyses at baseline, on-treatment and off-treatment assessments

'+' indicates that respondents using that language were more likely to report symptoms for that item compared with English and with other items in the same scale ($P < 0.001$ and ln odds ratio > 0.64).

'−' indicates that respondents using that language were less likely to score highly on that item.

'o' indicates there was no statistically significant DIF or that the magnitude of the DIF effect was less than 0.64.

'×' indicates that DIF analyses were not conducted because of insufficient sample size.

Adapted from Scott *et al.* (2009), with permission.

Items Q29 and Q30 were two questions about overall quality of life. These showed no DIF for any of the different languages. Item Q22 (Did you worry?) had higher scores in Germany, and item Q27 concerning social activities was scored lower in Denmark and in Germany. In general, there was good consistency between the three time-points, and there were no situations in which there was positive and negative DIF on the same item in the same population.

(a) Explain the meaning of uniform and non-uniform DIF.
(b) Why is the assessment of DIF an adequate method with which to validate an instrument after translation?
(c) Explain why the researchers were happy that they did not find a '+' and '−' in the same cell of their table.

Responsiveness

7.1 Introduction

The ultimate goal of medicine is to cure patients. Therefore, assessing whether the disease status of patients has changed over time is often the most important objective of measurements in clinical practice and clinical and health research. In Section 3.2.3, we stated that we need measurement instruments with an evaluative purpose or application to detect changes in health status over time. These instruments should be responsive. Responsiveness is defined by the COSMIN panel as 'the ability of an instrument to detect change over time in the construct to be measured' (Mokkink *et al.*, 2010a). In essence, when assessing responsiveness the hypothesis is tested that if patients change on the construct of interest, their scores on the measurement instrument assessing this construct change accordingly. The approach to assess responsiveness is quite similar as for validity, as we will show in this chapter. In Section 7.2, we will start by elaborating a bit more on the concept of responsiveness. We will discuss the relationship between responsiveness and validity, taking responsiveness as an aspect of validity, in a longitudinal context. We will also elaborate on the definition of responsiveness and the impact of this definition on the assessment of responsiveness.

Subsequently, in Sections 7.3 and 7.4 we will discuss two different approaches for assessing responsiveness: a criterion approach and a construct approach. The criterion approach is appropriate for situations in which there is a gold standard for the construct to be measured, and the construct approach is appropriate for situations in which there is no gold standard.

In this chapter, we will not only explain how responsiveness should be assessed, but also how it should not be assessed because there is much confusion about responsiveness in the literature. In Section 7.5 we will discuss some, in our opinion, inappropriate alternative measures, that are frequently used to assess responsiveness. We will explain why we consider these measures inappropriate in most situations. Several examples from different medical disciplines will be presented throughout the chapter.

Note that responsiveness is only relevant for measurement instruments used in evaluative applications (i.e. when the instrument is used in a longitudinal study to measure change over time). If an instrument is only used for discriminating between patients at one point in time, then responsiveness is not an issue.

7.2 The concept of responsiveness

7.2.1 Responsiveness as an aspect of validity

During the nineteen seventies and eighties, the concept of responsiveness first received attention in the medical literature on measurement issues (Deyo and Centor, 1986; Guyatt *et al.*, 1987). There have been major discussions about whether responsiveness should be considered as a separate measurement property, or as an aspect of validity. In Chapter 6, validity was defined as 'the degree to which an instrument truly measures the construct(s) it purports to measure'. This definition implies that if you want to measure change, a valid instrument should truly measure changes in the construct(s) it purports to measure. We therefore consider responsiveness as an aspect of validity. The only difference between validity and responsiveness is that validity refers to the validity of a single score (estimated on the basis of one measurement), and responsiveness refers to the validity of a change score (estimated on the basis of two measurements).

However, in analogy to the COSMIN panel, we treat responsiveness as a separate measurement property to emphasize this distinction between the validity of a single score and the validity of a change score. Both are important, and may lead to different results.

7.2.2 Definition of responsiveness

Many different definitions of responsiveness have been proposed in the literature over the past decades (Terwee *et al.*, 2003). Some of the proposed definitions differ only slightly from the COSMIN definition, but other definitions are based on very different points of view. There are two other points of view that we want to discuss.

First of all, some authors have defined responsiveness as 'the ability to detect change in general'. This could be any kind of change, but it is most often defined as a statistically significant change after treatment. For example, if a group of patients have a change in scores on the instrument under study over time (e.g. assessed with a paired t-test), it is concluded that the instrument is responsive. We consider the concept of detecting any change odd, because any change can refer to true change, but also to noise, or change in a different construct. Therefore, it is important to include in the definition the notion that the construct of interest has truly changed. To detect noise is not what we want, and the ability to detect change when there is no true change also makes no sense.

Secondly, some authors have defined responsiveness as 'the ability to detect clinically important change'. This definition requires a definition of what constitutes an important change. The importance of a change is not a responsiveness issue, because it concerns the interpretation of the change score, not the validity of the change score. Therefore, the term 'important' was not included in the COSMIN definition of responsiveness.

7.2.3 Implications for measuring responsiveness

Assuming that responsiveness is an aspect of validity, it is logical that the methodological principles for assessing responsiveness are similar to those used to assess validity. We follow the same strategies as presented in Chapter 6 on validity. The only difference is that in the present chapter we focus on the validity of change scores, while in Chapter 6 we focused on the validity of single scores. This has some important consequences for design and analyses, which will be discussed below.

Because we focus on change scores, a longitudinal study is required in which changes on the construct are expected to occur. In a responsiveness study, at least two measurements should be taken in order to calculate change scores. To determine whether the instrument under study can detect changes, the design should be chosen in such a way that it could be expected that at least some proportion of the patients would improve or deteriorate on the construct to be measured. Otherwise, if no change on the instrument is observed, it is difficult to decide afterwards whether the patients really did not change, or whether the measurement instrument was not responsive. For example, responsiveness can be assessed in patients with a chronic progressive disease, who are known to deteriorate over time, or in a study in which patients are given a treatment or some other kind of intervention known to induce a change on the construct to be measured. The principle is that when a patient group is expected to change on the construct to be measured, you want to show that the instrument can measure this change. The time-period between the two measurements can be short (e.g. a few weeks) or long (e.g. a period of months). This is not relevant, as long as it can be expected that during this time-period at least a proportion of the patients will improve or deteriorate on the construct to be measured.

In analogy to validity, assessing responsiveness consists of testing hypotheses. These hypotheses now concern the expected relationships between changes on the instrument under study and changes on other instruments that measure similar or different constructs, or expected differences between groups in changes on the instrument. For example, the responsiveness of a visual examination (the instrument under study) to measure shoulder range of motion in a group of patients with shoulder trauma could be assessed. To do this one could test the hypothesis that changes in shoulder range of motion over a period of 6 months, as estimated by the visual examination, will correlate highly (e.g. > 0.50 or perhaps even > 0.70) with changes in range of motion, as measured with an inclinometer. This is because an inclinometer is expected to measure the same construct as is measured with visual examination. If the hypothesis is not rejected, then visual examination is apparently a suitable method for the measurement of changes in shoulder range of motion in this population.

As indicated in Section 6.5.2, formulating hypotheses requires detailed knowledge of the construct (and its dimensions) that one intends to measure with the instrument under study and a conceptual model to hypothesize relationships with changes in other constructs. In addition, detailed knowledge is required about the other constructs being measured in the responsiveness study. As with validity, assessing responsiveness is a continuous process of accumulating evidence. It is not possible to formulate standards for the number of hypotheses that need to be tested. This depends on the construct to be measured, the study population and context, and the content and measurement properties of the instruments used for comparison. Sometimes negative results (e.g. a very low correlation between changes in similar instruments) may provide more convincing evidence for assuming that an instrument is not responsive than positive results (e.g. a moderate correlation between changes in similar instruments) for assuming that an instrument is responsive. One can therefore never conclude that an instrument *is* responsive.

Similar to validity, different approaches can be used, and the evidence from these approaches should be combined in order to draw conclusions about the degree of responsiveness of the instrument in a specific population and context. The two main approaches for assessing responsiveness are the construct approach and the criterion approach. These will be discussed in the following sections.

7.3 Criterion approach

When a gold standard for change is available, a criterion approach can be used to assess the degree to which changes in the scores on a measurement instrument are an adequate reflection of changes in scores on a 'gold standard'. When the occurrence of change is not assumed but measured, then the measurement instrument used as gold standard should be known to be responsive. This is comparable with assessing criterion validity, but the difference is that we now look at the criterion validity of change scores instead of single scores.

The general design of the criterion approach is almost identical to the design of criterion-related validation, and consists of the following steps:

(1) identify a suitable criterion (a gold standard for the construct of interest) and a method of measurement
(2) identify an appropriate sample of the target population in which the measurement instrument will ultimately be used
(3) define a priori the required level of agreement between changes on the measurement instrument and changes on the criterion
(4) obtain the changes in scores on the measurement instrument and the changes in scores on the gold standard, independently from each other, but over the same time period
(5) determine the strength of the relationship between changes in scores on the measurement instrument and changes in scores on the criterion

For more details of these requirements, see Section 6.4. Two additional remarks can be made here that are specific for assessing responsiveness:

With regard to step 1, we indicated in Chapter 6 that gold standards for patient-reported outcomes are very rare. There is only an acceptable gold standard for a shortened version of a patient-reported outcome. In that case, the original long version might be considered a gold standard. However, in many studies on the responsiveness of patient-reported outcomes a global rating scale (GRS) is used as a gold standard for measuring change. Patients are asked at follow-up, in a single question, to indicate how much they have changed (since baseline) on the construct of interest (e.g. on a five-point rating scale ranging from much worse, to much better). Such a GRS has high face validity, and may therefore be considered a reasonable gold standard for patient-reported outcomes, provided that the GRS assesses the same construct as the instrument under study. However, doubt has been expressed about the reliability and validity of such retrospective measures of change (Norman *et al.*, 1997). Therefore, some authors consider assessing responsiveness using a GRS to be a construct approach, rather than a criterion approach. This discussion illustrates that there is no clear cut-off point between a gold standard and silver, bronze or other standard. We consider a GRS to be a suitable criterion if the GRS measures the same construct as the instrument under study. If the GRS measures another construct (e.g. the GRS measures a general change in a patient's 'condition', while the instrument under study measures a narrower construct such as physical functioning), it is sensible to consider this as a construct approach, and relevant hypotheses should be formulated and tested (see Section 7.4).

Step 3 concerns criteria for the level of agreement between the scores of the measurement instrument and the gold standard that is considered to be acceptable. In Section 6.4 we stated that it is difficult to provide these criteria, and that correlations higher than 0.7 are sometimes reported to be acceptable. In responsiveness studies, which focus on agreement between change scores on the measurement instrument and change scores on the gold standard, lower correlations are often found. This can be explained by the fact that in order to obtain a change score two measurements of both the instrument under study and the gold standard are used. Each measurement is accompanied by a certain degree of measurement error. Therefore, lower correlations should be expected for the strength of the relationship between changes in the instrument scores and changes in the criterion scores.

Several statistical methods can be used for the criterion approach, depending on the level of measurement. Change scores on the instrument under study, as well as on the gold standard, can be dichotomous (change versus no change), ordinal (e.g. very much worse, a little worse, unchanged, a little better, very much better) or continuous (e.g. a change in score on a questionnaire). An overview of the statistical parameters used at various measurement levels of the gold standard and the measurement instruments was presented in Table 6.2. Correlations are often used when the gold standard is a continuous variable, or receiver operating characteristic curves (ROCs) when the gold standard is a dichotomous variable. The area under the ROC curve (AUC) is considered to measure the ability of an instrument to discriminate between patients who are considered to be improved (or deteriorated) and patients who are not considered to be improved (or deteriorated) according to the gold standard. An AUC of at least 0.70 is usually considered to be appropriate.

For the ROC method, there is an extra requirement with regard to the population. The sample should not only contain at least a proportion of patients who show change (see Section 7.2.3), but also a proportion who do not change.

7.3.1 Example of a continuous variable as gold standard

Leung *et al.* (2006) examined the responsiveness of the 2-min walk test (2MWT) as a measure of walking ability, in 45 patients with moderate to severe chronic obstructive pulmonary disease. Patients were asked to walk as far as they could at their own pace in 2 min, back and forth along a 30-m indoor corridor. The distance walked was recorded in metres. Each patient was asked to perform three 2MWTs with a rest-interval of about 20 min between tests. The longest distance walked was included in the analysis. As a criterion, they used the 6-min walk test (6MWT). Patients were asked to walk back and forth at their preferred pace along a corridor, attempting to cover as much ground as possible in 6 min. The distance walked was recorded in metres. Two 6-min walk tests were performed with an adequate recovery time between each test, and the longest distance walked was included in the analysis. The rationale for this study was that the 2MWT might be a useful alternative for the 6MWT, because the 6MWT is more exhausting for patients with severe chronic obstructive pulmonary disease (some patients with severe symptoms may not even be able to complete a 6MWT), and more time-consuming in a busy healthcare setting.

The 2MWT and the 6MWT took place at the start and at the end of a 5-week intensive pulmonary rehabilitation program. Responsiveness was assessed by calculating the correlation between the change in the distance walked in the 2MWT and the change in distance walked in the 6MWT. This correlation was 0.70, and the authors concluded that the responsiveness of the 2MWT was good.

A minor comment on this study is the moderate sample size ($n = 45$).

7.3.2 Example of dichotomous variable as gold standard

Spies-Dorgelo *et al.* (2006) examined the responsiveness of the 'hand and finger function' subscale of the Arthritis Impact Measurement Scales (AIMS-HFF) in patients with hand and wrist problems. This subscale contains five questions about limitations in hand and finger function while performing the following specific tasks: writing with a pen or pencil, buttoning up a shirt, turning a key, tying knots or shoelaces, and opening a jar. The items were summarized, and a total score was calculated, ranging from 0 (good functioning) to 10 (poor functioning). The study population consisted of 84 participants recruited in primary care for a longitudinal study on the diagnosis and prognosis of hand and wrist problems. At the 3-month follow-up, patients were asked to score the change in their ability to perform daily activities on a GRS. The seven response options were: (1) 'very much improved'; (2) 'much improved'; (3) 'a little improved'; (4) 'no change'; (5) 'a little deterioration'; (6) 'much deterioration'; (7) 'very much deterioration' (the latter three categories were combined in the analyses). This measurement of change was used as the criterion (gold standard) for the evaluation of responsiveness. A total of 76 patients completed the follow-up questionnaire. The authors first calculated the correlation between changes on the AIMS-HFF and the GRS. The observed Spearman's rho correlation was 0.52, which the authors considered to be moderate. Then they looked at mean changes in the AIMS-HFF scores for categories of improvement, as indicated on the GRS (Table 7.1).

Table 7.1 Changes in AIMS-HFF scores between baseline and 3-month follow-up for categories of improvement on the GRS

	n	Mean ± SD
Very much improved	16	1.47 ± 1.44
Much improved	11	2.18 ± 2.80
A little improved	6	1.10 ± 1.41
No change	34	−0.18 ± 1.36
Deterioration	9	−0.89 ± 2.33

Adapted from Spies-Dorgelo *et al.* (2006), with permission.

The authors stated that although self-reported improvement was associated with an improvement in scores on the AIMS-HFF, there was no gradual increase in scores over the categories of improvement.

Subsequently, they performed a ROC analysis. They considered patients who showed any improvement at all on the GRS as 'improved' ($n = 33$), and those reporting no change as 'stable' ($n = 34$). Those who reported any deterioration ($n = 9$) were excluded from this analysis. The AUC was then calculated as a measure of the ability of the AIMS-HFF to discriminate between those who had improved and those who remained stable according to the GRS. The AUC was 0.79, which the authors considered to be good.

A few remarks can be made about this study. First of all, although the total sample size of this study can be considered good ($n = 84$) and the amount of drop out was acceptable (eight patients, so there were 76 included in the responsiveness analysis), we observe that the sample sizes of the subgroups for the analyses are moderate ($n = 33$ versus $n = 34$ in the ROC analysis). Most of the subgroups, presented in Table 7.1, are very small. If these small subgroups were expected, the authors should have included more patients. The sample size of the various subgroups should therefore be taken into account when designing a responsiveness study.

Secondly, no explicit criteria were defined beforehand with regard to how high the AUC should be, or how much difference in change score on the AIMS-HFF was expected between the subgroups in Table 7.1. In the following section, we will demonstrate that defining explicit hypotheses makes the interpretation of the data more transparent.

7.4 Construct approach

If there is no gold standard available, the assessment of responsiveness relies on testing hypotheses, just like the assessment of construct validity described in Section 6.5.2. In the case of responsiveness, the hypotheses concern expected mean differences between changes in scores on the instrument in groups, or expected correlations between changes in scores on the instrument and changes in scores on other instruments known to have adequate responsiveness. One could also consider relative correlations, for example one may hypothesize that the change on instrument A is expected to correlate more with the change on instrument B than with the change on instrument C because the constructs being measured by instruments A and B are more similar than the construct being measured with instrument C.

Testing hypotheses is much less common in responsiveness studies than in validity studies. This may be due to the confusion in the literature with regard to how responsiveness should be assessed. Only after the achievement of consensus that responsiveness should be treated as an aspect of validity, did researchers start to apply the same strategies for assessing responsiveness.

As we stated in Section 6.5.2, specific hypotheses to be tested should be formulated a priori, preferably before the data collection and certainly before the data analysis. Without specific hypotheses, the risk of bias is high, because retrospectively it is tempting to think up alternative explanations for low correlations instead of concluding that an instrument may not be responsive. This is especially problematic when the researchers also are the developers of the instrument, or when they use the instrument as an outcome measure in their (clinical) studies. Another advantage of defining explicit hypotheses is that it makes interpretation of the data more transparent, because it enables quantification of the number of correlations of differences in accordance with the hypotheses. This will be shown in an example below.

Just like the hypotheses for testing validity, the hypotheses for testing responsiveness should include the expected direction (positive or negative) and the (absolute or relative) magnitude of the correlations or differences between the change scores. For example, one may expect a positive correlation of at least 0.50 between changes on two instruments that intend to measure the same construct. Or, one may expect that the change in score on instrument A correlates at least 0.10 points higher with the change in score on instrument B than with the change in score on instrument C (see example below). Or, one may expect a mean difference of 10 points on a scale from 0 to 100 in change scores on the instrument between two patient groups who are expected to differ in change on the construct to be measured. Without this specification of the expected differences or correlations, it is difficult to decide afterwards whether the hypothesis is confirmed or not.

One should not rely on P values of the correlations, because it is not relevant to determine whether correlations differ statistically significantly from zero. Instead, the responsiveness issue concerns whether the direction and magnitude of the observed correlation is similar to what was expected based on the construct being measured. One should therefore compare the observed magnitude of the correlation with the expected correlation. When assessing differences between changes in groups, it is also less relevant whether these differences are statistically significant (which partly depends on the sample size) than whether these differences are as large as was hypothesized.

Finally, it is important to note that to facilitate interpretation of the results, authors should provide arguments or evidence for their hypotheses (e.g. based on previous research findings).

Example of hypotheses testing

De Boer *et al.* (2006) assessed the responsiveness of the Vision-Related Quality of Life Core Measure (VCM1). The VCM1 measures vision-related quality of life, operationalized as feelings and perceptions associated with visual impairment. It consists of one unidimensional scale with nine items. A total score was calculated from 0 (lowest quality of life) to 100 (highest quality of life). The study population consisted of 329 visually impaired older men and women who participated in a 1-year follow-up study on the effect of low vision services on quality of life. The instruments used for comparison were: (1) the VF-14, which is a visual functioning questionnaire developed specifically for patients with cataracts (earlier studies have reported on

Table 7.2 Hypotheses for the responsiveness of the VCM1

	Hypotheses	Correlations	Confirmed
1	The correlation of change on the VCM1 with change on the VF-14 is 0.1 higher than the correlation of change on the VCM1 with the GRS	0.39 vs 0.19	Yes
2	The correlation of change on the VCM1 with change on the VF-14 is 0.2 higher than the correlation of change on the VCM1 with change in visual acuity	0.39 vs −0.02	Yes
3	The correlation of change on the VCM1 with change on the VF-14 is 0.3 higher than the correlation of change on the VCM1 with change on the EuroQol	0.39 vs 0.26	No
4	The correlation of change on VCM1 with the GRS is 0.1 higher than the correlation of change on VCM1 with change in visual acuity	0.19 vs −0.02	Yes
5	The correlation of change on the VCM1 with the GRS is 0.2 higher than the correlation of change on the VCM1 with the change on the EuroQol	0.19 vs 0.26	No
6	The correlation of change on the VCM1 with change in visual acuity is 0.1 higher than the correlation of change on the VCM1 with change on the EuroQol	−0.02 vs 0.26	No
	Total amount of hypotheses that were rejected		3/6

Adapted from De Boer *et al.* (2006), with permission.

the reliability, validity and responsiveness of the VF-14 in patients with cataract); (2) the EuroQol, which is a generic health-related quality of life questionnaire (De Boer *et al.* found adequate reliability in their study population, but other measurement properties (validity, responsiveness) have not been assessed in visually impaired patients); (3) a single global question (GRS) about perceived changes in eye condition; and (4) distance visual acuity. All measurements took place at baseline and after 5 months of follow-up, except for the GRS, which was only completed at follow-up. As a method for assessing responsiveness, the authors postulated specific hypotheses about the expected relationships between changes on the VCM1 and changes on the other instruments (see Table 7.2). For example, they expected that change scores of the VCM1 would correlate more with the GRS than with changes in visual acuity, because the GRS is an assessment of changes in the eye condition from the patient's perspective, as is the VCM1. They also expected the correlation of change on the VCM1 with change on the VF-14 to be higher than the correlation of change on the VCM1 with change on the EuroQol, because there is quite some overlap in the content of the questions in the VCM1 and VF-14. Responsiveness was considered to be high if less than 25% of the hypotheses were rejected, moderate if 25–50% were rejected and poor if more than 50% were rejected.

The percentage of hypotheses that were rejected for the VCM1 was 50%, which the authors considered to be moderate responsiveness. According to the authors, the moderate results were mainly due to the fact that correlations between changes on the VCM1 and changes in visual acuity (–0.02) were lower than expected. However, if the correlation with visual acuity would have been higher, the responsiveness might have been worse instead of better. Another explanation could be that the correlation between the changes on the VCM1 and changes in the EuroQol were greater than expected. The EuroQol was included in the three hypotheses that could not be confirmed.

However, when considering the correlations presented in Table 7.2, it can be concluded that the rather low correlation between changes in the VCM1 and changes on the VF-14 (which measures a similar construct) (0.39) and the low correlation between changes on the VCM1 and the GRS (0.19) indicate that the VCM1 might, indeed, not be very responsive.

A strong point of this study was that specific hypotheses were defined before the data collection, including the magnitude of the expected differences between the correlations. A limitation of this study is that the GRS focused on perceived changes in 'eye condition', which may not be the same as perceived changes in feelings and perceptions associated with visual impairment, as measured by the VCM1. This could be an alternative explanation for the low correlation between changes on the VCM1 and the GRS (0.19). If a global rating of change is used, we recommend that this question should be formulated in such a way that it measures the same construct as the instrument under study. If the instrument has subscales that measure different constructs, we recommend that multiple global ratings of change should be used, and that a specific question should be formulated for each construct measured. Another limitation of this study is that it provided little information about the measurement properties of the EuroQol in this population. A final limitation is that some hypotheses were dependent upon each other. Because the correlation between the VCM1 and EuroQol was higher than expected, hypotheses 3, 5 and 6 could not be confirmed.

7.5 Inappropriate measures of responsiveness

A number of other methods to assess responsiveness have been proposed in the literature, but we have not discussed these so far. However, some methods, such as effect sizes (ES), are widely used. In this section we will explain why these measures are not appropriate for the definition of responsiveness and therefore provide only limited evidence for responsiveness.

7.5.1 Effect sizes

Many studies assess responsiveness on the basis of ES. ES are usually calculated either as the mean change score in a group of patients, divided by the standard deviation (SD) of the baseline scores of this group, or as the mean change score in a group of patients, divided by the SD of this change score (also referred to as the standardized response mean (SRM)). These measures were developed as standardized measures of the magnitude of the effect of an intervention or other events that happened over time, expressing the magnitude of change in the amount of SDs. As a rule of thumb, the criteria proposed by Cohen (1977) are often used: ES of 0.20 are generally considered as small, ES of 0.50 are generally considered as moderate and ES of 0.80 are generally considered as large. Many authors interpret ES as measures of responsiveness, and conclude that their instrument is responsive if the ES is large.

For example, Johansson *et al.* (2009) used the Spinal Cord Index of Function (SIF) to measure changes in ability to perform various transfers (e.g. moving from bed to wheelchair or from wheelchair to shower chair) in non-ambulant patients with a spinal cord lesion participating in a rehabilitation program. The SIF consists of nine parameters, which are summarized in a total score, ranging from 9 to 54 points, with higher scores indicating better functioning. The ES, calculated as described above, was 9.1. They concluded: 'The effect size calculating the magnitude of change in ability to transfer, from the time of admission to the study until discharge, proved to be 9.1 for the SIF, showing a high magnitude of change, proving the instrument's responsiveness to changes'.

We do not agree with this conclusion. A high magnitude of change gives little indication of the ability of the instrument to detect change over time on the construct to be measured, because the observed change might be smaller than the true change in ability to transfer. Reasons why the true change may have not been detected by an instrument could be the occurrence of a ceiling effect or a lack of relevant items (lack of content validity). Furthermore, ES are highly dependent on the SD (of the baseline scores (ES) or the change scores (SRM)), and will therefore be higher in a relatively homogeneous population (ES) or if the variation in treatment effect is small (SRM). In this study, the SD of the baseline score was very small, which contributed to the large ES. Therefore, without a comparison instrument or strongly grounded hypotheses about the expected magnitude of the effects, the results provide very limited evidence of responsiveness.

ES are measures of the *magnitude* of the change scores, rather than the *validity* of the change scores. Therefore, ES should be considered inappropriate as parameters of responsiveness.

7.5.2 Paired *t*-test

Some authors use the *P* value obtained from a paired *t*-test as a measure of responsiveness. For example, Berry *et al.* (2004) investigated the responsiveness (which they called sensitivity to change) of the skin management needs assessment checklist (SMnac), to measure skin management ability in patients with spinal cord injury. They included 317 patients, who were measured twice, before and after a rehabilitation program. A paired-sample *t*-test was used to evaluate the responsiveness of the SMnac. There was a significant difference between the first and second SMnac scores ($P < 0.001$), so the authors concluded that the SMnac has high responsiveness.

We do not agree with this conclusion, because the *P* value from the paired *t*-test is a measure of the statistical *significance* of the change scores instead of the *validity* of the change scores. Statistical significance depends on the magnitude of change, the SD of the change scores, and the sample size.

Therefore, the paired *t*-test should not be considered as a good parameter of responsiveness.

7.5.3 Guyatt's responsiveness ratio

Guyatt *et al.* (1987) introduced a responsiveness ratio, defined as the minimal important change (MIC; which is the smallest change in score that patients consider important) on an instrument, divided by the SD of change scores in stable patients, to assess the likelihood of an instrument to detect a clinically important treatment effect:

$$Guyatt's\ responsiveness\ ratio = \frac{MIC}{SD_{change}}.$$

In Chapter 8, we will explain how this MIC value can be determined. We do not consider this ratio to be an appropriate parameter of responsiveness, because Guyatt's responsiveness ratio gives no information about the validity of the change scores (remember our definition of responsiveness referring to the validity of change scores). The numerator (MIC) is a measure of the *interpretability* of the change scores, and not the *validity* of the change scores. The denominator (SD of the change scores in stable patients) is an assessment of measurement error (closely related to the limits of agreement and the smallest detectable change, see Sections 5.4.2.2 and 5.6.2.2). Thus, neither the numerator nor denominator of this ratio reflects the validity of the change scores, and therefore we do not consider this ratio as a measure of responsiveness.

In fact, Guyatt *et al.* also acknowledged this in their article. They stated that 'demonstration of responsiveness is not sufficient to ensure the usefulness of an evaluative instrument. In addition, it must be shown to be valid.' They argued that an instrument can be responsive but the apparent improvement may represent change in a different construct such as satisfaction with medical care. Similarly, if an intervention of unknown effectiveness is administered and no change on the instrument is observed, it will be impossible, without knowing if other related measures have changed, to determine if the instrument is unresponsive or the intervention ineffective.

From this statement it can be concluded that Guyatt *et al.* make a distinction between responsiveness (which they define as the responsiveness ratio above) and validity, which they define as the validity of change scores. We, however, have incorporated validity within our definition of responsiveness, i.e. the validity of change scores. Therefore, we consider Guyatt's responsiveness ratio not as a measure of responsiveness. In Chapter 8 we will explain why we consider the concept of relating MIC to measurement error as a useful approach for assessing the interpretability of change scores.

7.5.4 Exceptions

In Section 7.5.1 and 7.5.2 we explained why ES and P values are considered to be inappropriate measures of responsiveness. However, if these measures are used in a construct validity approach with a priori defined hypotheses about the expected magnitude of the ES or changes, then the use of ES or P values is acceptable. An example of such a study is presented below.

Morris *et al.* (2009) examined the responsiveness of the Oxford Ankle Foot Questionnaire (OAFQ). The OAFQ measures child- or parent (proxy)-reported health status, and was developed for 5–16-year-old children with foot and ankle problems. The questionnaire includes 15 items; six items for the physical domain, four for the school and play domain, four for the emotional domain and one for the foot wear domain. The domain scores were calculated as the total of the item scores, and transformed to a percentage scale (0–100), with a higher score indicating better functioning.

Eighty children, between 5 and 16 years of age, who were seeking orthopaedic management for a foot or ankle problem, either at an elective outpatient clinic ($n = 55$) or a trauma unit outpatient clinic ($n = 25$), were included in the study. The children ($n = 78$ of 80) and one of their parents ($n = 80$) completed the OAFQ at baseline. At follow-up, 34 children and 37 parents from the elective group and 16 children and 16 parents from the trauma group completed the 2-month follow-up measurements.

The responsiveness of the OAFQ was assessed by determining changes in scores between baseline and follow-up, using paired t-tests. ES were also calculated as mean change, divided by the baseline SD. These were classified as large (0.8), moderate (0.5) or small (0.2). In addition to calculating these parameters, the authors defined specific hypotheses about the expected results. Their main hypotheses for responsiveness were that (1) there would be greater improvements in the scores of trauma patients than in the scores

Table 7.3 Mean (SD) change in the domain scores of the Oxford Ankle Foot Questionnaire

	Elective				Trauma			
				Effect				Effect
	n	Change	P value	size	n	Change	P value	size
Physical								
Child	34	9.8 (23.7)	0.022	0.4	16	43.2 (21.8)	<0.001	2.0
Parent	37	10.7 (27.1)	0.006	0.5	16	39.8 (28.8)	<0.001	1.7
School & Play								
Child	32	−0.3 (17.8)	0.924	0.0	16	45.2 (32.1)	<0.001	1.3
Parent	35	8.9 (23.0)	0.029	0.4	14	56.4 (29.1)	<0.001	1.6
Emotional								
Child	34	5.5 (17.0)	0.067	0.2	16	17.4 (23.0)	0.008	0.8
Parent	37	8.4 (19.6)	0.013	0.3	16	20.8 (21.4)	0.001	1.0
Footwear (single item)								
Child	34	2.2 (35.0)	0.716	0.1	16	56.3 (36.0)	<0.001	1.6
Parent	37	3.4 (34.4)	0.554	0.1	16	60.9 (54.0)	<0.001	2.2

of elective patients at follow-up, and (2) the ES would be greater for the physical domain than for the other domains, because this is the focus of orthopaedic management. The results are presented in Table 7.3.

All OAFQ scores are transformed to a percentage scale (0–100), with higher scores indicating better functioning. Some samples are smaller than 34 of 37 or 16 of 16 because of missing values. Table 7.3 was adapted with permission from Morris *et al.* (2009).

As expected, the ES in the domain scores were found to be substantially greater for trauma patients than for elective patients. All P values of changes in the trauma group were also much smaller than P values of changes in the elective group, even though the sample size of the trauma group was smaller. They did not test the difference between changes in the two groups for statistical significance. As hypothesized, the ES were greater for the physical domain than for the other domains, although not in all cases.

This example demonstrates that ES can be used to assess responsiveness, but *only* when specific hypotheses are tested (in this case concerning expected differences in changes between groups).

The approach would have been even better if the authors had defined in their hypotheses the magnitude of the expected differences in changes between the two groups and between the change scores of the different domains. Another limitation of this study is that the sample sizes of the two groups were rather small.

7.6 Other design issues

In Chapter 6 (Section 6.6) we provided some guidelines for sample sizes in validity studies and handling missing values. These guidelines also apply to studies on responsiveness. We also explained that when validation takes place during a clinical study, this could cause problems in the interpretation of results. For the same reason, one should be cautious when evaluating the responsiveness of a measurement instrument in the same study in which the instrument is used as an outcome measure. This will be demonstrated in the following example.

Turcot *et al.* (2009) measured tibial and femoral accelerations as a parameter of knee instability in 24 patients with knee osteoarthritis (OA) before and 2 weeks after a 12-week rehabilitation program (RP). Accelerations were measured in three directions: medial–lateral (ML), anterior–posterior (AP) and proximal–distal (PD), and expressed as the standard value of gravitational acceleration (g). ES were calculated as observed change/$SD_{\text{before RP}}$. The results are presented in Table 7.4.

The data show that the changes in AP acceleration were greater than the changes in ML and PD accelerations. The authors concluded that 'the results show that the estimation of knee acceleration parameters is responsive to gait changes in knee OA subjects by the reduction of accelerations, especially in AP direction'. However, at the same time they concluded that 'the significant AP acceleration reduction of 19% during the loading phase of gait suggests that the rehabilitation treatment proposed in this study could have benefits on knee OA gait by decreasing AP instability.' Now, what conclusion can be drawn from this finding? Does it tell us something about the quality of the instrument, or about the effect of the intervention? These two issues cannot be disentangled. The problem becomes even clearer in the interpretation of acceleration in the ML direction. Almost no change is observed. Does this mean that there is no effect in the ML direction, or

Table 7.4 Accelerations before and after rehabilitation in patients with knee OA

	Before RP		After RP			
Acceleration	Mean	SD	Mean	SD	ES	SRM
ML (g)	0.56	0.33	0.57	0.30	0.03	0.05
AP (g)	−0.88	0.42	−0.74	0.38	0.33	0.52
PD (g)	0.25	0.13	0.27	0.15	0.15	0.22

Adapted from Turcot *et al.* (2009), with permission.
g, the standard value of gravitational acceleration at sea level.

that the instrument is not responsive. It is impossible to answer this question. Therefore, responsiveness should be assessed in a study population in which it is known that at least some of the patients change on the construct to be measured.

Finally, it is worth noticing that the term responsiveness is also used in the medical literature, with a different meaning. Responsiveness also indicates the physiological response of body systems to stimuli such as drugs or hormones. For example, Olson *et al.* (2010) studied the effect of a high fat diet on mammary gland response to oestrogen. They investigated how obesity and increased adiposity, as a result of a fat diet, were associated with reduced mammary gland responsiveness to oestrogen in mice. Although this is related to measuring change (in this case, change in mammary gland response to oestrogen), the aim of such studies is not to assess the quality of a measurement instrument. When searching for responsiveness studies, for example in PubMed, it is inevitable that many such studies will be among those retrieved.

7.7 Summary

The ultimate goal of medicine is to cure patients. Therefore, the ability of measurement instruments to detect changes over time is a very important measurement property. The COSMIN panel defined responsiveness as 'the ability of an instrument to detect change over time in the construct to be measured'. Responsiveness is an aspect of validity. The only difference between validity and responsiveness is that validity refers to the validity of a single score, and responsiveness refers to the validity of a change score.

Although the results of assessing validity and responsiveness can differ, the basic methodological principles are the same. Responsiveness is, however, treated as a separate measurement property to emphasize that validity of both single scores and change scores is important, and may lead to different results. There is a lot of confusion in the literature about the concept of responsiveness, and over the past decades many different definitions and measures have been proposed.

Responsiveness should be evaluated in a longitudinal study in which at least some of the patients are known to change on the construct to be measured. Based on the analogy between validity and responsiveness, a construct approach and a criterion approach are distinguished. When a gold standard is available, changes on the instrument can be compared with changes on the gold standard. Several statistical methods can be used for this comparison, depending on the level of measurement. If there is no gold standard available, the assessment of responsiveness relies on testing hypotheses about expected mean differences between changes in groups of patients or expected correlations between changes in the scores on the instrument and changes in other variables. Hypotheses may also concern the relative magnitude of correlations. Specific hypotheses to be tested should be formulated a priori, preferably before the data collection. The statistical methods should be suitable for the specific hypotheses. Hypotheses testing is an ongoing process; the more specific the hypotheses are, and the more hypotheses tested, the more evidence can be gathered for responsiveness.

There are a number of parameters proposed in the literature to assess responsiveness that we consider inappropriate. ES and SRM are considered to be inappropriate because they are measures of the magnitude of the change scores, rather than of the validity of the change scores. The P value from the paired t-test is considered to be inappropriate because it is a measure of the statistical significance of the change scores, instead of the validity of the change scores. Finally, Guyatt's responsiveness ratio is considered to be inappropriate because the MIC refers to the interpretability of the change scores, and not to the validity of the change scores.

Evaluating the responsiveness of a measurement instrument in the same study in which the instrument is used as an outcome measure makes it impossible to draw any firm conclusions about responsiveness.

Assignment

Methods to assess responsiveness

In a study of 120 patients with low back pain, Deyo and Centor (1986) studied the responsiveness of two instruments to measure functional status: the 45-item Sickness Impact Profile Physical Dimension (SIP-PD) and a brief condition-specific 24-item scale derived from the SIP, now known as the Roland–Morris Disability Questionnaire (RDQ). (Only part of the data from this article are used in the assignment.) The RDQ was developed by selecting 24 items from the SIP, which were considered to be most relevant for patients with back pain. In addition, the phrase 'because of my back' was added to each statement to distinguish disability due to back pain from disability due to other causes. In this study the complete SIP (136 items) was administered. The SIP-PD score was calculated from 45 of the SIP items, and the RDQ score was calculated from 24 of the SIP items (21 items overlap). The patients completed the questionnaire at baseline and after 3 weeks of follow-up. At the same time-points spine flexion and degrees of straight leg raising were measured. At the 3-week follow-up, the patients rated their pain improvement on a 6-point ordinal scale, (1 = much worse, 2 = slightly worse, 3 = the same, 4 = slightly better, 5 = much better, 6 = pain entirely gone). The examining clinician made a rating of overall improvement on a similar scale, based on the patient's appearance, self-rating, and physical examination. The patients were also asked to indicate whether or not they had fully resumed all activities (*yes* or *no*). The SIP-PD scores range from 0 to 100, with higher scores indicating more dysfunction, and the RDQ scores range from 0 to 24, with higher scores indicating more dysfunction. Change scores were calculated for the SIP-PD and the RDQ by subtracting the follow-up score from the baseline score. A positive change score indicated improvement.

As a first method for assessing responsiveness, they correlated change scores on the SIP-PD and on the RDQ with change scores in spine flexion, degrees of straight-leg raising, with the six-point patient and clinician ratings of change, and with the answers to the question concerning full resumption of all activities. These correlations are presented in Table 7.5.

The results suggest that the RDQ is more responsive than the SIP-PD, because most correlations with the other instruments are higher, although

Table 7.5 Spearman's correlations between change scores

	Self-rated pain improvement	Clinician's rating of improvement	Change in spine flexion	Change in straight leg raising	Full resumption of all activities
SIP-PD	0.32	0.26	0.27	0.06	0.33
RDQ	0.41	0.30	0.29	0.003	0.38

Adapted from Deyo and Centor (1986), with permission.

the correlations were moderate. Based on these moderate correlations, the authors concluded that 'the functional scales may be relatively insensitive in detecting clinical changes'.

(a) What do you think about the authors' conclusion?

As a second method for assessing responsiveness, Deyo and Centor examined change scores after treatment by calculating change (in %) from baseline (defined as mean change divided by mean baseline score) and paired *t*-statistics. They first investigated changes for the entire patient sample, and subsequently for two subgroups: those who indicated that they had fully resumed all their activities and those for whom both patient and clinician indicated pain improvement on the six-point rating scale. For the latter analysis, the six-point scale was reduced to a dichotomous variable (improved/ not improved). The results are presented in Table 7.6.

Based on the differences in the paired *t*-statistic between the SIP-PD and the RDQ, the authors concluded that in each patient group the RDQ appeared to be less responsive than the SIP-PD (although the differences were small). They argued that these results were somewhat contradictory to the results of the first method, which suggested that RDQ was more responsive than SIP-PD.

(b) How do you explain the contradiction in results between Tables 7.5 and 7.6?

As a third method for assessing responsiveness, Deyo and Centor calculated ROC curves for each instrument, against two 'external criteria'

Table 7.6 Score changes among patients who improved, according to different criteria

	Entire patient sample ($n = 120$)			Patients who have fully resumed all activities ($n = 72$)			Patients who have improved ($n = 87$)		
	Mean change (SD)	Change %	Paired t-statistic	Mean change (SD)	Change %	Paired t-statistic	Mean change (SD)	Change %	Paired t-statistic
SIP-PD	7.9 (12.9)	27	6.73	11.4 (12.9)	60	7.47	10.2 (13.1)	55	7.26
RDQ	3.0 (5.2)	30	6.35	4.4 (5.4)	46	6.96	3.8 (5.3)	40	6.70

SIP scores range from 0 to 100, RDQ scores range from 0 to 24.
Adapted from Deyo and Centor (1986), with permission.

for improvement. As a first criterion, they selected those patients who had fully resumed all activities. As a second criterion, they selected those patients for whom both the patient and clinician indicated pain improvement.

They used two different external criteria because, in their opinion, there is no gold standard for functional status. Therefore, they chose to use an approach 'like establishing construct validity' to compare the instruments against several criteria. They argued that results consistent with several criteria increase the odds that the relative performance of several scales is correctly ranked.

The areas under the ROC curves are presented in Table 7.7.

Table 7.7 Areas under the ROC curves (with standard errors)

	Using 'fully resumed all activities' as criterion	Using 'patients who improved' as criterion
SIP-PD	0.68 (0.049)	0.59 (0.068)
RDQ	0.72 (0.047)	0.67 (0.068)

Adapted from Deyo and Centro (1986), with permission.

The authors concluded that the RDQ showed slightly better discriminative ability than the SIP-PD, although the difference between the scales was not statistically significant.

(c) How do you explain the contradiction in results between Tables 7.6 and 7.7?
(d) Do you consider the 'external criteria' for improvement adequate?
(e) If you had to repeat this study, how would you improve its design?

8

Interpretability

8.1 Introduction

After addressing the development of measurement instruments in Chapters 3 and 4 and evaluating measurement properties (i.e. reliability, validity and responsiveness) in Chapters 5–7, it is time to pay attention to the interpretability of the scores when applying the measurement instruments. For well-known instruments, such as blood pressure measurements and the Apgar score, the interpretability will cause no problems, but for new or lesser known instruments this may be challenging. This particularly applies to the scores for multi-item measurement instruments, the meaning of which is not immediately clear. For example, in a randomized trial on back pain carried out in the United Kingdom, the effectiveness of exercise therapy and manipulation was compared with usual care in 1334 patients with low back pain. The researchers used the Roland–Morris Disability Questionnaire (RDQ) to assess functional disability (UK BEAM trial team, 2004). The RDQ has a 0–24-point scale, with a score of 0 indicating no disability, and 24 indicating very severe disability. The mean baseline score for the patients with low back pain was 9.0. In the group who received usual care, the mean RDQ value decreased to 6.8 after 3 months, resulting in an average improvement of 2.2 points. This gives rise to the following questions: What does a mean value of 9.0 points on the 0–24 RDQ scale mean? In addition, is an improvement of 2.2 points meaningful for the patients? The primary focus of this chapter is on the interpretability of scores and change scores on a measurement instrument. In other words, the aim is to learn more about the measurement instrument, and not about the disease under study.

We start with an explanation of the concept of interpretability, and which issues should be addressed in relation to interpretability. We will discuss methods to assess and enhance the interpretability of single scores, and then discuss the interpretation of change scores. Two topics receive special attention in this respect: the concepts of minimal important change (MIC) and response shift.

8.2 The concept of interpretability

The COSMIN panel defined interpretability as 'the degree to which one can assign qualitative meaning – that is, clinical or commonly understood connotations – to an instrument's quantitative scores or change in scores'. In everyday words, it is the degree to which it is clear what the scores or change scores mean. Interpretability is not a measurement property, like validity and reliability, because it does not refer to the quality of an instrument. It refers to what the scores on an instrument mean. However, interpretability was considered to be sufficiently important by the COSMIN panel to be included in the COSMIN taxonomy (see Figure 1.1) (Mokkink *et al.*, 2010a). They remarked that interpretability often receives insufficient attention. A proper interpretability of a score is a prerequisite for the well-considered use of an instrument in clinical practice and research.

In the concept of interpretability, there are a number of different issues to consider:

- What is the distribution of the scores of a study sample on the instrument?
- Are there floor and ceiling effects?
- Are scores and change scores available for relevant (sub)groups (e.g. for normative groups, subgroups of patients or the general population)?
- Is the MIC or the minimal important difference known?

These issues will all be discussed, starting with an explanation of why the distribution of scores is important, how this is examined using classical test theory (CTT) and item response theory (IRT), and when floor and ceiling effects occur.

8.3 Distribution of scores of the instrument

8.3.1 Importance of examining the distribution of scores

A study of interpretability starts with an examination of the distribution of scores in the study sample. This, of course, also includes an extensive description of the study sample, in order to know for what kind of population the scores are interpreted. In Chapter 4, we discussed the importance of the distribution of the item and scale scores of a study sample. In the development phase of an instrument, the question is: does a measurement instrument fit the population? At this time, we are interested in the distribution of scores to learn more about the characteristics of the measurement instrument. This distribution is important for two reasons: for a proper interpretation of the scores of a measurement instrument, and also for a proper interpretation of the measurement properties.

First of all, the distribution of the scores of a study sample is important for a proper interpretation of the scores on a measurement instrument. The distribution of the scores over the scale, in terms of mean and standard deviations (SDs), or in proportional distribution over classes, provides information about the location of the study sample on the measurement instrument. The distribution shows whether the study sample has high or low scores, whether the sample is distributed over the whole range of the scale, or whether patients are clustered at some locations on the scale (i.e. homogeneous population). In the following section, we will give examples, using CTT and IRT. Using CTT, we can only learn about the interpretation of the measurement instrument if we have additional information about the study population. Sections 8.4 and 8.5 will show how this works for the interpretation of single scores and change scores, respectively.

Secondly, the distribution of scores of the study sample is important for a proper interpretation of the measurement properties. We have seen in Chapter 5 that reliability parameters are highly dependent on variation in the sample. A poor result in a reliability analysis may be due to a lack of variation of scores on the measurement instrument. This also applies to the interpretation of Cronbach's alpha. Note that also for the assessment of construct validity and responsiveness, hypotheses are often formulated in terms of expected correlations between scores on measurement instruments. These correlations also tend to be higher in more heterogeneous samples. Thus, knowledge about the distribution of the population scores over the measurement instrument affects the values of several measurement properties.

8.3.2 Examining the distribution of scores using classical test theory methods

Using CTT methods to examine the distribution of the scores over the scale may start with a simple presentation of mean and SDs of the scores, or median values and interquartile ranges (IQR) for continuous variables, and the numbers (%) in the various classes for ordinal or nominal variables. In addition, a histogram or some type of other visual presentation provides a clear insight into the distribution. It is important to know how the scores of the study sample are distributed over the scale, or whether there is a clustering of patients. This clustering is often found at the higher or lower end of the scale.

As an example, we use data from a RCT, carried out by Hoving *et al.* (2002) in which three types of conservative treatment for neck pain were compared. We present a histogram (in Figure 8.1) of the baseline scores on the Neck Disability Index (NDI) of 60 patients who were randomly allocated to receive manual therapy. The NDI consists of 10 items with response options 0–5, resulting in a scale with a theoretical range of 0–50, with higher scores indicating more severe disability. The mean baseline value for NDI in these 60 patients was 13.55, with SD of 6.96.

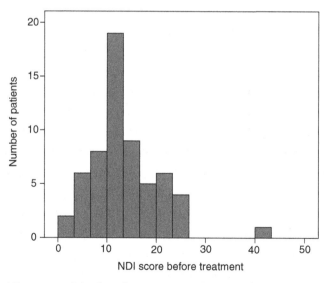

Figure 8.1   Histogram of the baseline scores on the NDI of 60 patients with non-specific neck pain that were allocated to manual therapy. Based on Hoving *et al.* (2002).

Most of the scores are at the lower end of the scale, indicating that most of the patients were only slightly disabled due to their neck pain at baseline. It can be seen beforehand that it will be difficult to detect large improvements in much of the sample, because of these low baseline scores.

Using CTT methods it is impossible to distinguish the sample characteristics from the measurement instrument characteristics. Additional information about the study population is necessary to make it possible to interpret the scores on the measurement instrument, as we will see in Sections 8.4 and 8.5.

8.3.3 Examining the distribution of scores using item response theory methods

Using IRT methods, information about the items and the study sample can be obtained at the same time (see Sections 2.5.2 and 4.6.2), thus enabling a distinction to be made between the instrument characteristics and study sample characteristics. A visual presentation of the position of the items (and their response categories) clearly shows whether there is a clustering of items at some ranges of the trait level, and large gaps between items at other ranges. The SF-36 Physical Scale has been examined with IRT analysis in a sample of patients with all kinds of chronic medical and psychiatric conditions who participated in the Medical Outcome Study (Haley *et al.*, 1994). Using the Rasch rating scale model for ordered response categories (Andrich, 1978), the location of the items was determined as presented in Figure 8.2.

There are no items between trait levels +1.5 and +3.5. This means that if patients improve in physical functioning in this range of the scale, the score on the measurement instrument would hardly change. Vice versa, the clustering of items around 0 implies that the score on the measurement instrument may change a lot with only a slight change in physical functioning. That would occur if we calculate the score on the SF-36 physical functioning scale as the total (or mean) item score. If the score is calculated by estimating the theta level (θ), the actual change on the trait level can be estimated more accurately, although the gain is usually small. In this IRT-based estimation of the score, the difficulty of the items, i.e. the unequal intervals between the items is taken into account. However, this estimation is rather complex,

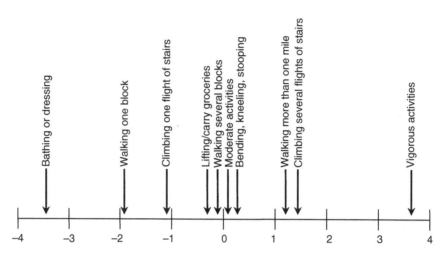

Figure 8.2   The distribution of the items of the SF-36 Physical Functioning Scale over the trait level in a sample of patients with chronic medical and psychiatric conditions. Adapted from Haley *et al.* (1994), with permission from Elsevier.

and beyond the scope of this book. For a further explanation we refer to Embretson and Reise (2000).

Using IRT methods the distribution of patients in the sample and of items can be shown on the same trait level, as presented in Figure 8.3 (the same as Figure 4.4 in Section 4.6.2) for the Neck Disability Index (NDI; Van der Velde *et al.*, 2009). This provides very useful information. Items at locations where there are no patients have no discriminative function in the sample. In addition, if there are hardly any items at the location where the largest part of the sample is found, patients can be insufficiently discriminated from each other. In Figure 8.3, one can see that there is much overlap in the location of the items and patients, with only a few items or response categories (thresholds) on the right side of the figure with little discriminative function.

8.3.4 Floor and ceiling effects

Floor or ceiling effects can occur when a high proportion of the total population has a score at the lower or upper end of the scale, respectively. Whether these effects do indeed occur, depends on the situation, which we will explain in this section.

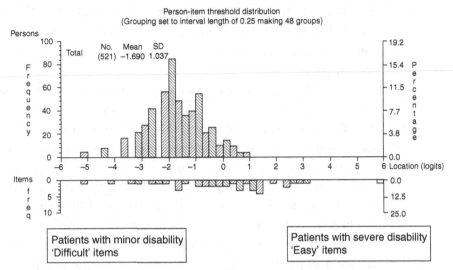

Figure 8.3   Distribution of subjects and item difficulties on the eight-item Neck Disability Index on a logit scale. Van der Velde *et al.* (2009), with permission.

In Chapter 4 (Section 4.6.3) we already drew attention to floor and ceiling effects when discussing the development of a measurement instrument. In the development phase, one can remedy floor and ceiling effects by including more items at the relevant end of the scale. Floor and ceiling effects are often encountered when an existing instrument is applied in a new target population.

Floor and ceiling effects pose the most problems in longitudinal analyses. This affects the responsiveness of an instrument, because patients who score at the end of the scale at baseline, say on the healthy side, can not show any further improvement. This means that when their health status further improves, this cannot be detected by the instrument. Whether there really is a floor or a ceiling effect depends on whether we want to discriminate patients in this group any further. A few examples will be presented to illustrate this.

Suppose we have an instrument to measure physical functioning before and after total knee replacement, and suppose that the most difficult item in this instrument is 'ability to walk 5 km'. A large proportion of the population will be able to do so some time after surgery, but we will not call this a ceiling effect if we want to label all these patients as having no functional disabilities. In that case, we are not interested in whether they are able to walk 40 km or run 5 km, so no new items are needed. Because we do not want to discriminate these patients any further, this is not considered to be a ceiling effect.

In an RCT, a clustering of patients at the higher end of the scale, corresponding to the most severe symptoms or worst stage of the disease, is often found at baseline. However, this is not a problem if the aim of the trial is to study the effects of interventions that will show improvements in these patients. They are expected to change in the direction of lower scores. However, if patients entering the trial already have rather low scores, as we saw in the example of the NDI in the Hoving RCT, there might be a problem, because if the intervention aims to lower the score further, there is not much room for improvement. So, let us take a look at what happened in the RCT on neck pain (Hoving *et al.*, 2002). Figure 8.4 shows a histogram of the scores after 7 weeks of manual therapy.

The patients had mild neck disability before the treatment (Figure 8.1), but more than 50% of the population who received manual therapy had a score below 10 after the treatment (Figure 8.4).

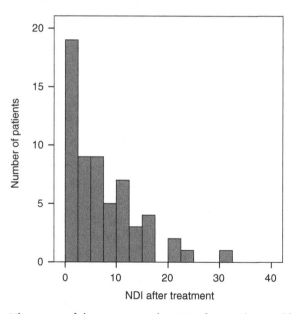

Figure 8.4   Histogram of the scores on the NDI of 60 patients with non-specific neck pain after 7 weeks of manual therapy treatment (Hoving *et al.*, 2002).

This is an interesting situation, because now there are two possibilities:

(1) If all patients scoring 0 (or less than 5) indeed experience no, or negligible neck disability, we do not say that there is a floor effect.
(2) However, if they still have neck disability, but the NDI does not pick this up, it is a shortcoming of the measurement instrument. This we define as a floor effect.

Let us take another look at Figure 8.3, which showed the distribution of the items of the NDI. Given that the study sample had low disability scores after the intervention, we can see in Figure 8.3 that there were sufficient items in this range of the scale (i.e. there were sufficient items that were difficult). Remember that patients who have no problems with the difficult items are patients with a low level of disability. So, at the lower end of the scale there were sufficient items to discriminate between patients, meaning that the patients with a low score had no problems. Assuming that the population in the Van der Velde study (described in Section 8.3.3) was, in terms of neck disability, similar to the Hoving study population (described in Section 8.3.2), we can now say that the low scores after treatment are not due to a floor effect, but that the patients really had low scores.

A ceiling effect might occur on the NDI when a patient starts with a trait level of 4 and deteriorates to a trait level of 5. In that range of the scale there are no items that can detect this change. This is then a ceiling effect. It is immediately clear that this would also affect the responsiveness of the scale: there is a change in health status that can not be detected by the measurement instrument.

Therefore, we must realize that when there are many patients at the lower or higher end of the scale we have to question whether this is a problem in terms of causing floor or ceiling effects, i.e. do we want to distinguish these patients further, and can we detect relevant changes in the direction of interest?

Note that a ceiling effect cannot occur if an instrument does not have a maximum score (e.g. the time needed to walk 10 metres).

8.4 Interpretation of single scores

In this section, we focus on the interpretation of single scores. Change scores will be discussed in the following section. Much can be learned about the interpretation of scores when the scores on a measurement instrument are presented for relevant (sub)groups. Relevant in this context may be the scores of a healthy population, or of the general population. In addition, scores of patients for whom the severity of the target condition or health status is known can help in the interpretation of scores. At the end of this section, we will show how IRT analysis can be used to obtain information about the meaning of single scores.

8.4.1 Using the norm scores of a general population

Norm values for a measurement instrument facilitate the interpretation of scores on the measurement instrument. The scores on a measurement instrument in the general population are usually considered to be norm scores. These scores can be used as reference values in the comparison of scores for varying disease groups. For example, Salaffi *et al.* (2009) compared the health status of patients with inflammatory rheumatic diseases (IRD), assessed with the SF-36, with the health status of a general population. The results are presented in Figure 8.5. The maximum score for each

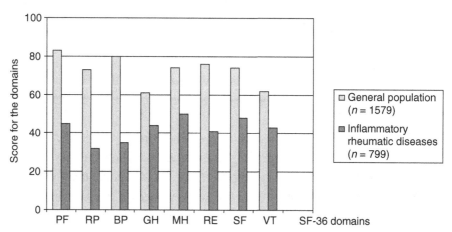

Figure 8.5   Comparison of the SF-36 health survey domain scores of patients with inflammatory rheumatic diseases (IRD) and general population normative data; higher scores represent a better health status. Physical functioning (PF), Role function – physical aspect (RF), Bodily pain (BP), General health perception (GH), Mental health (MH), Role function – emotional aspect (RE), Social functioning (SF), and Vitality (VT). Adapted from Salaffi *et al.* (2009), with permission.

of the eight SF-36 domains is 100. The lighter grey columns represent the scores of a general population, and the dark grey columns represent the scores of patients with IRD. This figure shows that the general population scored far less than 100 for the various SF-36 domains. Suppose one had found a score of 60 for the 'general health perception' domain. Without these norm scores of the general population one would consider a score of 60 to indicate that the patients with IRD perceive substantial health problems, but this figure shows that a score of 60 is normal for the general population.

8.4.2 Examining the scores of well-known groups

In the COSMIN definition of interpretability, it is said that the meaning of scores can be derived from clinical and commonly understood connotations (Mokkink *et al.*, 2010a). A nice example of how this works is provided by Wolfe *et al.* (2005) for the Health Assessment Questionnaire (HAQ), which ranges from 0 (no disability) to 3 (severe disability). To enhance interpretability of the scores, Wolfe *et al.* (2005) presented scores from the HAQ disability scale (HAQ-DI) for various subgroups of patients, including scores for working patients versus non-working patients, patients who were fully independent versus patients who were dependent on others, and patients with no knee or hip replacement versus patients with a knee or hip replacement. Figure 8.6 presents the HAQ-DI scores for these subgroups.

By observing these scores, clinicians and researchers working in this field get a feeling of what a score on the HAQ-DI means, because they have seen many patients with rheumatoid arthritis (RA) from the respective subgroups. In this way, the scores get a clinical connotation. Note that all comparisons in this example are cross-sectional, and should therefore not be interpreted in a longitudinal way, as we will see in Section 8.5.1.

8.4.3 Interpretations of the scores of item response theory-based instruments

Measurement instruments developed on the basis of IRT techniques, or that appear to satisfy an IRT model, have a clearer interpretation. That is because we have more information about the 'metrics' of the scale, and about the position of patients and items on this very scale.

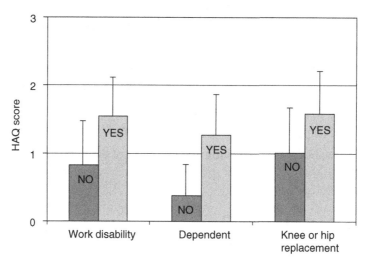

Figure 8.6   Mean scores (and SDs) on the HAQ-DI scale in various subgroups of patients with rheumatoid arthritis (RA). Based on Wolfe *et al.* (2005).

The positioning of patients among the items greatly facilitates interpretation of their scores, as can most easily be seen when looking at a Guttman scale we presented for 'walking ability' (see Table 2.2 in Chapter 2).

On the Guttman scale, as shown in Table 8.1, each item is scored as 0 (no, not able to) or 1 (yes, able to). Patients who have a total score of 4 on this scale are able to walk outdoors for 5 min, but not for 20 min. The scores can easily be interpreted from Table 8.1.

With the IRT method, as explained in Chapter 2 (Section 2.5) the item scores do not follow the hierarchy of the items as perfectly as on a Guttman scale. Therefore, we have to interpret the scores in terms of probabilities. However, as items and patients are located on the same scale, knowing the trait level of a patient makes it possible to locate the patient among the items (as shown in Figure 8.3).

The physical functioning scale of the SF-36 has been examined in an IRT analysis. A clear hierarchy of the items was found, although the fit of a Rasch model was not optimal (Haley *et al.*, 1994). In Figure 8.2, the locations of the items were presented. Using an IRT-based estimation of the scores, accounting for the different intervals between the items, it is possible to make a more accurate estimation of the physical functioning of patients than when using

Table 8.1 Six items on a fictitious 'Walking ability' scale with responses (0 or 1) from seven patients (A–G)

	Patients						
Walking ability	A	B	C	D	E	F	G
Stand	1	1	1	1	1	1	0
Walking, indoors with help	1	1	1	1	1	0	0
Walking, indoors without help	1	1	1	1	0	0	0
Walking, outdoors 5 min	1	1	1	0	0	0	0
Walking, outdoors 20 min	1	1	0	0	0	0	0
Running, 5 min	1	0	0	0	0	0	0
Sum-score	6	5	4	3	2	1	0

only the sum-score of the items. The correlation between the sum-score of the items and the IRT-based scores in the example of SF-36 physical functioning was very high (0.97–0.99) (McHorney *et al.*, 1997). Such high correlations are usually found (Skrondal and Rabe-Hesketh, 2004). This implies that calculating a total score of items with response options on an ordinal scale is not as fallacious as some authors want us to believe (Wright and Linacre, 1989). Therefore, it is not surprising that in IRT-based measurement instruments the actual value of θ (the trait level) is seldom determined. Instead, the scores of the items are simply added together, thereby ignoring the unknown size of the interval between the items (see Figure 8.2). However, if there are large gaps in the distribution of items at some locations of the scale and substantial clustering at other locations, an estimation of θ might be preferred.

8.4.4 Criteria for what is considered normal

By using an instrument, one becomes familiar with its scores, and there are many ways in which this works. Let us take the example of blood pressure. Nowadays, most clinicians and other healthcare workers know how systolic and diastolic blood pressure values should be interpreted. However, in the past when blood pressure measurement was in its infancy, one had to find out what was normal and what was abnormal. There are several ways (Fletcher and Fletcher, 2005) to define what is normal.

8.4.4.1. Based on the distribution of values of measurement instruments in the general population

We all know that growth charts are used in newborns to assess whether their length is long or short for their age, and in which percentile of the distribution they are positioned considering their weight-for-height at a specific age. Thus, normal and abnormal is defined by the distribution of scores in a general population: lowest 5% is considered 'too short' and highest 5% 'too long'. In this way it is possible to assess whether the infant is small or large, relative to the population norm, and what is even more important, whether the infant has a steady and healthy development (i.e. does not deviate too much from his or her own percentile line). In 2006, the World Health Organization published new norms for developed countries (WHO, 2006).

8.4.4.2. Based on elevated risk for disease

For blood pressure, the values at which the risk for cardiovascular diseases starts to increase has played a major role in defining the normal value for blood pressure. This can be read in the background document of the most recent US national guidelines on the prevention, detection, evaluation and treatment of high blood pressure (Chobanian *et al.*, 2003). However, the discussions about normal values for older people are interesting. We know that blood pressure increases with age, so according to the 'elevated risk' principle, almost all older people have high blood pressure. Because of reluctance to admit that more than half the population has high blood pressure, one may argue to change the norm values for older people (i.e. considering a higher cut-off point for abnormal blood pressure values in older persons). The latter reasoning is based on the 'distribution' principle.

8.4.4.3. Based on what is treatable

We have seen over time that blood pressure is being treated earlier (i.e. at lower values), because we now have medication/drugs for patients with slightly elevated blood pressure. This has lowered blood pressure values that are considered abnormal, and therefore, in this reasoning, 'abnormal' is defined as what can be treated.

8.5 Interpretation of change scores

8.5.1 Distinction between changes and differences

Before we discuss the interpretation of change scores, it is important to emphasize the distinction between changes and differences. To avoid confusion, we recommend to use the term 'difference' for cross-sectional comparisons between patients, and 'change' for intra-individual changes that are assessed longitudinally within patients over time. The reason why it is important to distinguish between changes and differences can be illustrated by looking again at the data in Figure 8.6, presenting HAQ-DI values for various subgroups of patients with RA. The group of patients with RA who did not have a knee or hip replacement have lower (i.e. more favourable) scores on the HAQ-DI than the group of patients with a knee or hip replacement. Interpreting these data in a longitudinal manner (i.e. as a change between pre-surgery and post-surgery assessments) would suggest that knee or hip replacement surgery leads to a deterioration in health status. However, the data show there are differences between groups of patients with RA, and these groups may differ in many respects. Before knee or hip replacement surgery, patients are probably younger, their duration of RA may be shorter and severity of RA is certainly less. The patients who have had knee or hip replacement surgery had such a severe stage of RA that surgery was indicated. Therefore, it is not surprising that they have a lower HAQ-DI score, even after surgery, than patients with no indication for knee or hip replacement surgery. It is well known, however, that knee or hip replacement surgery is a very effective therapy that leads to large improvement in health status. That is why we emphasize the distinction between changes and differences.

8.5.2 Relationship with change scores on other known instruments

The interpretability of change scores resembles, to a large extent, the interpretability of single scores. Again, we relate the changes observed with the instrument under study to changes observed with well-known instruments. Table 8.2 shows the change in scores on a numerical rating scale for pain intensity (ranging from 0 indicating no pain to 10 indicating the worst pain imaginable) of patients with low back pain, related to their score on a global rating scale (GRS), to indicate the perceived effect of the therapy they

Table 8.2 The mean change scores (SD) for pain intensity scored on a numerical rating scale (Pain-NRS) by patients with low back pain, according to their answer on the global rating of perceived change

Global perceived change	Number of patients $n = 438$	Change in Pain-NRS Mean$_{change}$ (SD$_{change}$)
Completely recovered	105	5.9 (2.6)
Much improved	219	4.1 (2.4)
Slightly improved	66	1.8 (2.0)
No change	28	0.7 (2.0)
Slightly worse	17	−0.4 (1.3)
Much worse	3	−2.3 (1.5)

De Vet *et al.* (2007), with permission.

had received. It shows that patients who reported no change in health status changed very little in pain intensity (de Vet *et al.*, 2007). A change in pain intensity of 2 points corresponded to a slight improvement, and patients who reported they had completely recovered had an average change of almost 6 points.

This example provides useful information on how change scores on the measurement instrument correspond to the magnitude of change, as perceived by patients. When interpreting change scores, two values are of special interest: the smallest detectable change (SDC) and the MIC.

8.5.3 Smallest detectable change

8.5.3.1 Smallest detectable change is based on measurement error

SDC is a concept closely related to the measurement error and the reliability of measurement instruments. We have already mentioned the term SDC in Chapter 5 on reliability (Section 5.6.2.2). It is important to note that not every change on a measurement instrument can be considered to be a real or true change. Small changes may be due to measurement error, i.e. they may be comparable in size or even smaller than the differences found when repeated measurements are performed in a stable population. Therefore, the SDC was defined in Section 5.6.2.2 as change beyond measurement error; this is a change that falls outside the limits of agreement of the Bland and Altman method. In formula, that is a change larger than $\bar{d} \pm 1.96 \times SD_{difference}$ or, in the absence of systematic differences, larger than $\pm 1.96 \times SD_{difference} = \pm 1.96 \times \sqrt{2} \times SEM$ (standard error of measurement). The limits of agreement give an indication of how much the scores can vary in stable patients. So, a change in scores within the limits of agreement or smaller than the SDC can be attributed to measurement error, and only outside the limits of agreement we can be confident these are statistically significant changes. Instead of SDC, the terms minimal detectable change, minimal real change or true change have also been used. The SDC is similar to the Reliable Change Index (RCI), defined by Jacobson and Truax (1991) as (pre-test score − post-test score)/$SD_{difference}$. $SD_{difference}$ equals $\sqrt{2} \times SEM$, and represents the spread of the distribution of change scores that would be expected if no true change had occurred. If RCI > 1.96 true change has occurred. The relationship of the SDC with measurement error implies that when using measurement instruments with a small measurement error, relatively small changes can already be identified as real changes. However, if the measurement error is large, changes on the measurement instrument must be substantial before we can be sure they are not due to measurement error.

In Section 5.4.2.1, we have seen that the SEM can be based on Cronbach's alpha and test–retest parameters. To determine the SDC, the SEM to be used should be based on test–retest parameters, and not on Cronbach's alpha. The reason for this is that Cronbach's alpha is assessed at a single point in time, and does not reflect the variation in scores when the measurement is assessed at different time-points. This variation may be due to biological variation in the patient. In addition, the mood of a patient while filling in a questionnaire may determine whether he/she gives more positive or negative answers in case of doubt. The variation may also be due to the measurement variation in the observer who might apply the criteria strictly or less strictly, or due to the different days of measurements, on which the observers or patients may vary in their concentration. If we consider changes in the course of a disease, patients have to be measured at different time-points, and the above-mentioned variations are at stake. Thus, for interpreting the change scores the assessment of measurement error based on a test–retest parameter is required. We can not stress strongly enough that it is not sufficient to base the SDC on Cronbach's alpha.

We stated in Chapter 5 (Section 5.8) that test–retest reliability should be assessed in a stable population. However, what *is* a stable population? By choosing a short time interval, we assume that the patient characteristics under study will not have changed. Sometimes patients are asked whether their characteristics have changed, and if so, they are excluded from the test–retest analysis.

Change scores are assessed over a specific time-period. In clinical research or practice, a change score is typically based on a pre-treatment score and a post-treatment score, with an interval as long as the duration of the treatment period. For practical reasons (i.e. saving an extra measurement after a short time interval for test–retest analysis), this longer time-interval might also be taken to perform the test–retest analysis, provided that the analysis only includes a stable population. The question 'Has your health status changed during this specific period?' is usually the leading question with which to define a stable group of patients. In that case, the SEM and the limits of agreement are assessed in patients who are considered to be stable over this longer period. Apart from the practical advantage, it makes sense to estimate measurement error over a longer time interval, because the changes we are considering also concern this longer interval. The validity of this approach needs further study.

The SD used to calculate the limits of agreement in these longitudinal situations is often referred to as SD_{change} instead of $SD_{difference}$. That is because this SD is derived from change data (shown in Table 8.2), and it concerns intra-individual changes over time in a stable group. As we stated in Chapter 5 (Section 5.8), the assumption in test–retest analysis is that the patients are stable, and the differences in scores are due to differences in measurements because of different raters, different days or biological variation. Therefore, in reliability analysis we used the term $SD_{difference}$. Note that $SD_{difference}$ and SD_{change} have the same function in the estimation of the limits of agreement.

8.5.3.2 Smallest detectable change in individual patients and in groups of patients

In Chapter 5 on reliability (Section 5.4.1.2), we explained the principles of reducing measurement error by performing repeated measurements and calculating average scores. Applying these average scores, the measurement error becomes smaller and this means that we can detect smaller changes beyond measurement error (i.e. the SDC becomes smaller). In Section 5.15, we extended this reasoning to the application of measurement instruments in groups of patients for research purposes. The fact that measurement error is reduced when measuring in groups of patients, implies that the SDC is reduced by a factor $\sqrt{n}$, when a group of n patients is studied. It also implies that in comparison with clinical research, in clinical practice greater changes are needed to be detected beyond measurement error, or as we saw in Section 5.15, more reliable measurement instruments are required, because decisions are taken on individual patients.

8.5.4 Minimal important change

8.5.4.1 The concept of minimal important change

The MIC is defined by the COSMIN panel as 'the smallest change in score in the construct to be measured which patients perceive as important'. For patient-reported outcomes (PRO), the MIC should be considered from the perspective of the patient. Determining the MIC for non-PRO instruments, a clinician's perspective of which change is minimally important could be relevant. For example, Bruynesteyn *et al.* (2002) evaluated criteria for the scoring of X-rays of hands and feet in patients with rheumatoid arthritis. They wanted to enhance the interpretation of a new scoring system for these X-rays and used the expert opinion of five experienced rheumatologists to determine which changes on hand and foot films they considered to be minimally important. From a clinician's perspective, a MIC may be one that indicates a change in the treatment or in the prognosis of the patient. The assessment of MIC has received much attention. In the interpretation of RCT results, two important questions need to be answered: Are the results statistically significant? Are they clinically relevant? To assess the relevance, the MIC might be of interest. Particularly in very large RCTs, small improvements in patients and small differences between trial arms become statistically significant, but then the question is: are such small improvements relevant for the clinicians or for the patients? In other words, what is the MIC? This question is relevant in research as well as in clinical practice.

8.5.4.2 Methods to determine minimal important change

There is no consensus on the best method to determine MIC. In this section, we will explain the most frequently used methods, but for an extensive overview of the existing methods, we refer to Crosby *et al.* (2003). In the literature, anchor-based and distribution-based approaches are distinguished. In this section we will describe the essentials of both approaches, and explain why we favour the anchor-based approach.

The anchor-based approach uses an external criterion, or *anchor*, i.e. a well interpretable measurement instrument to determine what patients or their clinicians consider as important improvement or important deterioration. Anchor-based methods assess which changes on the measurement instrument correspond with the MIC defined on the anchor.

An example of an anchor-based approach is the mean change method, in which the MIC is defined as the mean change in score on the measurement instrument in the subcategory of patients who are minimally importantly changed, according to the anchor. Looking at Table 8.2, the MIC of the Pain-NRS could, for example, be defined as the mean change in scores in patients who consider themselves to be 'slightly improved'. The MIC would then be 1.8 points.

Another anchor-based method is the receiver operating characteristic (ROC) method, which resembles the analysis of a diagnostic study. We mentioned the ROC method in Chapter 6 on validity (Section 6.4.1) to assess criterion validity. Using this approach to assess MIC, the health status measurement instrument at issue is considered as the diagnostic test, and the anchor functions as the gold standard. The anchor distinguishes patients with important improvement or deterioration from patients with no important change. The instrument's sensitivity is the proportion of importantly improved (or deteriorated) patients, according to the anchor, that are correctly identified as such by the health status measurement instrument (based on a specific cut-off value on the instrument). Its specificity is the proportion of patients with 'no important change' (according to the anchor) that is correctly identified as such by the health status measurement instrument. As the two groups of 'importantly changed' and 'not importantly changed' patients will overlap in their change scores on the measurement instrument, we will have to choose a cut-off point. In diagnostic studies, the optimal ROC cut-off point is often chosen, i.e. the value for which the sum of the proportions of misclassifications ([1-sensitivity] + [1-specificity]) is smallest. In analogy, the MIC is defined as this optimal ROC cut-off point. An example of the ROC method can be found in Section 8.5.4.3.

The advantage of anchor-based methods is that the concept of 'minimal importance' is explicitly defined and incorporated in the method. However, as will be explained later, these methods fail to take into account the variability of the scores of the instrument in the sample. For example, the mean change method only uses the mean value in that group, irrespective of how large the SD is. If the SD of this group had been 5.0 instead of 2.0 (in Table 8.2) then change values far from 1.8 may also occur in patients who said that they had slightly improved. The ROC method searches for the optimal cut-off points, irrespective of how much misclassification occurs.

Distribution-based approaches are based on distributional characteristics of the sample, and express the observed change in the measurement instrument under study to some form of variation to obtain a standardized metric. A frequently used parameter is the effect size, a parameter that relates the observed change to the sample variability (change/$SD_{baseline}$) (see Chapter 7, Section 7.5.1). One might, for example, state that an effect size of 0.5 would correspond to a MIC; in other words, the MIC is defined as 0.5 $SD_{baseline}$ (Norman *et al.*, 2003). However, it might seem odd to relate the change to the heterogeneity of the study population in which it is determined. This implies that a change might be considered important if it is observed in a homogeneous study sample, whereas the same magnitude of change would not be considered important if it was observed in a heterogeneous study sample.

Some authors relate the observed change to the SEM. Threshold values of $1 \times SEM$ and $1.96 \times SEM$ have been proposed to reflect MIC (Crosby *et al.*, 2003). Note that they link the MIC to a parameter of measurement error.

The major disadvantage of all methods that use the distribution-based approach is that they do not, in themselves, provide a good indication of the *importance* of the observed change. For that reason, in our opinion, they do not qualify as methods to assess MIC. Therefore, anchor-based methods are preferred.

Crosby *et al.* (2003) plead for a combination of anchor-based and distribution-based methods to take advantage of both an external criterion and a measure of variability. Agreeing with Crosby *et al.*, we designed a method that integrated both approaches, which we called the *visual anchor-based MIC distribution* (De Vet *et al.*, 2007). This method is presented in the next section.

8.5.4.3. The visual anchor-based minimal important change distribution method

We will first describe the three steps in this method, followed by an example.

Step 1: Divide the study sample according to the anchor

The visual anchor-based MIC distribution is based on the ROC method, as described above. Using an anchor, we divide the study sample into three groups: patients that have importantly improved, not importantly changed and importantly deteriorated patients.

Step 2: Plot the distribution of change scores

We then plot distributions of the change scores on the health status measurement instrument of these three groups (Figure 8.7). Distributions of the improved patients and deteriorated patients are presented on the left-hand side, and the distribution of the not importantly changed patients is presented on the right-hand side. The number of patients in the unchanged, improved and deteriorated group may differ. However, we do not want the sample sizes of these three groups to influence the curves and cut-off points. Therefore, the areas under the three curves should be made equal. This is achieved by using the proportional frequencies instead of the absolute numbers. We assess the MICs for improvement and for deterioration separately, because these might differ (Crosby *et al.*, 2003).

Step 3: Determine the cut-off point

In Figure 8.7, we see that the distributions overlap. For example, a change score of 0 occurs in the sample of patients who have importantly improved according to the anchor, but also in the sample of patients who are unchanged. Because of this overlap, the challenge is to find a cut-off point that leads to the minimal amount of misclassification. The shaded areas show the proportion of misclassified patients. We consider the optimal ROC cut-off point to be the MIC value. This is the value for which the sum of the shaded areas is smallest (i.e. in diagnostic terms, the value of [1-sensitivity] + [1-specificity] is smallest). On the left-hand side, we find false-negative misclassifications (i.e. according to the anchor patients have improved, but according to the cut-off value on the measurement instrument they have not improved). On the right-hand side, we find the false-positive misclassifications. According to the anchor, these patients have not changed, whereas according to the

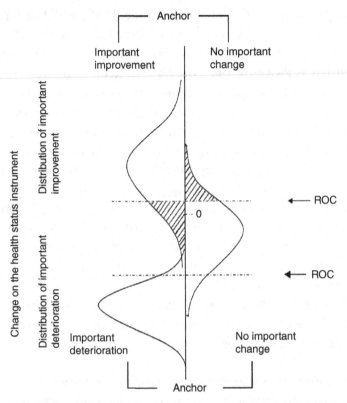

Figure 8.7   Graph of the anchor-based MIC distribution, with indication of the ROC cut-off point for improvement and deterioration. With kind permission from Springer Science+Business Media: De Vet *et al.* (2007).

cut-off value on the measurement instrument they seem to have improved. Note that proportions of misclassifications, instead of the absolute numbers of misclassified patients, are used to decide about the optimal cut-off points. That was the reason why we needed equal surfaces under the three curves in step 2. Note that the assumption for the optimal ROC cut-off point is that false-positive and false-negative results are equally weighted.

An example
We will illustrate the various steps with an example, determining the MIC for improvement for an instrument called the PRAFAB questionnaire (based on Hendriks *et al.*, 2008), which aims to assess the impact of stress

urinary incontinence (UI) in women. (The database and various steps in the analysis can be found at www.clinimetrics.nl) It consists of five items, which measure protection, amount, frequency, adjustment and body image, abbreviated as PRAFAB. The score for each item ranges from 1, indicating no problem, to 4, indicating severe problems. Therefore, the PRAFAB score ranges from 5 to 20 points, with a higher score indicating more problems. A total of 534 women with stress incontinence who received pelvic floor muscle training completed the PRAFAB questionnaire before treatment and after 12 weeks of treatment. After treatment, they also rated their condition on a GRS by answering the question: 'How does your current condition compare to how it was before you started the treatment?'. Patients were classified into nine distinct groups: 1 = completely recovered, 2 = much improved, 3 = moderately improved, 4 = slightly improved, 5 = unchanged, 6 = slightly deteriorated, 7 = moderately deteriorated, 8 = much deteriorated, 9 = worse than ever.

Table 8.3 shows the relationship between the scores on the GRS and the change in PRAFAB score; the correlation between the two scores was –0.88 (Spearman's correlation coefficient).

Step 1: Divide the study sample according to the anchor

Patients who had moderately improved, much improved or completely recovered were considered as 'importantly improved'. Patients who indicated no change or experienced a slight improvement or deterioration were considered as 'not importantly changed'. In Assignment 8.2, we ask you to repeat the analysis with another definition of important change.

Step 2: Plot the distribution of change scores

Figure 8.8 shows the distribution of the patient group who had importantly improved on the anchor on the left-hand side (scores 1, 2 and 3), and the distribution of the patient group with no important improvement (scores 4, 5 and 6) on the right-hand side. To obtain curves of similar size, the relative frequency distribution (proportion) of change scores on the PRAFAB for the 'importantly improved' group and the 'not importantly improved' group are used, as presented in Table 8.4. To obtain the left-hand curve, negative values should be given to change scores of the 'importantly

Table 8.3 The mean difference (T0 – T2) in the PRAFAB scores by GRS at 12 weeks follow-up for the total group of patients with stress urinary incontinence

Global rating scale	Number of patients $n = 534$	Change in PRAFAB score (T0 – T2) Mean$_{change}$ (SD$_{change}$)
1 Completely recovered	124	6.51 (1.84)
2 Much improved	86	4.52 (1.71)
3 Moderately improved	86	3.57 (1.33)
4 Slightly improved	49	2.55 (0.79)
5 Unchanged	139	0.82 (0.98)
6 Slightly deteriorated	39	−0.36 (1.06)
7 Moderately deteriorated	7	−2.29 (0.76)
8 Much deteriorated	3	−4.00 (1.73)
9 Worse than ever	1	−6.00 (–)
Importantly improved (1, 2, 3)	296	5.08 (2.09)
Not importantly improved (4, 5, 6)	227	0.99 (1.33)
Importantly deteriorated (7, 8, 9)	11	−3.09 (1.58)

Positive scores indicate an improvement of the impact of the incontinence.
Based on Hendriks *et al.* (2008), with permission.

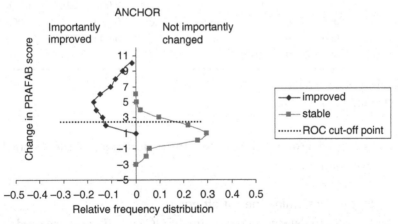

Figure 8.8   Distribution of change scores on the PRAFAB questionnaire of patients who reported an important improvement ($n = 296$) compared with those with no important improvement ($n = 227$) on the anchor (GRS). With kind permission from Springer Science+Business Media: De Vet *et al.* (2007).

Table 8.4 Change scores on the PRAFAB of 'importantly improved' and 'not importantly changed' groups, and corresponding values for sensitivity and specificity

Change score T0 – T2	'Importantly improved' group N	proportion	'Not importantly changed' group N	proportion	ROC cut-off point on PRAFAB	Sens	Spec	1-Sens	1-Spec	Sum of [1-Sens] + [1-Spec]
11	0	0.000	0	0.000	11.00	0.000	1.000	1.000	0.000	1.000
10	4	0.014	0	0.000	9.50	0.014	1.000	0.986	0.000	0.986
9	16	0.054	0	0.000	8.50	0.068	1.000	0.932	0.000	0.932
8	25	0.084	0	0.000	7.50	0.152	1.000	0.848	0.000	0.848
7	31	0.105	0	0.000	6.50	0.257	1.000	0.743	0.000	0.743
6	43	0.145	0	0.000	5.50	0.402	1.000	0.598	0.000	0.598
5	51	0.172	1	0.004	4.50	0.574	0.996	0.426	0.004	0.430
4	48	0.162	5	0.022	3.50	0.736	0.974	0.264	0.026	0.290
3	41	0.139	22	0.097	**2.50**	**0.875**	**0.877**	**0.125**	**0.123**	**0.248**
2	37	0.125	50	0.220	1.50	1.000	0.656	0.000	0.344	0.344
1	0	0.000	67	0.295	0.50	1.000	0.361	0.000	0.639	0.639
0	0	0.000	59	0.260	-0.50	1.000	0.101	0.000	0.899	0.899
-1	0	0.000	13	0.057	-1.50	1.000	0.044	0.000	0.956	0.956
-2	0	0.000	10	0.044	-2.50	1.000	0.000	0.000	1.000	1.000
-3	0	0.000	0	0	-3.50	1.000	0.000	0.000	1.000	1.000
-4	0	0.000	0	0	-4.50	1.000	0.000	0.000	1.000	1.000
-5	0	0.000	0	0	-5.50	1.000	0.000	0.000	1.000	1.000
-6	0	0.000	0	0	-6.50	1.000	0.000	0.000	1.000	1.000
-7	0	0.000	0	0	-7.00	1.000	0.000	0.000	1.000	1.000
Total	296	1.000	227	1.000						

Sens, sensitivity; Spec, specificity.
Based on Hendriks *et al.* (2008), with permission.

improved' group. This results in the typical graph of the anchor-based MIC distribution.

Step 3: Determine the cut-off point

In order to determine the optimal ROC cut-off point, we need information about sensitivities and specificities at all potential cut-off points. These are presented in Table 8.4, together with the sum of 1-sensitivity and 1-specificity (i.e. the proportion of misclassification). For example, when we take a cut-off value of 6.5 points, all patients who are 'not importantly improved' according to the anchor are correctly classified by the PRAFAB (i.e. the specificity is 1, and 1-specificity is 0). At this cut-off value of 6.5 points, the sensitivity is 0.257, meaning that about one-quarter of the 'importantly improved' group is correctly classified [(4 + 16 + 25 + 31)/296]. We also see that in Figure 8.8 the largest part of the distribution on the left-hand side is below 6.5 points. At a cut-off value of −0.5, the sensitivity is 1 (i.e. all patients who consider themselves to be importantly improved, according to the anchor, are correctly classified as improved by the PRAFAB). The specificity is 0.101 (23 of 227), and 1-specificity is 0.899, meaning that according to the anchor most of the 'not importantly changed' patients are falsely classified as importantly changed by the PRAFAB. The least misclassifications occur at a cut-off value of 2.5. (Note that 2.5 is not a change score that occurs by subtracting the pre- and post-PRAFAB scores. Using half scores is a characteristic of ROC analysis in SPSS. We did not try to change this because it facilitates interpretation of the MIC: a two-point difference is less than the MIC, while a three-point change exceeds the MIC.) The ROC graph (Figure 8.9) is obtained by plotting sensitivity versus 1-specificity at every possible cut-off point (i.e. change score) on the PRAFAB.

Using the change score of 2.5 as cut-off point, the sensitivity is 0.877 and the specificity is 0.875. This means that the PRAFAB can correctly distinguish between patients who consider themselves importantly improved on the GRS and those who do not. This also means that the PRAFAB is a responsive measurement instrument for this purpose (see Sections 7.3 and 7.4)

Interpreting the anchor-based minimal important change distribution

The anchor-based MIC distribution graph contains a number of interesting features. First, it shows how well an instrument distinguishes between patients who, according to the anchor, are importantly improved or importantly deteriorated from those with no important change. Figure 8.10 presents two examples of anchor-based MIC distributions.

On the left-hand side, we can see a high correlation between the anchor and measurement instrument. On the right-hand side, the correlation is much lower, which results in a much flatter curve, with much more overlap. Hence, in the left situation, the instrument is much better capable of

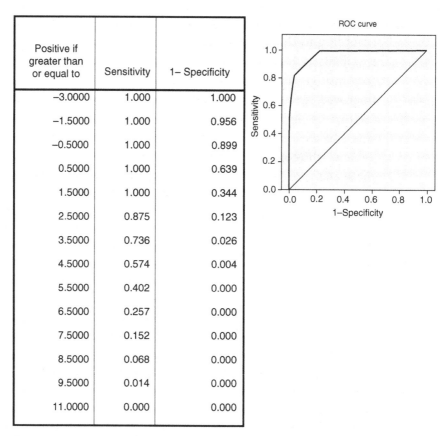

Positive if greater than or equal to	Sensitivity	1– Specificity
–3.0000	1.000	1.000
–1.5000	1.000	0.956
–0.5000	1.000	0.899
0.5000	1.000	0.639
1.5000	1.000	0.344
2.5000	0.875	0.123
3.5000	0.736	0.026
4.5000	0.574	0.004
5.5000	0.402	0.000
6.5000	0.257	0.000
7.5000	0.152	0.000
8.5000	0.068	0.000
9.5000	0.014	0.000
11.0000	0.000	0.000

Figure 8.9   ROC curve representing the sensitivity and 1-specificity at various change scores on the PRAFAB questionnaire. With kind permission from Springer Science+Business Media: De Vet *et al.* (2007).

distinguishing between patients who, according to the anchor, are importantly improved or importantly deteriorated and those that are not importantly changed. As can be seen in this figure, the value of the MIC is the same, so if the MIC value was presented without the graph, we would not see the underlying distributions.

Secondly, the graph of the anchor-based MIC distribution shows the consequences of a specific cut-off point for the amount of misclassification. The optimal ROC cut-off point minimizes the misclassification. However, there might be situations in which we consider false-positive misclassifications to be more severe than false-negative misclassifications. Suppose, for example,

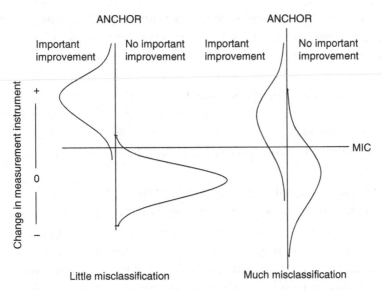

Figure 8.10 Two examples of anchor-based MIC distributions with the same MIC value, but different underlying distributions; left-hand side: little misclassification; right-hand side: much misclassification. Reprinted from De Vet *et al.* (2010), with permission from Elsevier.

that patients with stress UI who do not show an important improvement after pelvic floor muscle training are referred for surgery, and this is decided on the basis on their PRAFAB score. In this situation, we may be more reluctant to refer patients who do not need surgery than to deny surgery for patients who really do need it. In this case, we might give false positives more weight than false negatives. This means that the cut-off point in Figure 8.7 should be moved upwards. On the left-hand side of the figure (false negatives), we then can see how many more patients who actually need surgery will not receive it (or it will be postponed).

Thirdly, the visual anchor-based MIC distribution, as presented in Figure 8.7, shows differences in the location and shape of the curves of the 'improved' and 'deteriorated' patients. From such a graph, we can see whether the MIC values for deterioration and improvement differ. In Figure 8.7, even without numbers on the y-axis, it is evident that if the optimal ROC cut-off point was used, the MIC for deterioration is greater than the MIC for improvement. This means that negative changes in scores must be greater than positive score changes before patients report an important change. For a more elaborate discussion about the strength and limitations of this approach, we refer to De Vet *et al.* (2007; 2009).

8.5.4.4 Minimal important change is a variable concept

Now that we have discussed a number of methods to assess MIC values, and have seen which choices have to be made in this process, one can imagine a measurement instrument does not have a fixed MIC value.

Minimal important change depends on the type of anchor

All kinds of anchors can be used, from the perspectives of both the patient and the clinician, and even clinical outcomes can be used as an anchor. For example, haemoglobin level and response to treatment were used as anchors in the assessment of the MIC value for the anaemia and fatigue subscales of the functional assessment of cancer therapy (FACT) questionnaire (Cella *et al.*, 2002). These clinical outcomes might be a reasonable anchor for instruments assessing the functioning of patients, but less suitable as an anchor for instruments that assess the impact of disease on a patient's health-related quality of life (HRQL). From a patient perspective, a GRS (as presented in Tables 8.2 and 8.3) is often used as the anchor to assess perceived changes in (specific aspects of) health status. Such a GRS is closely linked to the phrase 'perceived important by patients' in the definition of MIC, and to the simple question patients are asked in clinical practice: 'Do you feel better?'.

However, critical remarks have been made about such a transition question, first with regard to its reliability (Norman *et al.*, 1997; Guyatt *et al.*, 2002), because it is only one question, and it tends to depend more on the most recent measurement than on the first measurement, which is an indication of recall bias. In our opinion, the patient's global rating of change is still a useful anchor with which to define MIC. However, we share these concerns, and therefore recommend that further research should be carried out to find a more appropriate anchor for the perspective of the patient.

Clinicians may differ from patients in their opinions about what is important. As a consequence, clinician-based anchors may result in different MIC values than patient-based anchors. Kosinski *et al.* (2000) used five different anchors to estimate the MICs for the SF-36 in patients with RA. They found different MIC values, depending on the anchor used, thus supporting the statement that the MIC depends on the type of anchor.

Minimal important change depends on the definition of 'minimal important change' on the anchor

In the definition of minimal importance on the anchors, some authors tend to emphasize 'minimal', while others stress 'important' (Sloan *et al.*, 2005). For example, studies using a patient GRS for perceived change as an anchor have used different definitions of 'minimal importance' for this anchor. Some defined a slight change on the anchor as 'minimally important', consisting of the categories 'a little worse/better' and 'somewhat worse/better'; other authors have defined 'minimal importance' as a greater change on the anchor, and have set the cut-off point for MIC between 'slightly improved' and 'much improved', or at 'moderate improvement'. There is no right or wrong in this respect: it is a decision made by patients about what they consider to be important. However, two remarks must be made. First, the decision about MIC is often taken by the researcher, and not by patients, because they decide which category they define as minimally important. Secondly, the reference standard is usually based on the 'amount' of change and, remarkably, little research has focused on the 'importance' of the change. Awaiting the results of further research, decisions will therefore remain arbitrary.

Minimal important change depends on baseline values and patient groups

Several studies have shown that the MIC value of a measurement instrument depends on the baseline score on that instrument (Crosby *et al.*, 2003). Patients with a high score at baseline (indicating higher severity) must often have a change of more points than patients with lower scores at baseline to indicate an important change. Therefore, percentage of change from baseline has been proposed as a more stable measure for MIC values than absolute changes. This dependence on severity of the disease is also found in comparisons of MIC values for different subgroups of patients. For example, Bruynesteyn *et al.* (2002) found different MIC values, depending on the disease activity (mild versus high disease activity).

Minimal important change depends on the direction of change

There is still discussion about whether the MIC for improvement is the same as the MIC for deterioration. In some studies the same MIC is reported for patients who improve and patients who deteriorate, but others studies have observed different MIC values for improvement and deterioration (Crosby *et al.*, 2003). Therefore, it is recommended to assess a separate MIC value for improvement and deterioration.

As the MIC is dependent on the above-mentioned factors, it is an illusion that the MIC of a measurement instrument will be a fixed value. Various authors have therefore suggested there should be a range of MIC values to account for this diversity. Moreover, it has been recommended that different anchors and different methods are used (Revicki *et al.*, 2008) to give reasonable limits to MIC.

We recommend an anchor-based method, and have explained that the visual anchor-based MIC distribution, in particular, gives a lot of extra information that is useful for the proper interpretation of a MIC value. It is wise to use different anchors, if available. However, it is important that the anchor reflects the construct that the instrument under study aims to measure. When the resulting range of MIC values is so large that it loses its clinical meaningfulness, it is better to interpret change scores by presenting MIC values for different anchors or for different situations, i.e. showing its diversity, rather than hiding it.

8.5.5 Distinction between the smallest detectable change and the minimal important change

We have defined SDC as 'the smallest change that can be detected by the instrument, beyond measurement error'. MIC was defined as the smallest change in score in the construct to be measured that is perceived as important by patients, clinicians or relevant others. Considering these definitions, it is clear that these are different concepts. Confusion on this issue has been generated by the use of distribution-based methods to assess the MIC value. Some of the distribution-based methods that have been proposed as parameters for MIC are conceptually more closely related to the SDC than to the

MIC. Wyrwich *et al.* (1999) evaluated whether the $1 \times$ SEM criterion can be applied as a proxy for MIC. Wyrwich (2004) showed that if the cut-off point for 'minimal importance' on the anchor is set between 'no change' and 'slightly changed' (i.e. the first category above no change), the value of the MIC approximates the value of the SEM. As we saw in Section 5.3, the SEM is a parameter of measurement error. Therefore, linking changes to the SEM refer more to detectable change beyond measurement error (i.e. SDC), than to important change.

Norman *et al.* (2003) performed a systematic review of 38 studies, including 62 effect sizes, and observed, with only a few exceptions, that MICs for HRQL instruments were close to an effect size of 0.5 (i.e. half an SD). They explained their findings of 0.5 SD by referring to psychophysiological evidence that the limit of people's ability to discriminate is approximately 1 part in 7, which is very close to half an SD. Thus, this criterion of 0.5 SD may be considered as a threshold of detection, and therefore corresponds to an SDC, rather than to MIC.

It is important to make the distinction between MIC and SDC. Assessing the MIC by a parameter of SDC is like saying that what we cannot detect is not important (by definition) (De Vet and Terwee, 2010). A direct consequence of this reasoning is that all measurement instruments are adequate, because they all can detect MIC, but we know that this is not true. Such a reasoning would impede further improvement of measurement instruments. For a better interpretation of change scores, both the SDC and the MIC are important benchmarks on the scale of the measurement instrument. Moreover, appreciating the distinction, we can answer the important question: is a measurement instrument able to detect changes as small as the MIC value?

Figure 8.11 shows how changes should be interpreted in various situations. Figure 8.11(a) represents the situation that the SDC value is smaller than the MIC. In other words, the measurement error is sufficiently small to detect MIC values at the individual level. Change values lying between the SDC and MIC are considered statistically significant but not important. Figure 8.11(b) represents the situation that SDC is larger than MIC. Change values lying between the MIC and SDC are considered important by patients, but are not statistically significant, i.e. they cannot be distinguished from measurement error.

It is interesting to discuss Guyatt's responsiveness ratio again at this point. As shown in Chapter 7 (Section 7.5.3) Guyatt's responsiveness ratio relates

(a)

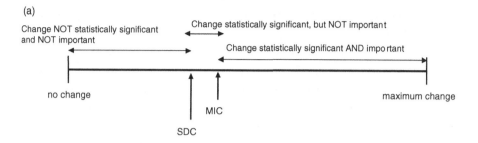

(b)

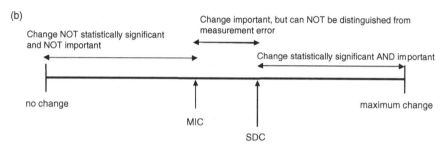

Figure 8.11 (a) Interpretation of change when MIC is larger than SDC. (b)Interpretation of change when MIC is smaller than SDC. Reprinted from De Vet and Terwee (2010), with permission from Elsevier.

the MIC to the SD_{change} in a stable group of patients. We argued that Guyatt's responsiveness ratio is an inadequate measure of responsiveness because it lacks to assess the validity of change scores. However, Guyatt's responsiveness ratio is quite informative for the interpretability of a measurement instrument. As $SDC = 1.96 \times SD_{change}$, it can be shown that if the Guyatt responsiveness ratio is larger than 1.96, then the MIC value lies outside the limits of agreement, and thus is larger than the SDC. Thus, Guyatt's responsiveness ratio relates the MIC to the measurement error, in a similar way as we do in Figure 8.11.

Many authors use the Guyatt responsiveness ratio with observed change in the numerator instead of MIC. In that case, the formula of Guyatt responsiveness ratio resembles the formula for RCI as discussed in Section 8.5.3.1. However, there is a conceptual difference, for the RCI is used to provide information on the magnitude of change, while the Guyatt responsiveness ratio (with MIC in the numerator) gives information on the interpretability of the measurement instrument.

Returning to our example of the PRAFAB, we can compare the MIC value of 2.5 with the SDC. In this population, we had no data on test–retest analysis with a very short interval. Therefore, we calculated the SDC based on the patient group who experienced no change in impact of urine incontinence over the 12-week period. Table 8.3 shows that there were 139 patients in this category. They showed a mean change of 0.82 points and SD of 0.98. Calculating the SDC as $1.96 \times SD_{change}$ amounts to 1.92. This means that the SDC is smaller than the MIC. Therefore, the PRAFAB is able to detect MIC at individual level. It has to be noted that for most measurement instruments the SDC is greater than the MIC. This implies that these instruments are not able to detect MIC at individual level on the basis of single measurements. However, taking the mean value of multiple measurements will make these instruments suitable for application in clinical practice. As noted in Sections 5.15 and 8.5.3.2, these instruments are often very suitable for research purposes, where the measurement error is reduced when groups of patients are studied.

8.5.6 Response shift

Now that we have learned more about the interpretation of change scores, we will discuss response shift. In clinical practice and research, patients are often monitored over time, and they are repeatedly measured to assess the clinical course of their disease or their health status. During these longitudinal assessments, characteristics should be measured with the same measurement instruments. For example, MRI scans are used, among other things, for identifying changes in brain tissue of patients with multiple sclerosis. The MRI techniques are improving continuously over time. Among other things, new contrast agents are used to detect a wider array of metabolites, new criteria and rating scales are proposed to increase sensitivity while maintaining the specificity. Usually it is known when changes in the procedures or scoring methods have occurred. It goes without saying that for an appropriate evaluation of the progress of multiple sclerosis the same techniques should be used over time. This also holds if disease progression is evaluated by PRO measures. However, in the case of PROs, subtle changes may occur that are much more difficult to detect. These subtle changes concern altered ways in which patients perceive their health status, and interpret and respond to questions, based on cognitive psychological mechanisms. This is called response shift.

Response shift can occur in all patient-reported measures. It was defined by Sprangers and Schwartz (1999) as a change in the meaning of self-evaluation of a target construct as a result of:

(1) redefinition of the target construct (reconceptualization)
(2) change in the respondent's values (reprioritization, i.e. change in importance of domains substituting the target construct) or
(3) change in the respondent's internal standards of measurement (scale recalibration).

In order to illustrate these rather abstract descriptions, we will provide an example of each.

During the clinical course of their disease, there may be a change in the way patients assess their situation. This is illustrated by the following example. Let us consider patients who suddenly become wheelchair-bound because of a spinal cord injury. At first, they will probably rate their health status as very poor because of losing their walking ability. However, after a while, they might have accepted their physical limitations to some extent, and have possibly set new goals and challenges. They will then rate their perceived health status as better, whereas in reality their health condition has not changed.

(1) *Reconceptualization.* One can imagine that being wheelchair-bound they totally ignore walking ability in their assessment, i.e. they define health status in such a way that walking ability is no longer part of it. This is called reconceptualization. Thus, the construct that they assess has changed.

(2) *Reprioritization.* When asked about their health status, other aspects than walking ability have become more important. For example, they may consider social contacts more important than they did in the past. This is an example of reprioritization.

(3) *Scale recalibration.* Suppose that these patients also develop decubitus. At the first assessment, patients have rated the severity of their pain with a score of 7 on a 10-point scale. Between the first and second assessment, some of these patients might suffer more pain than they have ever experienced before. At the second assessment, these patients might score their pain as 9 or 10. However, they realize that their pain during

the first assessment was much lower than 7 points (e.g. only 4 or 5 points on the 10-point scale) if they had used the same reference framework as they used now. This is called scale recalibration.

In all these examples, the construct that is measured (1 and 2) or the scale that is used to rate the response (3) has changed over time in the patient's mind. As can be seen from the definition, response shift can occur in all patient-reported measurements, and especially when patients are asked to make an overall assessment. For example, the question 'Do you have difficulty with a long walk?' requires careful consideration: the patient has to think about what 'difficulty' is and about what is meant by 'a long walk'. These undefined formulations can result in different interpretations over time. The question 'Can you walk for 10 minutes?' requires less consideration and evaluation, and is therefore less prone to response shift (Schwartz and Rapkin, 2004).

8.5.6.1 A conceptual model of response shift

The original conceptual model proposed by Sprangers and Schwartz (1999), presented in Figure 8.12, shows how response shift affects ratings of perceived quality of life as a results of changes in health status. Although it has been adapted and extended, resulting in even more complex models (Rapkin and Schwartz, 2004), the original model gives much insight into what response shift is and what causes it. Note that this model refers to quality of life measurements, but also applies to other patient-reported measurements.

The model has five components: the catalyst, the antecedents, mechanisms, response shift and perceived quality of life. The catalyst is a change in health status. The antecedents refer to stable patient characteristics, which may affect the patients' assessments and responses on how the change in health status has affected their perceived quality of life. Examples are age, education, expectations and personality characteristics such as optimism, sense of control and self-esteem. For example, an optimistic patient might consider a slight decrease in physical functioning to have less impact on health status than a pessimistic patient might do. The mechanisms encompass the more dynamic processes that might affect a patient's rating of perceived quality of life, such as coping, reprioritizing goals and reframing expectations.

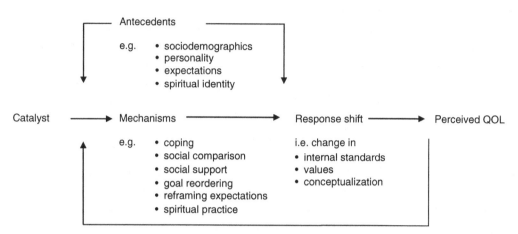

Figure 8.12 A theoretical model of response shift and perceived quality of life. Reprinted from Sprangers and Schwartz (1999), with permission from Elsevier.

An example of the latter is an answer that is often heard: 'considering my age, or considering the stage of my disease, I am doing quite well'. These specific mechanisms of adaptation lead to response shift. The mechanisms refer to behavioural, cognitive and affective processes to accommodate the change in health status. They can be seen as coping mechanisms applied to deal with a change in health status. Patients do this by reconceptualizing and reprioritizing their health status (i.e. domains of health status that are heavily affected are completely neglected, or considered to be less important, respectively). Patients may also change their scaling. If they expect their health status to become worse, they recalibrate their scale to leave room for further deterioration.

8.5.6.2 Assessment of response shift

In the following section, we will describe a number of methods that are helpful to determine response shift. For a complete overview, we refer to Barclay-Goddard *et al.* (2009).

Qualitative methods

Much insight into response shift is obtained by means of qualitative methods. Interviewing patients provides direct information about how they interpret questions and how they choose their answers. From cognitive psychology and survey methodology, it is known that at least four actions are required from respondents in order to answer a question: they must comprehend the question, retrieve necessary information from memory, decide on which information is needed to answer the question, and respond to the question or choose the adequate response option (Tourangeau *et al.*, 2000). It has been shown that the response shift takes place during all four actions required to answer a question (Bloem *et al.*, 2008).

The 'three step test interview', combining a 'think aloud' method and a cognitive interview is a suitable method for this type of qualitative research. It starts with patients completing the questionnaire while thinking aloud. In the second step, the interviewer asks questions concerning the items about which the patient was apparently thinking, without talking. In the third step, the aim is to collect more information about the cognitive processes. For example: Which information was taken into consideration? How did the weighing up process go? What was the point of reference? We refer to Westerman *et al.* (2008) and Bloem *et al.* (2008) for illustrative examples of such qualitative analyses of response shift.

Quantitative methods

The first method to be described is the 'then-test'. Suppose, the patient first completes a questionnaire about health status (the pre-test) and after some time when the patient's health status has changed, a second questionnaire is completed (the post-test). At the post-test measurement, the patient is asked to complete the questionnaire again for his pre-test health status. This is called the 'then-test'. Hence, the 'then-test' is a retrospective assessment of the pre-test, which is assessed at the same time as the post-test. As both the 'then-test' and the post-test take place at the same time, it is assumed that the same standards, values and concepts will be used, thus accounting for response shift. The difference between the 'then-test' and the pre-test is referred to as the response shift effect.

Jansen *et al.* (2000) tried to quantify the response shift in the Rotterdam Symptom Checklist by using the 'then-test' in patients before and after radiotherapy for breast cancer. Significant scale recalibration effects were observed in areas of fatigue and overall quality of life. A 'then-test' embedded in qualitative research provides an enormous amount of information about adaptive mechanisms used in the responses to questions (Westerman *et al.*, 2008).

Individualized measures

In Chapter 3, we mentioned the SEIQOL-DW as a measurement instrument to individually weigh the importance of domains in HRQL. The patients are asked to quantify the relative importance of all domains. Over time, reprioritization is reflected by a change in the magnitude of the domains chosen, and reconceptualization occurs when one domain is completely neglected at a second assessment.

Although these methods can indicate that a response shift has occurred in a particular patient, they can not easily be converted into a numerical value of the response shift effect.

Factor analysis

We have seen in Chapter 6 on validity (Section 6.5.2) that confirmatory factor analysis tests the factor structure of a construct. In Section 6.5.3.3, we discussed how factor analysis could be used to test measurement invariance after the translation or cultural adaptation of a questionnaire. Using data from the pre-test and post-test, factor analysis can also be used to test whether, and to what extent, response shift has occurred. In fact, it is the assessment of measurement invariance (see Chapter 6, Section 6.5.3.3) over time. Confirmatory factor analysis quantifies the three mechanisms of response shift: reconceptualization, reprioritization and recalibration. Reconceptualization means that some domains disappear, or that new domains appear. In factor analysis, this implies a change in the number of factors found. Reprioritization means a change in the importance of various domains. This is expressed in different factor loadings in the two data sets, i.e. the importance of the items has changed. Scale recalibration might also take place. This aspect of response shift can be detected with factor analysis, by testing whether the mean values of the variables change, i.e. testing the equivalence of the intercepts. In addition to indicating which element of response shift has occurred, confirmatory factor analysis is able to distinguish the response shift from true changes. However, the performance and interpretation of such a confirmatory factor analysis is quite complex, and therefore beyond the scope of this book. We refer to Oort, for details about the theory (Oort, 2005) and application (Oort et al., 2005).

Which method do we prefer?

The quantitative and qualitative methods complement each other. The qualitative methods and individualized measures provide insight into the mechanisms of response shift, but only the 'then-test' and factor analysis provide insight into the magnitude of the effect. The 'then-test' gives an overall estimate of the effect, while factor analysis is able to specify which parts are due to reconceptualization, reprioritization and recalibration. Furthermore, factor analysis is able to distinguish between response shift and true changes in the construct. Therefore, factor analysis is preferable for quantitative analysis. To obtain more knowledge about which mechanisms are involved in response shift, a qualitative analysis is indispensable. Therefore, we recommend using a combination of qualitative and quantitative methods.

8.5.6.3 Interpretation of response shift

A point of debate concerning response shift is whether or not one should adjust for response shift. Some researchers tend to do this, because they regard response shift as bias. In our opinion, adjustment for response shift is not always necessary. For example, suppose we are studying patients with cancer. People in the environment clearly observe that the patients' health status is deteriorating. However, patients themselves do not report any deterioration in perceived general health status, as scored for instance with the SF-36. Should the patient's answers be doubted? We have to keep the construct under study in mind: health status as observed by other people is a construct that differs from the patient's own perceived health status, in which coping and adaptation may play a role. If perceived health status is what we want to assess, then adjustment is not necessary in our opinion.

In some cases, achieving response shift may be the actual aim of the treatment. For example, in rehabilitation medicine, some patients can not recover, in the sense that their physical condition can not be improved. However, much improvement in perceived health status can be gained by learning alternative ways of movement, by resetting goals or by learning to accept limitations and focusing on the remaining possibilities. Thus, inducing response shift is the aim of many interventions in the field of rehabilitation medicine.

To a certain extent, response shift can be avoided by careful formulation of questions, which can be made more specific and leave less room for variation in interpretation by the patients. For instance, instead of asking about long walks, one can specify a 10-km walk. Furthermore, specifying the point of reference deters patients from choosing their own point of reference, as patients can do in different ways (Fayers *et al.*, 2007).

The concept of response shift and its mechanisms in health assessment is relatively new. Therefore, issues such as meaning, assessment and interpretation of response shift are still under discussion.

8.6 Summary

The interpretability of a score is the degree to which one can assign qualitative meaning to an instrument's scores or change in scores. Interpretability is not considered to be a measurement property, but it is an important requirement for the intelligent use of a measurement instrument.

A study on interpretability starts with examining the distribution of the scores in the target population. Knowing the variation of scores in the population helps us to interpret some measurement properties, such as reliability and responsiveness. Furthermore, the distribution may reveal clustering of scores, which often occurs at the extremes of the scale and indicates a lack of discriminative ability of patients at that range of the scale. Whether or not this clustering causes floor or ceiling effects depends on the purpose of the measurement. Floor and ceiling effects occur when we want to distinguish these clustered patients' scores from each other, and when we want to detect change in the direction in which there is no further room for improvement or deterioration. In this latter case, the responsiveness of the instrument will be affected. Floor and ceiling effects often occur when the measurement instrument is applied to another target population than that for which it was originally developed.

IRT analysis is more powerful than CTT analysis if we wish to examine the distribution of scores on a scale, because with IRT the location of items as well as patients can be presented on the same scale. This reveals various important interpretation issues: it shows whether there is a clustering of patients' scores, whether there is a clustering of items and whether there is sufficient overlap between the locations of the items and the patients. Furthermore, with IRT analysis an inherent interpretation of a patient's score is possible, because it indicates which items the patient probably can and cannot do. In CTT analysis, other measurement instruments are needed to facilitate the interpretation of the scores.

It is informative to know the scores of relevant subgroups of patients, for example, the scores of patients who visit their general practitioner versus the scores of hospitalized patients. When using these measurement instruments, we become more familiar with scores in various groups of patients, and can more easily learn the meaning of the scores. For the interpretation of change scores, we can follow the same strategy of comparison of instruments and subgroups with clinical or commonly understood connotations. We stressed the importance of distinguishing between the interpretation of changes within patients and the difference between patients.

With regard to the change scores of measurement instruments, there are a few benchmarks of special interest: the SDC and MIC. We defined the SDC as the smallest change that can be detected by the instrument, beyond measurement error, and the MIC was defined as the smallest change in score in the construct to be measured that patients perceive as important.

We discussed a number of methods that can be used to assess MIC values, and explained the visual anchor-based MIC distribution method in detail. This method requires us to choose about an adequate anchor and to define minimal importance on that anchor. Furthermore, it provides extra information about the consequences of the chosen MIC value. Appreciating and acknowledging the distinction between MIC and SDC enhances the interpretation of the change scores on a measurement instrument.

Response shift is another interpretability issue. It can occur when patient-reported measurement instruments are administered over time. Response shift is defined as a change in the meaning of self-evaluation of a target construct as a result of a change in the respondent's internal standards, values and conceptualization of the construct. Response shift is often the result of adaptation to a change in health status.

We presented a number of methods that can be used to assess response shift and discussed their interpretation. Suggestions on how to avoid response shift were also made. At first sight, response shift seems to cause bias. However, adjustment is not always necessary. When carefully considering the construct to be measured and appreciating the way in which patients perceive their health status, it can be concluded that the patient's response is exactly the answer that was asked for.

A proper interpretability of a score is a prerequisite for well-considered use of an instrument in clinical practice and research.

Assignments

1. Distributions

The Multidimensional Fatigue Inventory (MFI-20), aims to assess fatigue in patients, and consists of five domains: general fatigue, physical fatigue, mental fatigue, reduced motivation and reduced activity (we discussed the MFI-20 in Section 3.2.1). Each domain contains four items scored on a five-point Likert scale, resulting in a range for the total score of 4–20, with 20 indicating the highest degree of fatigue. Lin *et al.* (2009) validated the MFI-20 for use in a US adult population sample. They included three study samples: 292 patients with chronic fatigue syndrome (CFS) satisfying at least four CFS symptoms (CFS-like), 269 chronically unwell patients and 222 well persons.

Table 8.5 presents some data about the distribution of three of the five MFI domains in these three study samples.

(a) What kind of information does this table provide about the interpretability of the MFI-20?
(b) Is the information on the distribution of the domains informative?
(c) Did floor or ceiling effects occur?

2. Determining the minimal important change for the PRAFAB questionnaire, using the anchor-based minimal important change distribution method

In Section 8.5.4.3, when determining the MIC for the PRAFAB questionnaire we considered the patients who scored moderately improved, much improved and completely recovered as 'importantly improved'.

What is the MIC value if the patients who scored slightly improved on the anchor are included in the group of 'importantly improved' patients (i.e. when the cut-off point on the anchor for importantly improved is laid between the categories 'no change' and 'slightly improved')? The deteriorated group is omitted from this analysis. The data set 'PRAFAB.sav' can be found on the website www.clinimetrics.nl.

(a) Determine the mean change values in the nine categories of the GRS.

Table 8.5 Descriptive statistics for three of the five MFI-20 subscales for the three study samples

	All	CFS-like	Chronically unwell	Well
General fatigue				
Mean	12.90	16.38	12.84	8.42
SD	4.68	2.73	3.93	3.59
25%	9.00	15.00	10.00	6.00
Median	14.00	17.00	13.00	8.00
75%	17.00	18.00	16.00	11.00
Range	4–20	6–20	4–10	4–20
% at floor	3.45	0	1.49	10.31
% at ceiling	6.13	13.01	3.36	0.45
Physical fatigue				
Mean	10.85	13.63	10.39	7.77
SD	4.36	3.79	3.76	3.36
25%	7.00	11.00	8.00	5.00
Median	11.00	14.00	10.00	7.00
75%	14.00	16.00	13.00	10.00
Range	4–20	4–20	4–20	4–19
% at floor	6.39	0.34	5.60	15.25
% at ceiling	2.81	6.51	1.12	1
Reduced activity				
Mean	9.25	11.32	9.06	6.76
SD	4.16	4.37	3.75	2.67
25 %	6.00	8.00	6.00	5.00
Median	8.00	11.00	8.00	6.00
75%	12.00	15.00	12.00	8.00
Range	4–20	4–20	4–20	4–16
% at floor	11.49	3.77	8.96	24.66
% at ceiling	2.43	5.14	1.49	0

Lin *et al.* (2009), with permission.

(b) Determine the distribution of the change scores (T0 – T2) in the 'importantly improved' group, and the distribution of the change scores (T0 – T2) in the 'non-changed' group (present absolute numbers and relative frequencies).

(c) Determine the optimal ROC cut-off point.

(d) Draw a graph in Excel or another program to get a graph of the anchor-based MIC distribution.

3. Response shift

Dempster *et al.* (2010) reported on a study that assessed HRQL among people attending cardiac rehabilitation. In total, 57 patients completed the assessments before (pre-test) and after (post-test) a 10-week rehabilitation program that consisted of a supervised physical exercise program and presentations on health education such as a healthy diet and stress management. Because the authors were interested whether response shift occurred in these assessments they included the SEIQOL-DW in their study and also used a then-test approach.

SEIQOL-DW is a quality of life measurement instrument, in which the individual patient determines the importance of the various domains. For this purpose, the total HRQL is represented by a circle. The patient mentions the five areas of life (e.g. health, family, work or social life) that are most important to him/her. For the direct weighting, the patient, with help from the researcher, divides the circle into five pie-segments according to the relative importance of these five areas of life, with percentages (%) that add up to 100%. Then the patient rates the quality of these five areas on a vertical 0–100 VAS. The ultimate SEIQOL-DW score is calculated as the sum of the score for each of the five areas, multiplied by the percentage of relative importance of that area (i.e. Σrelative weight × VAS score).

The information from the SEIQOL-DW and the then-test was obtained by interviews. The maximum score of the SEIQOL-DW is 100 indicating optimal HRQL, and lower values indicate less HRQL.

The authors analysed whether the life areas mentioned by the participants differed between pre-test and post-test, indicating a change over time. They presented all this in Table 8.6 as an illustration.

(a) About which mechanism of response shift does this table provide information?

(b) Please comment on how the data are presented.

The authors calculated an intraclass correlation coefficient (ICC) to evaluate whether the relative importance of the life areas was similar at the pre-test

Table 8.6 Life areas (or cues) nominated by participants ($n = 57$)

Areas of life	Pre-test frequency	%	Post-test frequency	%
Family	52	91.2	48	84.2
Hobby	30	52.6	22	38.6
Social life	29	50.9	26	45.6
Work	27	47.4	20	35.1
Health	26	45.6	39	68.4
Home	18	31.6	15	26.3
Relationship	17	29.8	13	22.8

Adapted from Dempster *et al.* (2010) with permission.

and post-test. The authors do not clearly describe how they dealt with the fact that persons might have changed one or more of their five life areas. It appears that they worked with 'areas of life' numbered 1–5, irrespective of whether these areas were the same in the pre-test and post-test assessment. The ICC value was 0.74.

(c) About which mechanism of response shift does the ICC value provide information?

(d) Which data would you have liked to be presented instead of the ICC value.

The instruction for the then-test was as follows: 'I would like you to look again at these five important life areas. This time I would like you to show me how you now think you were doing in each of these five areas when we first met. I am not asking you to try and remember how these important life areas were functioning, but rather how, when looking back today, you think they were functioning when we first met …' . The authors then compared the then-test score with the pre-test score.

(e) Considering this instruction, about which mechanism of response shift does the difference between the pre-test and then-test scores provide information?

The actual values for the SEIQOL-DW (Σrelative weight $\times$ VAS score) for the five important areas for HRQL were not presented in the paper by Dempster *et al.* (2010). They presented only the differences between the pre-test and post-test scores and the differences with the then-test. It appeared that the then-test score was lower than the pre-test score: difference: −9.56 (SD = 18.07; $P < 0.001$). The post-test score was slightly higher than the pre-test score: difference +5.09 (SD = 17.08; $P = 0.028$), indicating an improvement in HRQL.

(f)   How large is the effect of the rehabilitation programme with and without taking response shift into account? (It might be helpful to assume a certain value for the pre-test score, e.g. 64.)

(g)   Which mechanisms of response shift are included in the difference between the post-test and the pre-test? (Note that this question differs from Assignment 3(e)

(h)   Would you label the response shift as bias in this study?

Systematic reviews of measurement properties

9.1 Introduction

Systematic reviews are made for many different types of studies, such as randomized clinical trials (RCTs), observational studies and diagnostic studies. Researchers, doctors and policy-makers use the results and conclusions of systematic reviews for research purposes, development of guidelines, and evidence-based patient care and policy-making. It saves them a considerable amount of time in searching for literature, and reading and interpreting the relevant articles. For the same purposes, more and more systematic reviews of studies focusing on the measurement properties of measurement instruments are being published. The aim of such reviews is to find all the existing evidence of the properties of one or more measurement instruments, to evaluate the strength of this evidence, and come to a conclusion about the best instrument available for a particular purpose. They may also result in a recommendation for additional research.

In this chapter, we will describe the global structure of a systematic review of measurement properties. In such a review the content of measurement instruments is described, the methodological quality of the studies focusing on the measurement properties is critically appraised, and results concerning the quality and appropriateness of the instruments for a specific purpose are summarized. The method of conducting a systematic review consists of the 10 steps described in Table 9.1. We will discuss each step separately in the following sections of this chapter. It should be noted, however, that some aspects of the methodology are still under development.

Table 9.1 Ten steps to conduct a systematic review of measurement properties

(1) formulate a research question
(2) perform a literature search
(3) formulate eligibility criteria
(4) select articles
(5) evaluate the methodological quality of the included studies
(6) extract the data
(7) compare the content
(8) data synthesis – evaluate the evidence for adequate measurement properties
(9) draw an overall conclusion of the systematic review
(10) report on the systematic review

9.2 Research question

9.2.1 Types of systematic reviews

Systematic reviews of measurement properties may be based on different research questions, i.e. to find and evaluate:

1. all available studies on the measurement properties of *one measurement instrument*. For example, a systematic review of the measurement properties of the Western Ontario and McMaster Universities Index of Osteoarthritis (WOMAC) (McConnell *et al.*, 2001).

2. all available studies on the measurement properties of a selection of the *most commonly used measurement instruments* that aim to measure a particular construct in a particular population. For example, a systematic review of the measurement properties of the five most commonly used tests to measure walking ability in patients with cardiorespiratory disorders (Solway *et al.*, 2001).

3. all available studies on the measurement properties of *all available measurement instruments that aim to measure a particular construct in a particular population*. For example, a systematic review of all currently available quality-of-life measurement instruments suitable for use in palliative care (Albers *et al.*, 2010).

4. all available studies on the measurement properties of *all available measurement instruments (without specifying the construct to be measured) in a particular patient population*. For example, a systematic review of outcome measures for psoriasis (Ashcroft *et al.*, 1999).

Some systematic reviews aim to make an inventory of measurement instruments (e.g. of all available measurement instruments for a particular construct or of all those used in RCTs). Such reviews primarily focus on the use of the measurement instruments and not on their quality. Therefore, they are not considered to be systematic reviews of measurement properties.

9.2.2 Key elements of the research question

Four key elements should be included in the research question: (1) the construct of interest or the name(s) of the measurement instrument(s) of interest; (2) the population of interest (3) the type of measurement instrument of interest (e.g. imaging techniques, laboratory tests, observation scales, performance-based instruments, interviews or questionnaires, etc.); and (4) the measurement properties on which the review focuses. An example of a research question is: 'What are the measurement properties of pain observation scales used in or developed for older adults with severe cognitive impairments, communication difficulties or both' (Van Herk *et al.*, 2007).

Whether to restrict the systematic review to one or to several measurement instruments depends on the purpose of the review and the amount of information available. If there is a lot of available evidence concerning many instruments, it may become too extensive and complex to conduct a review including all measurement instruments. Therefore, one might choose to conduct a review of the two or three instruments most commonly used to measure the construct of interest. If the interest lies in the quality of one particular instrument, or the quality of a particular version (e.g. only the self-administered version of a questionnaire or the Dutch version of a questionnaire), it might be more appropriate to conduct a systematic review of the measurement properties of the (version of the) instrument of interest. If it is the intention to decide on the best available measurement instrument, no instruments should be excluded, and all measurement properties should be included.

9.2.3 Systematic reviews to select the best measurement instrument

Most systematic reviews focus on all measurement properties of the included instruments. However, there are also reviews that focus on only one measurement property (e.g. a review of the reliability of functional MRI) (Bennett and Miller, 2010), or a review of the construct validity of instruments measuring impairments in body structures and function in patients with rheumatic disorders (Swinkels *et al.*, 2006). These reviews are not suitable for selecting the best instrument, because not all of the measurement properties are evaluated.

This chapter focuses on systematic reviews of measurement properties that aim to select the best measurement instrument available for a particular purpose. In order to make a well-considered choice, in such a review it is important to evaluate the measurement properties of all, or at least the most important, measurement instruments. Unlike systematic reviews of RCTs or diagnostic studies, which usually focus on one outcome (effect size or diagnostic accuracy), a systematic review of measurement properties focuses on many outcomes, i.e. the various measurement properties. The evidence for the various measurement properties may be provided by different sets of studies. This means, that, in fact, a systematic review of measurement properties consists of several systematic reviews, i.e. one for each measurement property. Therefore, conducting such a review can be quite complex and time-consuming, but they are well worth the effort – for the individual researcher and for the research community as a whole. To find out whether a systematic review on measurement properties of instruments measuring a specific construct in a specific population exists, a list of published systematic reviews is available at www.cosmin.nl.

9.3 Literature search

An adequate literature search is of utmost importance for a systematic review in order to find all the available evidence. A suboptimal search might miss important articles, and could even lead to wrong conclusions. A good literature search for systematic reviews of measurement properties is challenging, because studies on measurement properties are difficult to find. This is due to: (1) a large variation in the terminology used for measurement properties; (2) a sometimes incomplete and often unpredictable indexing of the primary studies; and (3) poorly reported abstracts of studies on measurement properties.

9.3.1 Databases

As is the case in reviews of other types of research, not all relevant articles will be found in one database. It is therefore recommended to search more databases. We recommend using at least MEDLINE (e.g. using the PubMed interface) and EMBASE (Exerpta Medica Database). In addition, databases focusing on specific professional organisations can be searched (e.g. CINAHL, Cumulative Index to Nursing and Allied Health Literature), which is a resource for nursing and allied health literature, or subject-specific databases, such as PsycINFO or SportDiscus, which are resources for psychological literature, and sports and sports medicine journals, respectively.

9.3.2 Build a search strategy

A search strategy should contain searches for several characteristics of the studies of interest. These correspond to a certain extent with the key elements of the research question (see Section 9.2.2) and consist of a collection of search terms for the following characteristics: (1) construct of interest; (2) target population; and (3) measurement properties. For each of these characteristics a comprehensive list of possible synonyms should be made, consisting of index terms (such as 'MeSH terms' (Medical Subject Headings) in MEDLINE and EMTREE terms in EMBASE) and free text words (i.e. words in the title or abstract). These synonyms for each characteristic should be combined with the conjunction 'OR'. The searches for these three characteristics should then be combined with the conjunction 'AND', to obtain the list of references that should be used to select the relevant articles. Selecting adequate search terms and building the search strategy should be carried out by an expert on the specific construct in close co-operation with a medical information specialist.

1: Construct of interest

Examples of search terms for the construct 'activities of daily living' in MEDLINE are: 'activities of daily living' as MeSH term, complemented by the following search terms as free text words: instrumental activities of daily living, instrumental ADL, IADL, extended ADL, complex ADL, advanced ADL, functional ability, everyday functioning and activities of daily living (Sikkes *et al.*, 2009). If the aim of the review is to evaluate the quality of one specific measurement instrument, or a selection of commonly used instruments, terms for the construct can be replaced by the name(s) of these measurement instrument(s).

2: Target population

The search terms for the target population can be similar to the terms used in a review on RCTs. For example, for a review of patients with neck pain the search terms for the target population could be: neck[MeSH] OR 'neck pain'[MeSH] OR 'neck injuries'[MeSH] OR 'whiplash injuries'[MeSH]. The target population does not necessarily have to be a patient population. For example, a specific age group of the general population may be of interest (e.g. children). The search terms for this target population could, for example, include: child*[tw] OR schoolchild*[tw] OR infan*[tw] OR adolescen*[tw] OR pediatr*[tw] OR paediatr*[tw] OR neonat*[tw] OR boy[tw] OR boys[tw] OR boyhood[tw] OR girl[tw] OR girls[tw] OR girlhood[tw] OR youth[tw], etc. The indication [tw] in MEDLINE recognizes the specific term in the title, abstract and MeSH index. A specific setting can also be chosen to define the target population. For example, in a review of measurement instruments suitable for use in the palliative care setting (Albers *et al.*, 2010), the following search terms were used: palliative OR terminal OR 'end of life' OR 'limited life' OR 'hospice care' OR 'after-hours care'.

3: Measurement properties

To identify all studies that focus only on measurement properties, a highly sensitive (sensitivity 97.4%) methodological search filter has been developed for use in MEDLINE through PubMed (available via Terwee *et al.*, 2009). This search filter reduces the number of records that need to be read to identify one study on measurement properties from 87 (without the filter) to 23 (with the filter).

You may notice that *type of measurement instrument*, which was one of the four key elements of the research question, is not used as a basis for search terms. Possible terms for the type of measurement can be questionnaire, interview, performance test, laboratory test or scan, but no search terms for the type of instrument are included because this could result in a high risk of missing relevant articles. Many studies on measurement instruments do not use these specific terms, but use terms such as 'measure', 'method' or 'instrument' instead. These are such broad terms that they can not be used as search terms, because they would result in too many irrelevant articles. Therefore, we advise against the use of search terms indicating the type of measurement instrument.

In addition to the search strategy described above, we recommend that an additional search be performed, including the names of the instruments found in the initial search. These names can be combined, using the AND conjunction, with terms for the target population and the measurement properties.

We discourage the use of time limits or language restrictions in the search, because the aim is to find all relevant evidence for the quality of the included measurement instruments. Studies conducted many years before can still provide this evidence, and there is no reason to exclude these studies. An exception could be if one is interested in imaging techniques, and some of the older techniques may have become obsolete. Language restrictions are not recommended, but for practical reasons, the review is often restricted to articles written in languages in which the researchers are fluent. Note that a distinction should be made between the language in which the article is written and the language of the measurement instrument under study (if the instrument is based on written items, or an instruction text is included).

9.3.3 Reference checking

We recommend that the reference list of the articles identified with the electronic literature search should be checked to search for additional relevant studies. If many new studies are found through this method, this is an indication that the initial literature search was not adequate, and that even more studies might have been missed. We would then recommend that the search strategy should be improved and the initial search repeated.

9.3.4 Publication bias

Publication bias occurs when studies in which the quality of the measurement instrument under study was found to be poor are not published. There is no registration of studies of measurement properties, as there is for RCTs. Therefore, it is not yet possible to determine the impact of publication bias on the results of a systematic review of measurement properties.

9.4 Eligibility criteria

The search strategy will typically yield many records, because the aim of the search is to identify all articles that are possibly relevant, and broad search terms are used. The next step is now to define strict inclusion and exclusion criteria that will be used to select relevant articles. We recommend that at least the following inclusion criteria should be applied (again using the four key elements in the research question):

(1) instruments should aim to measure the construct of interest
(2) the study sample should be selected from the target population of interest
(3) the study should concern the type of measurement instrument of interest
(4) the aim of the study should be to develop a measurement instrument or evaluate one or more of the properties of an instrument.

A number of remarks can be made with regard to these inclusion criteria. As in the literature search, if the aim of the review is to evaluate the quality of one specific measurement instrument, or a selection of commonly used instruments, the first inclusion criteria can be replaced by the name(s) of these instrument(s).

If one is only interested in, for example, the German version of an instrument, this should be clearly stated in the research question and, consequently, an additional inclusion criterion can be formulated. In order to find all relevant information about the measurement properties of an instrument, articles on the development of that instrument must be included. This is because the articles often contain relevant information about the construct that is measured with the instrument, a description of the content (necessary in step 7 'comparing the content'), and other information that is needed to evaluate the content validity of the instrument. Therefore, we should not restrict the review to studies focusing on measurement property evaluation.

It is often possible to obtain a considerable amount of indirect evidence on the measurement properties of an instrument (e.g. from studies in which the instrument of interest is used in the validation process of another instrument, or in an RCT or other longitudinal study in which indirect evidence for responsiveness might be found). However, we recommend excluding such studies from the review for two reasons. First of all, it is very difficult to find all of these articles in a manageable and structured way, and secondly, it is often difficult to interpret the evidence for validity or responsiveness provided in these studies, because no hypotheses about these properties have been formulated or tested in them.

9.5 Selection of articles

An initial selection is made by applying eligibility criteria to all titles and abstracts found in the search. It is recommended that at least two researchers screen all titles and abstracts. They should independently assess the eligibility of the studies and discuss their assessments. When in doubt about the eligibility of a study, we recommend that the full text article is retrieved, and together with the full text articles likely to meet the inclusion criteria, be screened for eligibility. This should again be done by two researchers independently, who afterwards discuss their assessments and achieve consensus about inclusion or exclusion, if necessary because of disagreement, with the help of a third researcher.

The search should be carefully documented. The names of the databases that were searched, as well as the interface used to search the databases, such as PubMed or OVID for searching MEDLINE, should be documented. It is also important to document the date of the search, the exact search terms and any limitations (e.g. language or age restrictions) that were applied. Moreover, it is often necessary to update the search before submitting or publishing the review. The same search strategy should then be used again. It is valuable for readers to know which search terms were used in order to assess the comprehensiveness of the search strategy. Therefore, we recommend that the search strategy is made available for readers in an appendix or on a website. The date of the searches in each database should be described in the methods section of the article. Software such as Reference Manager or Endnote is very useful to manage references found in each database.

Next, we recommend careful documentation of records that were initially selected (i.e. based on title and abstract), the full text articles that were retrieved and articles included in the review. It is also useful to document reasons for the exclusion of retrieved full text articles, particularly in the case of doubtful articles, because journals sometimes require this information. Moreover, if the same article is found again, for example when updating the review, or if the search is performed in another database, it saves time if you have noted why a specific article was already excluded. We recommend that all information about the search and selection process is presented in a flow chart. Figure 9.1 presents an example of such a flow chart of a systematic review in which the aim was to find all studies reporting on measurement properties of quality of life instruments suitable for use in palliative care (Albers *et al.*, 2010).

9.6 Evaluation of the methodological quality of the included studies

It is important to evaluate the methodological quality of studies in which measurement properties are assessed. If a study meets the standards for good methodological quality, the risk of bias is minimal. 'Risk of bias' instruments have been developed for RCTs (e.g. the Delphi list) (Verhagen *et al.*, 2001) and for diagnostic studies (e.g. the QUADAS list) (Whiting *et al.*, 2003). In an international Delphi study, we developed the COSMIN checklist, which can be used to evaluate the methodological quality of studies on measurement properties (Mokkink *et al.*, 2010b). The checklist was specifically developed for studies on health-related patient-reported outcomes, but it can also be used to assess the quality of studies on other kinds of measurement instruments. It can be used to assess whether a study meets the standard for good methodological quality with regard to the following measurement properties: internal consistency, reliability, measurement error, content validity, construct validity (i.e. structural validity, hypotheses testing and cross-cultural validity), criterion validity and responsiveness. It contains standards for studies that apply classical test theory (CTT), as well as for studies that apply item response theory (IRT). It includes a specific box that contains general requirements for articles in which IRT methods are applied (IRT box). In addition, the checklist contains standards for studies on interpretability, which was not considered a measurement property, though an important characteristic of a measurement instrument (see also Chapter 8). The standards apply to aspects of the study design and statistical methods. Another box contains general requirements for the generalizability

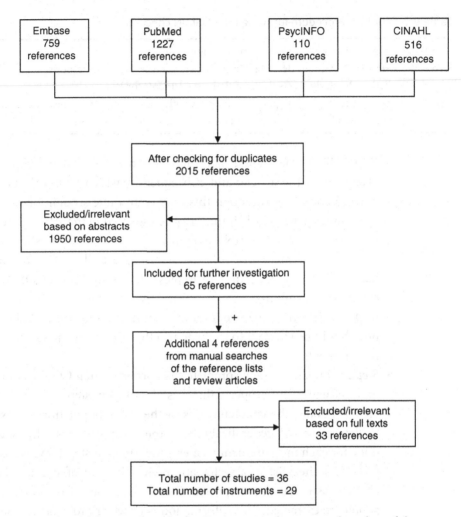

Figure 9.1   Flow chart of the search and selection process of a systematic review of the measurement properties of quality of life instruments for palliative care. Albers *et al.* (2010), with permission.

of results (Generalizability box). In Section 9.7 we discuss the generalizability of results. The COSMIN checklist and manual can be found at www.cosmin.nl.

To assess the quality of a study on measurement properties using the COSMIN checklist, a four-step procedure should be followed, as described in Table 9.2.

Table 9.2 Four-step procedure for using the COSMIN checklist

Step 1: determine which measurement properties are evaluated in the article
Step 2: if the statistical methods described in the article are based on item response theory (IRT), determine whether the study meets the specified requirements for IRT
Step 3: evaluate the methodological quality of the study with regard to the properties identified in step 1
Step 4: assess the generalizability of the results with regard to the properties identified in step 1

- *Step 1*: First, you should determine which measurement properties are evaluated in the article, and consequently, which COSMIN boxes you need to complete. Although this may seem quite straightforward, it can be complex, particularly if the terminology used in the article differs from that used in the COSMIN taxonomy. As a reviewer, you should decide which measurement properties are assessed, regardless of the terminology used in the included studies. Examples can be found at the COSMIN website (www.cosmin.nl).
- *Step 2*: If IRT methods are used in a study, the requirements in the IRT box should be checked to evaluate whether the study meets the specified requirements.
- *Step 3*: You should now complete the corresponding COSMIN boxes for each measurement property that was identified in step 1.
- *Step 4*: Finally, the characteristics of the study population are extracted to determine the generalizability of the study findings. This should be done for each measurement property identified in step 1. When using the COSMIN checklist in a systematic review, instead of stating whether a characteristic has been reported, the actual values of the characteristics should be extracted. This information is necessary to evaluate the generalizability of the results and to assess (dis)similarities of the studies in the process of data synthesis (see Section 9.7.2).

A detailed description of how to use the checklist, a rationale for each item, and suggestions for scoring the items, are provided in the COSMIN manual (www.cosmin.nl).

Example: Mazaheri *et al.* (2010)

The Foot and Ankle Ability Measure (FAAM) is a 29-item questionnaire to assess functional limitations in patients with varying leg, foot and ankle disorders. It is divided into two subscales: activities of daily living (ADL, 21 items) and sports (eight items). We will show how the COSMIN checklist can be used to evaluate the methodological quality of this study.

The first step is to determine which measurement properties are evaluated. In this article, internal consistency, reliability, measurement error and construct validity (i.e. hypotheses testing) were evaluated. No IRT methods were used, so the IRT box (step 2) does not need to be completed. The third step is to complete the COSMIN boxes for each measurement property evaluated in the article. For this article, four boxes (internal consistency, reliability, measurement error and hypotheses testing) need to be completed. In this example, we only focus on the assessment of reliability (the results of the other measurement properties are not shown here). In Figure 9.2 relevant parts of the article can be found. We will demonstrate how we would

---

Introduction

... Although the FAAM has been shown to have a good evidence of psychometric properties, its additional validation in other cultures is needed in order to compare and contrast assessments made in different countries. Therefore, the purpose of the study was to cross-culturally adapt and validate the Persian version of FAAM in a group of patients with foot and ankle disorders.

Methods

Participants and design

During a 1-year period, a consecutive sample of native Persian speaking outpatients with a range of foot and ankle disorders referred to 1 Orthopaedic and 4 Physical Therapy clinics in Tehran, and Isfahan, participated in the study. Patients were included in the study if the cause of their foot and ankle disorder was musculoskeletal in origin. Patients with a history of knee, hip or back pain during the last 3 months, systematic inflammatory rheumatic disease, neurological or vascular conditions, cancer, diabetes mellitus, alcohol abuse and psychiatric disorders were excluded from the study. Of 93 patients who were identified as eligible to participate in the study, all patients agreed to participate and completed the questionnaires. Most of the patients (78.5%) were diagnosed as having lateral ankle sprain. [...]. All patients received a region specific questionnaire, FAAM, and a generic one, Short-Form 36 Health Survey (SF-36), in the first visit. The questionnaires were completed in the clinic waiting room. To evaluate test-retest reliability, a sample of 60 subjects completed the FAAM 2–6 days after the first visit in the same location. To ensure that the health status remained stable between repeated measurements, all patients were explicitly asked by telephone contact that "Has your status changed over the last days since you filled out this questionnaire?". Three possible responses were: (1) no; (2) yes changed for the better and (3) yes changed for the worse. Sixty out of ninety-three patients responded "no" to the question.

Figure 9.2   Adapted from Mazaheri *et al.* (2010), with permission from Elsevier.

Instruments

The FAAM is a 29-item questionnaire divided into two subscales: activities of daily living (ADL) with 21 items and SPORTS with 8 items. Each item is scored on a 5-point Likert scale representing different levels of difficulty (no difficulty at all, slight difficulty, moderate difficulty, extreme difficulty, and unable to do). The ADL and SPORTS subscales have a total score of 84 and 32, respectively. The scores are transformed to percentages with higher scores indicating a higher level of functional status for each subscale. ...

Assessment of psychometric properties

... test-retest reliability was assessed using two-way random effects model of intraclass correlation coefficient (ICC2,1). ICC ≥0.70 were considered satisfactory for test-retest reliability. ...

Results

... Only 23 of 2697 (93 x 29) items (0.85%) were missing for the FAAM data. If the number of missing values were one or two for a subscale, they were substituted with the mean value. More than two missing values for a subscale were considered invalid....

Table II
Descriptive statistics and number (%) of patients reporting the worst possible score (floor effect) and the best possible score (ceiling effect) for the subscales of FAAM (N = 93)

FAAM subscales	Mean	SD	Range	Floor effect n (% of patients)	Ceiling effect n (% of patients)
ADL	69.19	21.97	4.74–100	0	2 (2.2)
SPORTS	41.67	25.13	0–93.75	7 (7.5)	0

In the sample of 60 patients who participated in the test-retest analysis, ADL and SPORTS subscales had mean (SD) scores of 68.69 (23.79) and 38.15 (25.64) for the test session and mean (SD) scores of 68.83 (23.04) and 38.70 (25.45) for the retest session, respectively. No significant difference between test and retest mean scores was obtained, indicating absence of any systematic change. The ICC (95% CI) for the ADL subscale was 0.98 (0.97-0.99). The ICC (95% CI) for the SPORTS subscale was 0.98 (0.97-0.99). ...

Discussion

... Another limitation of this study may be the short length of time (i.e., 2-6 days) between two measurements for test-retest reliability which increases the memory effects of first administration of the instrument on the performance of subsequent administration. ...

... The results of the present study must be generalised cautiously, because the population represents a sample with young age, with a prevalence of males and with a dominant diagnosis of lateral ankle sprain. ...

Figure 9.2 (*cont.*)

complete the COSMIN box for reliability, and explain our ratings. The fourth step will be discussed in Section 9.7.2.

First, we will show how the reliability box should be completed in this example (Table 9.3); secondly, we give our rationale for the answers; and thirdly, we explain how we come to a conclusion about the methodological quality of the study.

Table 9.3 Reliability box of the COSMIN checklist

Box B. Reliability

Design requirements		Yes	No	?
1	Was the percentage of missing items given?	☑	☐	
2	Was there a description of how missing items were handled?	☑	☐	
3	Was the sample size included in the analysis adequate?	☑	☐	☐
4	Were at least two measurements available?	☑	☐	
5	Were the administrations independent?	☑	☐	☐
6	Was the time interval stated?	☑	☐	
7	Were patients stable in the interim period on the construct to be measured?	☑	☐	☐
8	Was the time interval appropriate?	☐	☑	☐
9	Were the test conditions similar for both measurements (e.g. type of administration, environment, instructions)?	☑	☐	☐
10	Were there any other important flaws in the design or methods of the study?	☐	☑	

Statistical methods		yes	no	NA	?
11	For continuous scores: Was an intraclass correlation coefficient (ICC) calculated?	☑	☐	☐	
12	For dichotomous/nominal/ordinal scores: Was kappa calculated?	☐	☐	☑	
13	For ordinal scores: Was a weighted kappa calculated?	☐	☐	☑	☐
14	For ordinal scores: Was the weighting scheme described (e.g. linear, quadratic)?	☐	☐	☑	

Mokkink *et al.* (2010b), with permission.

The rationale for our answers is as follows:

(1) The percentage of missing items for the test data of the 93 patients who completed the baseline questionnaire was reported (i.e. 0.85%). There was no description of the percentage of missing items in the retest administration. We have ignored that in our rating.

(2) Depending on the number of missing items per patient in a subscale, the authors either substituted the missing value with the mean value, or they considered it invalid. Although they do not make it explicit, it is highly likely that they imputed the missing value with the mean value of other items from the patient's subscale. If more than two items in a subscale were missing, they probably considered the subscale score as missing. However, as the percentage of missing data was very low, different ways of handling missing data (e.g. ignoring or imputing missing items) will not have had any major consequences for the results.

(3) A total of 60 patients were included in the reliability analysis. We consider a sample size of 60 patients appropriate for the analyses of reliability.

(4) For each patient, data on two administrations were available.

(5) It was not described whether the administrations were independent, although we assumed that they were, because it is very uncommon that patients receive their answers to the first administration when they complete the second administration. However, due to the short time interval between the two administrations, the patients might have remembered their previous answers.

(6) The time interval was between 2 and 6 days.

(7) The patients were asked by telephone whether their status had changed during the days since they filled in the questionnaire. Patients who answered 'no' were included in the test–retest analysis. It should be noted that 'status' is somewhat vague; it would have been better if they were explicitly asked whether there was any change in their functional limitations due to their foot or ankle disorder.

(8) We consider a time interval of 2–6 days to be somewhat short, as the authors also acknowledge, because patients might have remembered their previous answers.

(9) Patients were asked to complete the same questionnaire again in 'the same location' (i.e. in the waiting room of the same clinic in which they had completed the first questionnaire).

(10) The study seems to be carefully designed and analysed, with no major flaws.

(11) The subscale scores are considered continuous; therefore, ICCs were calculated. The authors even explicitly described which type of ICC they calculated (see Section 5.4.1): a two-way random effects model of intraclass correlation coefficient (ICC 2.1) refers to $ICC_{agreement}$ (Shrout and Fleiss, 1979).

(12) Items 12–14 were not applicable for this study.

Now that we have completed each item of the reliability box, we need to come to an overall conclusion about the methodological quality of this reliability study. In general, when all items are satisfactorily answered, the methodological quality of a study is considered to be good. If one or more items have a negative score, the quality of the study is affected. In this case, we considered the time interval between test and retest to be inappropriate, and conclude that the methodological quality of the assessment of the measurement property reliability in this study is suboptimal. In Sections 9.9.2 and 9.9.3 we explain how the methodological quality is taken into account in the data synthesis. A scoring system to obtain a total score (excellent, good, fair, poor) for the methodological quality of a study for each measurement property is still under development. Up-to-date information regarding the COSMIN scoring system can be found on our website www.cosmin.nl.

9.7 Data extraction

The next step in conducting a systematic review is to extract relevant information from the included articles. The data should be preferably extracted by at least two independent researchers, using a data-extraction form specifically developed or adapted for each review. This form should contain items concerning: (1) the general characteristics of the instrument; (2) the characteristics of the study sample; and (3) the results with regard to the measurement properties.

9.7.1 General characteristics of the instrument

General characteristics of the instruments that need to be extracted are: a description of the construct to be measured and its conceptual framework (see Chapter 2), type of instrument (e.g. laboratory test, performance-based

Table 9.4 Characteristics of format and practicalities of a multi-item questionnaire

Format
(1) the number of items and (sub)scales in the questionnaire
(2) the number and type of response categories (i.e. nominal, ordinal, interval or ratio)
(3) the recall period in the questions (e.g. 1 week, 4 weeks, 6 months)
(4) the scoring algorithm (e.g. how total scores and subscores are calculated and how missing items are handled)
(5) the average time needed for administration
(6) the mode of administration (e.g. self-report, interview, diary)
(7) the target population for whom the questionnaire was originally developed (e.g. age, gender, health status)
(8) how a full copy of the questionnaire can be obtained
(9) the instructions given to those who complete the questionnaire
(10) the available versions and translations of the questionnaire

test or self-report instrument), format and practicalities of the instrument (e.g. technical specifications of positron emission tomography scans, tasks to be performed in a performance-based test, number of questions and dimensions of a questionnaire or interview and its language version), information about feasibility, costs or time needed to administer, etc. Much of this information can usually be found in articles describing instrument development.

In Table 9.4, we suggest several characteristics of the format and other practicalities that could be extracted for a multi-item questionnaire.

If the instrument(s) under study concern(s) a performance-based test, it is useful to extract information such as the number of activities to be performed, facilities required to perform an activity, description of the activities, and instructions for supervisors. For imaging techniques, information about technical requirements, procedures and types of tracers used are relevant. The descriptive information can be used to compare the instruments with regard to content and practicalities. In Section 9.8, we will explain the content comparison in more detail.

9.7.2 Characteristics of the study population

Important characteristics of the study population are age, gender, disease characteristics, setting, country, patient selection methods and response

Table 9.5 Characteristics of the study population extracted using the generalizability box of the COSMIN checklist

Generalizability box

	Data
Was the sample in which the instrument was evaluated adequately described?	$n = 60$
1 Median or mean age (with standard deviation or range)?	Not reported
2 Distribution of gender?	Not reported
3 Important disease characteristics (e.g. severity, status, duration) and description of treatment?	Not reported
4 Setting(s) in which the study was conducted (e.g. general population, primary care or hospital/ rehabilitation care)?	Clinics for orthopaedics and physiotherapy
5 Countries in which the study was conducted?	Tehran and Isfahan, Iran
6 Language in which the instrument was evaluated?	Persian
7 Was the method used to select patients adequately described (e.g. convenience, consecutive or random)?	Consecutive
8 Was the percentage of missing responses (response rate) acceptable?	Response 100%

Mokkink *et al.* (2010b), with permission.

rate. The reason why this information should be extracted is to make it possible to determine the type of population to which the results of a study on measurement properties can be generalized and to assess the (dis)similarities of study populations and settings in the process of data synthesis (Section 9.9). Note that item 7 in Table 9.4 referred to the target population for which the measurement instrument was developed. Here we refer to the study population in which the measurement instrument properties were tested.

We use the Mazaheri *et al.* (2010) study introduced in Section 9.6 to illustrate how the generalizability box of the COSMIN checklist can be used to assess generalizability of the results in the reliability study. Table 9.5 presents the results, and below we comment on each item.

1–3. The demographic and clinical characteristics of all 93 patients were described in the Mazaheri *et al.* (2010) article. However, a sample of 60 patients was used for the assessment of test–retest reliability. This sample differed from the total one in their responses to the question about change in status. It is unclear whether the demographic and clinical characteristics of the stable subgroup differed from the characteristics of the total sample. For example, the test–retest sample could have been younger, or had a higher level of education. This is unknown, and therefore, the COSMIN items 1–3 are scored to be 'not reported'.

4–6. The patients were recruited from one orthopaedic and four physical therapy clinics in Tehran and Isfahan, two big cities in Iran. They all received the Persian version of the questionnaires.

7. The patients were selected consecutively.

8. All patients agreed to participate in the study, thus the response rate was 100%.

Overall, we can conclude that the generalizability is suboptimal.

Item 5, concerning the country in which the study was conducted, and item 6, concerning the language version, is particularly important for studies on patient-reported outcomes (PROs).

9.7.3 Results of the measurement properties

To evaluate the quality of the measurement instrument itself, information on its measurement properties should be extracted, i.e. the results of the analyses of each of the measurement properties. For example, the values of Cronbach's alpha, kappa values, limits of agreement, correlations between (change) scores, the results of the factor analysis or the area under the ROC curve. The accompanying confidence intervals and the sample size used in each analysis are also relevant, and should be extracted.

9.8 Content comparison

When choosing between different health measurement instruments, one of the methods that can help when deciding on the best available measurement instrument for a particular purpose is a content comparison. Content

Table 9.6 Content of patient self-report instruments to measure chemotherapy-induced nausea and vomiting

Item	MANE	MANE-FU	INVR	FLIE	FLIE 5-day recall	CINE-QLQ	MAT	NV5[a]
Nausea	•	•	•	•	•	•	•	•
Vomiting	•	•	•	•	•	•	•	•
Retching			•			•		•
Anticipatory	•	•	[b]			•		•
Acute	•	•	•	•	•	•	•	•
Delayed			[b]	•[c]	•	•	•	•
Occurrence		•	•	•	•	•	•	•
Frequency	•	•	•			•	•	•
Intensity	•	•						•
Duration	•	•	•				•	•
Interference with function			•	•	•	•		•
Anti-emetics		•				•		•

Adapted from Brearley *et al.* (2008), with permission.

[a] With additional tools.

[b] Not specifically designed to capture, but could be used – instrument would need to be administered on multiple occasions.

[c] Initial delayed up to 3 days post-chemotherapy.

MANE, Morrow Assessment of Nausea and Emesis; MANE-FU, later version of MANE; INVR, Index of Nausea, Vomiting and Retching; FLIE, Functional Living Index-Emesis; CINE-QLQ, Chemotherapy-induced Nausea and Emesis Quality of Life Questionnaire; MAT, Multinational Association of Supportive Care in Cancer (MASCC) Assessment Tool; NV5, Osoba nausea and vomiting model (plus additional tools).

comparison is a useful tool to see the differences in content between several questionnaires or several performance-based tests. For example, Brearley *et al.* (2008) compared the content of eight self-report instruments to measure chemotherapy-induced nausea, vomiting and retching (CINVR). They examined, among other things, which aspects of CINVR were covered by the eight instruments. Table 9.6 shows which instruments include items concerning the different phases (anticipatory, acute and delayed), domains (nausea, vomiting and retching) and characteristics of the complaints (occurrence, frequency, duration, and intensity).

9.9 Data synthesis: evaluation of the evidence for adequacy of the measurement properties

In this step we need to take all the evidence per measurement property of an instrument into consideration, which means that we will somehow have to combine results from different studies. The measurement properties of an instrument in one population or setting may be different to those in another population or setting. We have seen that reliability parameters depend on the heterogeneity of the sample, and that a measurement instrument should be validated for different target populations. Therefore, the results with regard to measurement properties can only be generalized to populations that are similar to the study sample in which the measurement properties have been evaluated. This implies that when a measurement property has been evaluated in different studies we need to consider the (dis)similarities in populations and settings in the various studies, and the (dis)similarities of the results, and decide which studies can reasonably be combined. Next, we decide on whether to perform a quantitative combination of the results or to draw a conclusion about the measurement property in a qualitative manner. In the end, we have to decide from the combined results of the various studies whether the measurement property is adequate. Criteria for adequacy will be presented in Section 9.9.4

9.9.1 Homogeneity of the study characteristics

Combining the results of different studies concerning a measurement property is only possible if the studies are sufficiently similar with regard to study population and setting, the (language) version of the instrument that is used, and the form of administration. In Section 6.2, we stated that the FDA considered these to be new situations requiring new validation studies (FDA Guidance, 2009, pp. 20–1). To assess the similarities of different study populations, the data extracted with the generalizability box are indispensable. As in the case of systematic reviews of RCTs, no standard rules can be formulated about which factors should be taken into account and what is sufficiently similar, and it is up to the researcher to decide what is clinically sensible to combine. An example is presented in Assignment 9.2.

Next, data synthesis should take place for each measurement property. There are two options for data synthesis: quantitative analysis (statistical pooling) or qualitative analysis (best evidence synthesis). We will discuss both options.

9.9.2 Quantitative analysis (statistical pooling)

Statistical methods exist for pooling the following statistical parameters: Cronbach's alphas, correlation coefficients (intraclass, Spearman, Pearson), standard errors of measurement (SEMs) and minimal important change (MIC) values. The existence of a method, however, does not in itself guarantee that pooling is justified; other requirements must also be met. Pooling should only be performed if there are several studies available that are sufficiently similar to be able to combine their results. This similarity applies not only to design characteristics (i.e. homogeneity of the study characteristics, as discussed in Section 9.9.1), but also to statistical homogeneity (i.e. similarity) of the results concerning the measurement property under study, (e.g. differences in ICCs). When conflicting or very different results are found in the included studies, pooling should not be performed. Another requirement is that the studies should at least be of fair methodological quality. Low-quality studies are often excluded in systematic reviews because the results of these studies may be biased. We know of only a few reviews that have performed statistical pooling of the results of measurement properties (e.g. Avina-Zubieta *et al.*, 2007; Garin *et al.*, 2009). More research is needed on the methodology of statistical pooling of the data from studies on measurement properties.

9.9.3 Qualitative analysis (best evidence synthesis)

Pooling is not an option when studies do not seem sufficiently similar, or when quantitative data is not available (e.g. for assessing content validity). However, we still have to come to a conclusion about the measurement property. In that case, best evidence synthesis can be performed. This is a qualitative analysis in which the following characteristics are taken into consideration: the methodological quality of the studies, consistency of the results, and homogeneity of the studies. Based on these characteristics, the level of evidence can be determined. For example, when a low score for a reliability parameter (e.g. ICC < 0.4) is found in a number of studies of good methodological quality, then there is strong evidence that the measurement instrument has low reliability, but when a high internal consistency is found in a number of studies of fair quality, there is only moderate evidence of high internal consistency. For reviews focusing on measurement properties, such levels of evidence are still under development. It is clear, though, that they are not so straightforward, and are different for each measurement property. Sometimes, evidence from different studies should be combined, as will be shown below. Although it is a qualitative analysis, information about how the methodological quality is classified, how the consistency of the results is assessed and how the homogeneity of the studies is determined should be described in as much detail as possible. In other words, the way in which the levels of evidence are established should be described.

Internal consistency

In order to be able to assess the internal consistency of a measurement instrument adequately, it is necessary to have information about the unidimensionality of the scales (i.e. from factor analyses) and about the Cronbach's alpha. This information may come from different studies. To obtain a rating of 'strong evidence for good internal consistency', three requirements should be met: (1) subscales should be shown to be unidimensional; (2) high Cronbach's alphas should be found in a number of studies of good methodological quality; and (3) results should be consistent. For example, when three studies are found that show the same subscales, and all studies show Cronbach's alphas between 0.85 and 0.90 for each subscale, it can be concluded that there is strong evidence for good internal consistency.

Reliability

There is strong evidence for the reliability of the instrument if a number of studies that are of good methodological quality have consistent results. If inconsistent results are found, the evidence becomes weaker. The evidence is also weaker when high reliability parameters are only found in studies of fair methodological quality. When deciding about the clinical homogeneity of reliability studies, one should also consider design issues, for example, the expertise of the observers. Note that in case of observer variation, a distinction can be made between evidence for intra-observer and inter-observer reliability when a large number of studies is available.

Measurement error

To evaluate the measurement error, it is necessary to have information about the smallest detectable change (SDC) as well as on the MIC. Again, this information may come from different studies. For strong evidence, the SDC should have been calculated (or, if possible, deduced from the data reported in an article) in a number of studies that are of good methodological quality. In addition, consistent findings of the MIC value should be obtained from a number of good quality studies. Next, an estimate should be made as to whether the SDC is smaller or larger than the MIC. Ideally, this should be based on comparing the pooled estimate of the SDC with the pooled estimate of the MIC. Alternatively, a qualitative assessment should be made. When the SDC is smaller than the MIC, important change can be distinguished from measurement error.

Content validity

Different aspects of content validity can be evaluated in different studies. There is strong evidence for good content validity if all four aspects have been adequately evaluated with positive results in good quality studies (i.e. there is evidence that all items are considered to be relevant for the construct, purpose and target population, and the instrument is considered to be comprehensive). There is weaker evidence if only two or three aspects have been evaluated (i.e. the items are to be considered relevant for the construct or target population).

Construct validity and responsiveness (hypotheses testing)

Validation is an ongoing process, and the results of different studies can be combined to obtain a complete list of all hypotheses that have been tested and to consider the number and types of hypotheses that have been confirmed or rejected. For example, one could use the criterion that 75% of the hypotheses should be confirmed to indicate adequate validity, as suggested by Terwee *et al.* (2007). In a systematic review, this criterion is not applied to each individual study, but to the combined results from all studies of sufficient methodological quality and similarity with regard to the study characteristics. Thus, all the evidence from all included studies will be combined for the assessment. How the strength of the hypotheses should be taken into account, needs to be studied in more detail.

9.9.4 Adequacy of the measurement properties

Criteria for adequacy should be applied to the combined results of the included studies. There are no consensus-based criteria available for the adequacy of a measurement property. We have given suggestions for such criteria throughout the book, even though they are arbitrary. Nunnally and Bernstein (1994) proposed a Cronbach's alpha between 0.70 and 0.90 as a measure of good internal consistency. In our experience, however, many good (subscales of) questionnaires have higher Cronbach's alphas. We give a positive rating for internal consistency if factor analysis has been applied and Cronbach's alpha is between 0.70 and 0.95 (see Section 4.5.2). For reliability, an ICC value of 0.70 is considered acceptable (Nunnally and Bernstein, 1994), but values greater than 0.80 or even greater than 0.90 are much better (see Section 5.6). For an adequate measurement error, the SDC should be smaller than the MIC value (see Section 8.5.5). For construct validity, based on hypotheses testing we arbitrarily decided that 75% of the hypotheses should be confirmed.

Other researchers may have good reasons to differ from our suggestions, but the reasons for applying stricter or more lenient criteria should be explained. Quality criteria for measurement properties were suggested by Terwee *et al.* (2007). These criteria combine standards for the methodological quality of studies with criteria for the adequacy of the study results. Nowadays, we recommend that the COSMIN checklist should be used to assess the methodological quality of studies (as explained in Section 9.6), but the criteria suggested by Terwee *et al.* could be applied to assess the adequacy of the measurement properties. Although these criteria were developed for (multi-item) health status questionnaires, they can also be applied to performance-based tests and other measurement instruments. As the criteria for the adequacy of measurement properties are continuously being improved and refined, we refer to our website www.cosmin.nl for up-to-date criteria.

9.10 Overall conclusions of the systematic review

To draw an overall conclusion about quality of an instrument to measure a specific construct, or to select the *best* measurement instrument for a particular situation, all measurement properties should be considered together.

The number of studies in which the measurement properties of the instrument is investigated, the methodological quality of these studies, and (the consistency of) the results of the studies should be taken into account. Conclusions should be drawn from studies with sufficient homogeneity (i.e. similarities with regard to the construct measured), the purpose of the study and the study population.

It is important that the conclusions of the review are fully transparent and justified. Therefore, reviews should present in detail the methods and criteria used in the data-synthesis process, i.e. how they combined information about the methodological quality and the results of various studies.

Throughout this book, we have emphasized that one cannot talk about *the* quality of a measurement instrument in general, but that this should always be considered within the context of a specific study population and purpose. This should also be made explicit in the systematic review. It should first be expressed in the research question, and then in the inclusion and exclusion criteria. During data extraction it is important to assess the study population characteristics (generalizability) for each measurement property separately, in order to be able to assess the (dis)similarities of the study populations. This eventually has consequences for the data synthesis and conclusions of the review. Thus, a systematic review may conclude that a measurement instrument is (the most) appropriate to measure a construct in one specific population or setting, but make no judgement about its use in other situations. Therefore, the key elements of the research question should be reflected in the review conclusions.

For most reviews performed until now, the conclusion is that there is insufficient evidence on most of the measurement properties. This does not mean that these are poor measurement instruments, it just means that there are no studies or only low-quality studies in which their measurement properties are assessed. Thus, the results of a systematic review also clearly reveal gaps in research. When instrument content seems promising, but its measurement properties are inadequately investigated, the conclusion can be drawn that more and better research on its measurement properties is needed. Note that measurement instruments with low content validity are not worthwhile enough to be examined further. In this way, a systematic review can set the agenda for further research on measurement properties.

9.11 Report on a systematic review of measurement properties

Guidelines for reporting systematic reviews have been published in the PRISMA Statement (available on www.prisma-statement.org). PRISMA stands for Preferred Reporting Items for Systematic Reviews and Meta-Analyses. It is a 27-item checklist, representing a minimum set of items for reporting in systematic reviews and meta-analyses. Although the PRISMA Statement focused on randomized trials, it can also be used as a guideline for reporting systematic reviews of other types of research, such as systematic reviews of measurement properties. In these guidelines, important issues about the title, abstract, introduction, methods, results, discussion and funding of the study are included.

The requirements on reporting of methods have been covered in the preceding sections. This section focuses on data presentation and, in particular, gives examples of tables that can be presented in the results section of a systematic review article. A systematic review of measurement properties should, at least, give information about the following issues: (1) results of the literature search and selection of the studies; (2) methodological quality of the included studies; (3) characteristics of the included measurement instruments; (4) characteristics of the included study populations; (5). adequacy/results of the measurement properties; and (6) the conclusion about the best measurement instrument. On each of these issues we will remark briefly, give an example or refer to the corresponding section in this chapter. For more examples we refer again to www.cosmin.nl.

1: Results of the literature search and selection of the studies
The results of the literature search and selection of the studies can best be summarized in a flow chart as presented in Figure 9.1. The PRISMA Statement also includes an example of such a flow chart. Note that in a systematic review on measurement properties the number of studies that provides relevant information may vary per measurement property. However, instead of drawing a flow chart for each measurement property, usually the flow chart includes all studies providing any information on one or more measurement properties.

2: The methodological quality of each study
The methodological quality of each study should be presented per measurement property. As an example, we present a table about questionnaires to measure neck pain and disability (own data).

Table 9.7 Methodological quality per measurement property for each study evaluating the Neck Disability Index

Study	Internal consistency	Measurement error	Reliability	Content validity	Structural validity	Hypotheses testing	Responsiveness
NDI							
Study 1				poor		poor	
Study 2			poor				poor
Study 3		fair	fair				fair
Study 4		poor	poor				fair
Study 5	poor	poor				poor	poor
Study 6	excellent				good	good	
Study 7				poor		fair	
Study 8						good	poor
Study 9							fair
Study 10	fair	poor	poor				poor
Study 11	fair				fair	poor	
Study 12	poor		poor	fair		fair	poor
Study 13			poor				good

In Table 9.7 the 13 studies that presented information on the Neck Disability Index (NDI) are shown. The rating of the methodological quality of these studies ranged from excellent, good, moderate to poor. These scores were obtained by using a preliminary (self-developed) scoring system based on the COSMIN checklist (see www.cosmin.nl). For many measurement properties in this study, only fair or poor studies are available. This weakens the ability to draw strong conclusions on the quality of the measurement properties of the NDI.

3: Characteristics of the included measurement instruments

An example of a table with instrument's characteristics, derived from a review by Bot *et al.* (2004b) on shoulder disability questionnaires, is presented in Table 9.8. Note that the target population refers to the population for which the measurement is developed, while the study population refers to the population in which the measurement properties were evaluated. For example, the Disabilities of the Arm, Shoulder, and Hand Scale (DASH) is developed as a generic measure for patients with all kinds of

Table 9.8 Description of characteristics of shoulder disability questionnaires

Questionnaire	Target population	Domains	Number of scales	Number of items	Number of response options	Range of scores	Time to administer (min)
SDQ-UK	Shoulder symptoms	Physical, emotional, social	1	22	2	0–22	?
SIQ	Shoulder instability	Pain symptoms, physical, emotional	1	12	5	12–60	?
OSQ	Shoulder operation	Pain, physical	1	12	5	12–60	?
SDQ-NL	Soft tissue, shoulder disorders	Pain, physical, emotional	1	16	3	0–100	5–10
RC-QOL	Rotator cuff disease	Pain symptoms, physical, emotional, social	1	34	VAS	0–100	?
DASH	Upper extremity	Pain symptoms, physical, emotional, social	1	30	5	0–100	<5

Adapted from Bot *et al.* (2004b), with permission.
SDQ-UK, Shoulder Disability Questionnaire UK version; SIQ, Shoulder Instability Questionnaire; OSQ, (Oxford) Shoulder Questionnaire; SDQ-NL, Shoulder Disability Questionnaire Dutch version; RC-QOL, Rotator Cuff Quality of Life Measure; DASH, Disabilities of the Arm, Shoulder, and Hand Scale; VAS, visual analogue scale.

upper extremity disorders, but Bot *et al.* (2004b) only selected studies in which the measurement properties of the DASH were examined in patients with shoulder disability, the topic of their review. If different versions of the same instrument are included in the systematic review this should become

Table 9.9 Characteristics of included study populations in the review on health-related quality of life instruments for adults with diabetes

Instrument	Country	n	Mean age (year)	Gender (%male)	Diabetes type/treatment (*n*)	Duration (year)
ADS	USA	200	58.4	100	Insulin (132)	15
ADDQol	UK, Bromley	102	61.6	54	Insulin/diet (38) tablet/diet (33), diet (30)	7.3
	UK, Cambridge	52	52.4	54	Insulin/diet (32) Tablet/diet (14), diet (6)	12.7
	Portugal	100	61.3	46	Type 2 (73), Type 1 (27)	12
D-39	USA	516	52.4	46.5	Type 1 (159), Type 2 (330)	14.2
		165	61.7	44.8	Type 1 (31), Type 2 (128)	11.5
		262	55.3	35.5	Type 1 (25), Type 2 (218)	10.1

Adapted from El Achhab *et al.* (2008), with permission.

ADS, appraisal of diabetes scale; ADDQol, audit of diabetes-dependent quality of life; D-39, diabetes-39.

clear in the table on the instruments' characteristics (see SDQ-UK and SDQ-NL in Table 9.8).

For multi-item instruments a content comparison of the included instruments, as presented in Table 9.6, may sometimes be helpful.

4. Characteristics of the study population

By constructing a table about the characteristics of the study samples, one has to keep in mind that this table should contain all information that is important for the generalizability of the results and to decide about similarities or dissimilarities of study samples for data synthesis. For the readers it should be clear why certain subgroups have been considered in the review. For example, when some studies have included patients with acute shoulder complaints, and other studies patients with chronic complaints, the evidence on the reliability of the instruments might be presented for acute and chronic patients separately.

Table 9.9 presents the study population characteristics in a systematic review on health-related quality of life instruments for patients with diabetes (El Achhab *et al.*, 2008). Important characteristics are the country where the study is performed, sample size of the study, age and gender distribution of the population, type of diabetes and type of treatment and duration of the disease. Using the COSMIN generalizability items as guidance, we can easily see that information is missing on setting, language of the questionnaire (although the country is mentioned), method of patient selection and percentage of missing values. This table shows whether the samples are similar or not, and helps in deciding about the proper way of data synthesis.

5: Results for the measurement properties

In order to provide full information and transparency it is recommended to present the full results separately for the measurement properties found in each study. An example of such a presentation can be found in Marinus *et al.* (2002) who evaluated the reliability, validity and responsiveness of quality-of-life measures for use in patients with Parkinson's disease. They found 21 studies addressing five scales, one of which was the questionnaire called Parkinson LebensQualität (PLQ), a German Parkinson quality of life questionnaire. The results of the studies assessing the measurement properties of the PLQ can be found in Table 9.10.

The tables presenting the results of each measurement property may become huge, especially when there is a large number of studies and, for example, when a large number of hypotheses have been tested to assess construct validity in some studies. Therefore, these overview tables may be presented in an appendix or on a website (see, for example, Bot *et al.*, 2004b who published two appendices on a website). These tables are important to publish for reasons of transparency, because they contain the raw data that are later summarized by the authors in the process of data synthesis. When readers would like to make other choices in the data synthesis process, these tables provide the information to do so.

6: Conclusion about the best measurement instrument

In order to come to a transparent conclusion of the review we recommend presenting an informative overview, listing all measurement instruments and a score for each measurement property. An example is shown in Table 9.11 (own data), presenting the results of a systematic review on the measurement properties of eight neck-specific questionnaires measuring pain or disability in patients with non-specific neck pain.

Table 9.10 Results of measurement properties of health-related quality of life scales for Parkinson's disease

| Scale | Reliability | | Validity | | | |
	Internal consistency	Test–retest	Content	Construct	Factorial	Responsiveness
PLQ	Alpha Total scale: 0.95	Total scale: $r = 0.87$	++	*Generic health-related quality of life scales*: EORTC QLQ 30: $r = 0.67$ ($n = 111$)	9 subscales, 1 or 2 factors/ subscale > 50% variance	2-week interval No external criterion
	Alpha subscales: 0.62–0.87			*Disease-specific measures:*	Depression	($n = 16$)
	Correlation subscale – total scale:	Subscales: $r = 0.69–0.86$		H and Y: $r = 0.27$, NS ($n = 21–29$) SES: $r = -0.27$, NS, ($n = 21–29$)	Physical achievement Leisure	
	$r = 0.73–0.86$ ($n = 405$)	($n = 65$; 14 days)		*Other measures:* Quality of life VAS: $r = 0.28$, NS ($n = 21–29$) ADL scale: $r = 0.73$ ($n = 111$)	Concentration Social integration Insecurity Restlessness Activity limitation Anxiety	

n, number of patients; alpha, Cronbach's alpha; r, Pearson; ++, adequate; PLQ, Parkinson Lëbensqualität; SES, Schwab and England scale; H and Y, Hoehn and Yahr staging; NS, not significant.
Adapted from Marinus *et al.* (2002), with permission.

An overall score for each measurement instrument and each measurement property is presented. In this overall score, the methodological quality of the study and the results of the measurement properties are combined. For example, a score of +++ for internal consistency of the NDI means there

Table 9.11 Quality of measurement properties per questionnaire

Question-naire	Internal consistency	Measurement error	Reliability	Content validity	Structural validity	Hypothesis testing	Respon-siveness
NDI	+++	?	-	+	CE	+++	CE
NPDS	?	NA	?	?	+	+	+
NBQ	?	?	?	NA	NA	+	+
NPQ	?	?	?	?	NA	+	++
WDQ	++	?	?	?	+	?	+
CNFDS	?	NA	?	?	NA	+	+
CNQ	NA	NA	+	?	NA	+	NA
CWOM	?	NA	NA	NA	NA	+	+

+++ or –, strong evidence positive/negative result; ++ or –, moderate evidence positive/negative result; + or –, limited evidence positive/negative result; CE, conflicting evidence; ?, unknown, due to poor methodological quality; NA, no information available.

is consistent evidence from multiple studies of good methodological quality for good internal consistency of this questionnaire. There was conflicting evidence from multiple studies of fair quality for the responsiveness of this questionnaire. Additional studies on responsiveness of the NDI are required. Methods and criteria used in the process of data synthesis (i.e. how information on the methodological quality and results of various studies was combined) should be clearly described.

In some studies, the authors report the outcome for the quality of the studies and for the results of a study, separately. An example of this was provided by Marinus *et al.* (2002). In addition to the raw data on measurement properties, shown in Table 9.10, they gave per measurement instrument, overall ratings of each measurement property combining multiple studies. They gave ratings of the results of each measurement property (i.e. before the slash) and ratings of the methodological quality of these studies (i.e. behind the slash) (Table 9.12). These overall ratings for quality and results are some kind of qualitative summary of the studies. In the article, they refer to certain standards to assess the quality of the studies and criteria to rate the results of the measurement properties for individual studies, but information about how they combined these when more studies examined the same instrument was lacking.

Table 9.12 Quality assessment table

Scale	Internal consistency	Test–retest reliability	Content validity	Construct validity	Responsiveness
PDQ-39	+++/+++	+++/+++	++/+++	+++/+++	++/+
PDQL	+++/+++	0	++/++	+++/+++	0
PIMS	+++/+++	+++/+++	?/–	?/–	0
PLQ	+++/+++	+++/+++	++/+++	+/++	–/–

+++/+++: signs before the slash refer to results of validity, reliability and responsiveness testing and signs behind the slash refer to thoroughness (strength of evidence) of validity, reliability and responsiveness testing.
Results of validity, reliability and responsiveness testing: 0, no numerical results reported; ?, results not interpretable; –, poor results; + fair results; ++, moderate results; +++, good results.
Thoroughness of validity, reliability and responsiveness testing: 0, no reported evidence; ?, results not interpretable; –, poor evidence; +, fair evidence; ++, moderate evidence; +++, good evidence.
Marinus *et al.* (2002), with permission.

In order to grade the evidence on each measurement property the quality of the studies should be integrated with the results of the studies. However, the methodology to do this is not well developed yet. For future developments see www.cosmin.nl.

9.12 State of affairs

On several occasions in this chapter, we have stated that the methodology of systematic reviews on measurement properties is still under development. Nevertheless, as the number of such systematic reviews is increasing rapidly, we wanted to give the reader some guidance on how to perform these reviews. This last section describes the state of affairs and at the same time puts forward the research agenda for the near future.

With the development of the COSMIN checklist (Mokkink *et al.*, 2010b) an instrument to assess the methodological quality of studies on measurement properties has become available. However, a rating system to classify the methodological quality of the studies as excellent, good, fair or poor quality is still in development. Moreover, methods to combine evidence on measurement properties from different studies are not well worked out yet.

It is evident though that these methods may differ per measurement property. More work needs to be done on the methodology of data synthesis for measurement properties, and this holds for statistical pooling as well as for best evidence syntheses.

Lack of good reporting of primary studies is a problem when conducting a systematic review. Poorly reported studies will limit the reader's ability to assess the methodological quality of a study. Therefore, in the fields of RCTs or diagnostic research, reporting guidelines for primary studies are developed, such as the CONSORT statement (Schulz *et al.*, 2010), or the STARD statement (Bossuyt *et al.*, 2003). Reporting guidelines for studies on measurement properties do not exist, yet. However, much information about relevant items can be deduced from the COSMIN checklist. In other words, the COSMIN checklist can be used as a guide when preparing a publication of a study evaluating measurement properties.

9.13 Comprehensiveness of systematic reviews of measurement properties

A systematic review on measurement properties consists of a collection of separate systematic reviews per measurement property. That these are separate reviews becomes visible in the number of studies that contribute data to each measurement property, a separate set of items (COSMIN box) per measurement property to appraise the methodological quality of the studies and separate methods of data synthesis per measurement property. However, to draw conclusions about the choice of the best measurement instrument in a particular situation, the results of multiple measurement properties should be taken into account. Therefore, a systematic review usually contains information on all measurement properties.

To demonstrate the extensiveness of these reviews we compare them with reviews of RCTs. To draw a conclusion about the best intervention for a specific health problem, a systematic review should summarize and combine the evidence on the effectiveness, the costs and on side-effects of all available interventions. However, usually only effectiveness or only side-effects are studied. Moreover, usually only one or two interventions are studied and not all available interventions. So to make a decision on the best intervention, information is needed from different systematic reviews.

In contrast, in systematic reviews of measurement properties all information to decide on the best instrument is provided in one review. However, if much evidence is available it is better to write an informative review on a few measurement instruments, or separate reviews for each measurement property than to write a superficial mega-review that lacks much relevant information.

9.14 Summary

A systematic review of measurement properties aims to find all evidence on the measurement properties of one or more measurement instruments, to evaluate this evidence and to come to a conclusion about the quality of each measurement instrument. When the aim is to select the best instrument available for a particular purpose, all instruments and all measurement properties should be included in the review. In a review on measurement properties the content of the instruments is described, the methodological quality of the studies on measurement properties are critically appraised and reported, and the results on the measurement properties are summarized. The research question of the review contains as key elements the construct and target population of interest, type of measurement instrument, and measurement properties on which the review focuses.

In order to identify all relevant articles a number of databases should be used, including MEDLINE and EMBASE, and the search terms should include all synonyms for the construct of interest and the target population. A sensitive methodological search filter to identify studies on measurement properties in MEDLINE through PubMed is available. Based on the abstracts or full articles of the retrieved references, relevant articles are selected by applying strictly formulated inclusion and exclusion criteria, by two reviewers independently of each other. This process of searching and section should be documented in a flow chart.

The next step is the appraisal of the methodological quality of studies evaluating measurement properties, for which the COSMIN checklist can be used. This checklist contains items to appraise the methodological quality of the assessment of each measurement property, items to consider the generalizability and items to appraise the quality of IRT methods when they are used.

Data extraction includes characteristics of the instruments, characteristics of the study populations, and results of the measurement properties. Characteristics of the study populations are important to consider the generalizability of the results and later on, to judge the (dis)similarities of the study populations included in the review. In case of multi-item instruments, characteristics of the instrument may be supplemented by a content comparison.

Before data synthesis, first the homogeneity of the study characteristics should be considered. Only results of similar study populations should be combined. This can be done by statistical pooling or by a best evidence synthesis. For both strategies, methods are still under development. The adequacy of the measurement properties should be considered for the combined set of studies. Sometimes evidence for the results of one measurement property is found in different studies (e.g. some studies evaluate the data structure of the instrument, while others provide data on the internal consistency of the (sub)scales).

To draw an overall conclusion on the quality of a measurement instrument to measure a specific construct or to select the *best* measurement instrument for a particular situation, the number of studies in which the measurement properties of the instrument is investigated, the methodological quality of these studies on measurement properties, and consistency of the results of those studies should be taken into account.

Conclusions should be drawn over studies with sufficient homogeneity (i.e. similarities with regard to construct measured, purpose and study population). When insufficient data are available to draw conclusions about the measurement instruments, the review often provides guidance for further research. The key elements of the research question should be reflected in the review conclusions.

Reports of systematic reviews of measurement properties should include: (1) results of the literature search and selection of the studies; (2) methodological quality of the included studies; (3) characteristics of the included measurement instruments; (4) characteristics of the included study populations; (5) raw data on the measurement properties; (6) results of the data synthesis; and (7) conclusion about the best measurement instrument. Extensive tables can be placed in appendices or on a website.

Assignments

1. Evaluate the methodological quality of a study with the COSMIN checklist

At www.clinimetrics.nl you find a link to the open access paper of Van den Bergh *et al.* (2009).

Read the article and rate the methodological quality of the study, using the COSMIN checklist. For instructions to complete the COSMIN checklist we refer to the COSMIN manual to be found at www.cosmin.nl.

2. Data synthesis of eight studies on the reliability of one instrument

This exercise might be good to perform with two people or in a small group to have some discussion.

The Quebec Back Pain Disability Scale (QBPDS) is a self-report questionnaire that aims to measure disability in patients with non-specific low back pain, developed by Kopec *et al.* (1996). Disability was defined as: 'any restriction or lack of ability to perform an activity in a manner or within the range considered normal for a human being'. The QBPDS consists of 20 items, regarding difficulty experienced while performing simple tasks in six domains (bed/rest, sitting/standing, ambulation, movement, bending/stooping, handling large/heavy objects). The items are scored from 0 to 5, and summarized in one total score. A full copy of the questionnaire can be found on our website www.clinimetrics.nl.

Eight studies have been published on the reliability of the QBPDS total score in different patient populations and countries. We have summarized the characteristics of the studies and study populations, the methodological quality of the studies, and results of the studies in a number of tables. Go to the website www.clinimetrics.nl to download and read the document 'Tables for Assignment 2 Chapter 9.pdf'. You don't need to read the articles for this assignment, but you can find the references on the website.

Read Table 9.13 (www.clinimetrics.nl). In this table the characteristics of the eight included studies are described in terms of study population, duration of complaints, age and gender, country and setting in which the study was performed.

(a) What are the main important differences between the studies and which studies do you consider sufficiently similar to be synthesized?

The methodological quality of each study was assessed using box B (reliability) of the COSMIN checklist. For this study, we used a special version of the COSMIN checklist, with a four-point rating scale, which is described in Table 9.14 (www.clinimetrics.nl). Each item was scored as excellent, good, fair or poor. This four-point rating system allows to determine a total quality score per box. The quality score is obtained by taking the lowest rating of any item in the box. Thus, if one item is scored 'poor', the quality rating of the study will be 'poor', regardless of the ratings of other items.

Read Table 9.15 (www.clinimetrics.nl). In this table, you will find the scores for each COSMIN item on the four-point rating scale. A description is provided in addition to the scores. Moreover, for each study a total quality score is provided.

(b) How would you deal with differences in the methodological quality of the studies in your data synthesis?

Read Table 9.16 (www.clinimetrics.nl). In this table, the results of the eight studies are presented with values for the ICCs that were found.

(c) Do you consider the results of the measurement properties consistent or not?

Read Table 9.17 (www.clinimetrics.nl). In this table you will find a description of levels of evidence that can be applied to combine the results of different studies.

(d) Which level of evidence would you apply to the results of these eight studies?

(e) What would be your overall conclusion about the reliability of the QBPDS?

References

Aaronson, N. K., Muller, M., Cohen, P. D., *et al.* (1998). Translation, validation, and norming of the Dutch language version of the SF-36 Health Survey in community and chronic disease populations. *Journal of Clinical Epidemiology*, **51**, 1055–68.

Albers, G., Echteld, M. A., De Vet, H. C., *et al.* (2010). Evaluation of quality-of-life measures for use in palliative care: a systematic review. *Palliative Medicine*, **24**, 17–37.

Andrich, D. (1978). A rating formulation for ordered response categories. *British Journal of Mathematical and Statistical Psychology*, **26**, 31–44.

Apgar V. (1953). A proposal for a new method of evaluation of newborn infants. *Anesthesia and Analgesia*, **32**, 260–7.

Ashcroft, D. M., Wan Po, A. L., Williams, H. C. and Griffiths, C. E. (1999). Clinical measures of disease severity and outcome in psoriasis: a critical appraisal of their quality. *British Journal of Dermatology*, **141**, 185–91.

Atkinson, M. J. and Lennox, R. D. (2006). Extending basic principles of measurement models to the design and validation of Patient Reported Outcomes. *Health and Quality of Life Outcomes*, **4**, 65.

Avina-Zubieta, J. A., Alarcon, G. S., Bischoff-Ferrari, H. A., *et al.* (2007). Measurement of fatigue in systemic lupus erythematosus: a systematic review. *Arthritis Care Research*, **57**, 1348–57.

Barclay-Goddard, R., Epstein, J. D. and Mayo, N. E. (2009). Response shift: a brief overview and proposed research priorities. *Quality of Life Research*, **18**, 335–46.

Baron, G., Tubach, F., Ravaud, P., Logeart, I. and Dougados, M. (2007). Validation of a Short Form of the Western Ontario and McMaster Universities Osteoarthritis Index function subscale in hip and knee osteoarthritis. *Arthritis and Rheumatism*, **57**, 633–8.

Beaton, D. E., Bombardier, C., Guillemin, F. and Bosi-Ferraz, M. (2000). Guidelines for the process of cross-cultural adaptation of self-report measures. *Spine*, **25**, 3186–91.

Bennett, C. M. and Miller, M. B. (2010). How reliable are the results from functional magnetic resonance imaging. *Annals of the New York Academy of Sciences*, **1191**, 133–55.

Berry, C., Kennedy, P. and Hindson, L. M. (2004). Internal consistency and responsiveness of the Skin Management Needs Assessment Checklist post-spinal cord injury. *Journal of Spinal Cord Medicine*, **27**, 63–71.

Bland, J. M. and Altman, D. G. (1986). Statistical methods for assessing agreement between two methods of clinical measurement. *Lancet*, **i**, 307–10.

Bland, J. M. and Altman, D. G. (1999). Measuring agreement in methods comparison studies. *Statistical Methods in Medical Research*, **8**, 135–60.

Bloem, E. F., Van Zuuren, F. J., Koeneman, M. A., *et al.* (2008). Clarifying quality of life assessment: do theoretical models capture the underlying cognitive processes? *Quality of Life Research*, **17**, 1093–102.

Bollen K. and Lennox R. (1991). Conventional wisdom on measurement: a structural equation perspective. *Psychological Bulletin*, **110**, 305–14.

Bolton J. E. and Humphreys B. K. (2002). The Bournemouth Questionnaire: a short form comprehensive outcome measure. II. Psychometric properties in neck pain patients. *Journal of Manipulative and Physiological Therapeutics*, **25**, 141–8.

Borsboom, D., Mellenbergh, G. J. and van Heerden, J. (2004). The concept of validity. *Psychological Review*, **111**, 1061–71.

Bossuyt, P. M., Reitsma, J. B., Bruns, D. E., *et al.* (2003). Towards complete and accurate reporting of studies of diagnostic accuracy: The STARD Initiative. *Annals of Internal Medicine*, **138**, 40–4.

Bot, S. D., Terwee, C. B., Van der Windt, D. A. W. M., *et al.* (2004a). Internal consistency and validity of a new physical workload questionnaire. *Occupational and Environmental Medicine*, **61**, 980–6.

Bot, S. D., Terwee, C. B., Van der Windt, D. A., *et al.* (2004b). Clinimetric evaluation of shoulder disability questionnaires: a systematic review of the literature. *Annals of Rheumatic Diseases*, **63**, 335–41.

Bradburn, N., Sudman, S. and Wansink, B. (2004). *Asking Questions: the definitive guide to questionnaire design – for market research, political polls, and social and health questionnaires*. Revised edition. San Francisco: Jossey-Bass, A Wiley Imprint.

Brearley, S. G., Clements, C. V. and Molassiotis, A. (2008). A review of patient self-report tools for chemotherapy-induced nausea and vomiting. *Supportive Care in Cancer*, **16**, 1213–29.

Brouwer, C. N. M., Schilder, A. G. M., Van Stel, H. F., *et al.* (2007). Reliability and validity of functional health status and health related quality of life questionnaires in children with recurrent acute otitis media. *Quality of Life Research*, **16**, 1357–73.

Browne, J. R., Boyle, C. A., McGee, H. M., McDonald, N. J. and Joyce, C. R. B. (1997). Development of a direct weighing procedure for quality of life domains. *Quality of Life Research*, **6**, 301–9.

Bruynesteyn, K., Van der Heijde, D., Boers, M., *et al.* (2002). Determination of the minimal clinical important difference in rheumatoid arthritis joint damage of the Sharp/Van der Heijde and Larsen/Scott scoring methods by clinical experts and comparison with the smallest detectable difference. *Arthritis and Rheumatism*, **46**, 913–20.

Campbell, D. T. and Fiske, D. W. (1959). Convergent and discriminant validation by the multitrait-multimethod matrix. *Psychological Bulletin*, **56**, 81–105.

Cella, D., Eton, D. T., Lai, J. S., Peterman, A. H. and Merkel. D. E. (2002). Combining anchor-based and distribution-based methods to derive minimal clinically important differences on the Functional Assessment of Cancer Therapy (FACT) Anemia and Fatigue scales. *Journal of Pain and Symptom Management*, **24**, 547–61.

Cella, D., Gershon, R., Lai, J. S. and Choi, S. (2007). The future of outcome measurement: item banking, tailored short-forms, and computerized adaptive testing. *Quality of Life Research*, **16** (Suppl 1), 133–41.

Chobanian, A. V., Bakris, G. L., Black, H. R., *et al.* and the National High Blood Pressure Education Program Coordinating Committee. (2003). Seventh report of the joint national committee on prevention, detection, evaluation, and treatment of high blood pressure. *Hypertension*, **42**, 1206–52.

Cieza, A and Stucki, G. (2005). Content comparison of health related quality of life (HRQOL) instruments based on the international classification of functioning, disability and health (ICF). *Quality of Life Research*, **14**, 1225–37.

Cohen, J. (1960). A coefficient of agreement for nominal scales. *Educational and Psychological Measurement*, **20**, 37–46.

Cohen, J. (1968). Weighted kappa: nominal scale agreement with provision for scaled disagreement or partial credit. *Psychological Bulletin*, **70**, 213–30.

Cohen, J. (1977). *Statistical Power Analysis for the Behavioural Sciences*. New York: Academic Press.

Collins, D. (2003). Pretesting survey instruments: an overview of cognitive methods. *Quality of Life Research*, **12**, 229–38.

Cortina, J. M. (1993). What is coefficient α? An examination of theory and applications. *Journal of Applied Psychology*, **78**, 98–104.

Crocker, L. and Algina, J. (1986). *Introduction to Classical and Modern Test Theory*. Belmont, CA: Wadsworth.

Cronbach, L. J. and Meehl, P. E. (1955). Construct validity in psychological tests. *Psychological Bulletin*, **52**, 281–302.

Crosby, R. D., Kolotkin, R. L. and Williams, G. R. (2003). Defining clinically meaningful change in health-related quality of life. *Journal of Clinical Epidemiology*, **56**, 395–407.

De Boer, M. R., Moll, A. C., De Vet, H. C., *et al.* (2004). Psychometric properties of vision-related quality of life questionnaires: a systematic review. *Ophthalmic and Physiological Optics*, **24**, 257–73.

De Boer, M. R., Terwee, C. B., De Vet, H. C. W., *et al.* (2006). Evaluation of cross-sectional and longitudinal construct validity of two vision-related quality of life questionnaires: the LVQOL and VCM1. *Quality of Life Research*, **15**, 233–48.

De Groot, V., Beckerman, H., Lankhorst, G. J. and Bouter, L. M. (2003). How to measure comorbidity: a critical review of available methods. *Journal of Clinical Epidemiology*, **56**, 221–9.

Dempster, M., Carney, R. and McClements, R. (2010). Response shift in the assessment of quality of life among people attending cardiac rehabilitation. *British Journal of Psychology*, **15**, 307–19.

DeVellis, R. F. (2006). Classical test theory. *Medical Care*, **44** (Suppl), 50–9.

De Vet, H. C. W. and Terwee, C. B. (2010). The minimal detectable change should not replace the minimal important difference. *Journal of Clinical Epidemiology*, **63**, 804–5.

De Vet, H. C. W., Knipschild, P. G., Schouten, H. J. A., *et al.* (1992). Sources of interobserver variation in histopathological grading of cervical dysplasia. *Journal of Clinical Epidemiology*, **45**, 785–90.

De Vet, H. C. W., Adèr, H. J., Terwee, C. B. and Pouwer, F. (2005). Are factor analytical techniques used appropriately in the validation of health status questionnaires? A systematic review on the quality of factor analysis of the SF-36. *Quality of Life Research*, **14**, 1203–18.

De Vet, H. C. W., Terwee, C. B., Knol, D. L. and Bouter, L. M. (2006). When to use agreement versus reliability measures. *Journal of Clinical Epidemiology*, **59**, 1033–9.

De Vet, H. C. W., Ostelo, R. W., Terwee, C. B., *et al.* (2007). Minimal important change determined by a visual method integrating an anchor-based and a distribution-based approach. *Quality of Life Research*, **16**, 131–42.

De Vet, H. C. W., Terluin, B., Knol, D. L., *et al.* (2010). Three ways to quantify uncertainty in individually applied 'minimally important change' values. *Journal of Clinical Epidemiology*, **63**, 37–45.

De Winter, A. F., Heemskerk, M. A., Terwee, C. B., *et al.* (2004). Inter-observer reproducibility of measurements of range of motion in patients with shoulder pain using a digital inclinometer. *Biomed Central Musculoskeletal Disorders*, **5**, 18.

Deyo, R. A. and Centor, R. M. (1986). Assessing the responsiveness of functional scales to clinical change: An analogy to diagnostic test performance. *Journal of Chronic Diseases*, **39**, 897–906.

Drummond, M. F., Sculpher, M. J., Torrance, G. W., O' Brien, B. J. and Stoddart, G. L. (2005). *Methods for the Economic Evaluation of Health Care Programmes*. 3rd edition. Oxford: Oxford University Press.

DuBeau, C. E., Levy, B., Mangione, C. M. and Resnick, N. M. (1998). The impact of urge incontinence of quality of life: importance of patients' perspective and explanatory style. *Journal of the American Geriatrics Society*, **46**, 683–92.

Edwards J. R. and Bagozzi R. P. (2000). On the nature and direction of relationships between constructs and measures. *Psychological Reviews*, **5**, 155–74.

Eid, M., Nussbeck, F. W., Geiser, C., Cole, D. A., Gollwitzer, M. and Lischetzke, T. (2008). Structural equation modeling of multitrait-multimethod data: different models for different types of methods. *Psychological Methods*, **13**, 230–53.

El Achhab, Y., Nejjari, C., Chikri, M. and Lyoussi, B. (2008). Disease-specific health-related quality of life instruments among adults diabetic: a systematic review. *Diabetes Research and Clinical Practice*, **80**, 171–84.

Embretson, S. E. and Reise, S. P. (2000). *Item Response Theory for Psychologists*. London: Lawrence Erlbaum.

Euser, A. M., Dekker, F. W. and Le Cessie, S. (2008). A practical approach to Bland-Altman plots and variation coefficients for log transformed variables. *Journal of Clinical Epidemiology*, **61**, 978–82.

Fayers, P. M. and Hand, D. J. (1997). Factor analysis, causal indicators, and quality of life. *Quality of Life Research*, **6**, 139–50.

Fayers, P. M. and Machin, D. (2007). *Quality of Life. The assessment, analysis and interpretation of patient-reported outcomes*. 2nd edition. Chicester, UK: Wiley.

Fayers, P. M., Hand, D. J., Bjordal K. and Groenvold M. (1997). Causal indicators in quality of life research. *Quality of Life Research*, **6**, 393–406.

Fayers, P. M., Langston, A. L., Robertson, C. and the PRISM Trial Group. (2007). Implicit self-comparisons against others could bias quality of life assessments. *Journal of Clinical Epidemiology*, **60**, 1034–9.

FDA Guidance for Industry. (2009). *Patient-reported Outcome Measures: Use in medical product development to support labelling claims.* Silver Spring, USA: US Department of Health and Human Services, Food and Drug Administration.

Feinstein, A. R. (1987). *Clinimetrics.* New Haven, MA: Yale University Press.

Fleiss, J. L. (1981). *Statistical Methods for Rates and Proportions.* 2nd edition. New York: Wiley.

Fleiss, J. L. and Cohen, J. (1973). The equivalence of weighted kappa and the intraclass correlation coefficient as measures of reliability. *Educational and Psychological Measurement*, **33**, 613–9.

Fletcher, R. H. and Fletcher, S. W. (2005). *Clinical Epidemiology: the essentials.* Baltimore, MD: Lippincott, Williams and Wilkins.

Floyd, F. J. and Widaman, K. F. (1995). Factor analysis in the development and refinement of clinical assessment instruments. *Psychological Assessment*, **7**, 286–99.

Garin, O., Ferrer, M., Pont, A., *et al.* (2009). Disease-specific health-related quality of life questionnaires for heart failure: a systematic review with meta-analyses. *Quality of Life Research*, **18**, 71–85.

Gerritsen, D. L., Steverink, N., Ooms, M. E. and Ribbe, M. W. (2004). Finding a useful conceptual basis for enhancing the quality of life of nursing home residents. *Quality of Life Research*, **13**, 611–24.

Giraudeau, B. and Mary, J. Y. (2001). Planning a reproducibility study: how many subjects and how many replicates per subject for an expected width of the 95 per cent confidence interval of the intraclass correlation coefficient. *Statistics in Medicine*, **20**, 3205–14.

Gregorich, S. E. (2006). Do self-report instruments allow meaningful comparisons across diverse population groups? Testing measurement invariance using the confirmatory factor analysis framework. *Medical Care*, **44** (Suppl), 78–94.

Guyatt, G., Walter, S. and Norman, G. (1987). Measuring change over time: Assessing the usefulness of evaluative instruments. *Journal of Chronic Diseases*, **40**, 171–8.

Guyatt, G. H., Kirshner, B. and Jaeschkle, R. (1992). Measuring health status: what are the necessary properties? *Journal of Clinical Epidemiology*, **12**, 1341–5.

Guyatt, G. H., Norman, G. R., Juniper, E. F. and Griffith, L. E. (2002). A critical look at transition ratings. *Journal of Clinical Epidemiology*, **55**, 900–8.

Hahn, E. A., Cella D., Chassany, O., *et al.* and the Clinical Significance Consensus Meeting Group. (2007). Precision of Health-Related Quality of Life data compared with other clinical measures. *Mayo Clinics Proceedings*, **82**, 1244–54.

Haley, S. M. McHorney, C. A. and Ware, J. E. (1994). Evaluation of the MOS SF-36 Physical Functioning scale (PF-10): I. Dimensionality and reproducibility of the Rasch Item Scale. *Journal of Clinical Epidemiology*, **47**, 671–84.

Hawthorne, G., Osborne, R. H., Taylor, A. and Sansoni, J. (2007). The SF36 Version 2: critical analyses of population weights, scoring algorithms and population norms. *Quality of Life Research*, **16**, 661–73.

Hays, R. D., Morales, L. S. and Reise, S. P. (2000). Item response theory and health outcomes measurement in the 21st century. *Medical Care*, **38** (Suppl), II28–II42.

Hendriks, E. J. M., Bernards, A. T. M., De Bie, R. A. and De Vet, H. C. W. (2008). The minimal clinical important change of the PRAFAB-questionnaire in women with stress urinary incontinence: results from a prospective cohort study. *Neurourology and Urodynamics*, **27**, 379–87.

Hildebrandt, V. H., Bongers, P. M., Van Dijk, F., Kemper, H. C. and Dul, J. (2001). Dutch Musculoskeletal Questionnaire: description and basic qualities. *Ergonomics*, **44**, 1038–55.

Hoopman, R., Terwee, C. B., Muller, M. J. and Aaronson, N. K. (2006). Translation and validation of the SF-36 Health Survey for use among Turkish and Moroccan ethnic minority cancer patients in The Netherlands. *European Journal of Cancer*, **42**, 2982–90.

Hoopman, R., Terwee, C. B. and Aaronson, N. K. (2008). Translated COOP/WONCA charts found appropriate for use among Turkish and Moroccan ethnic minority cancer patients. *Journal of Clinical Epidemiology*, **61**, 1036–48.

Hoving, J. L., Koes, B. W., De Vet, H. C., *et al.* (2002). Manual therapy, physical therapy, or continued care by a general practitioner for patients with neck pain. A randomized, controlled trial. *Annals of Internal Medicine*, **136**, 713–22.

Hu, L. and Bentler, P. M. (1999). Cutoff criteria for fit indexes in covariance structure analysis: conventional criteria versus new alternatives. *Structural Equation Modelling*, **6**, 1–55.

Hustvedt, B. E., Svendsen, M., Løvø, A., *et al.* (2008). Validation of ActiReg® to measure physical activity and energy expenditure against doubly labelled water in obese persons. *British Journal of Nutrition*, **100**, 219–26.

Jacobson, N. S. and Truax, P. (1991). Clinical significance: a statistical approach to defining meaningful change in psychotherapy research. *Journal of Consulting and Clinical Psychology*, **59**, 12–9.

Jansen, S. J. T., Stiggelbout, A. M., Nooij, M. A., Noordijk, E. M. and Kievit, J. (2000). Response shift in quality of life measurement in early-stage breast cancer patients undergoing radiotherapy. *Quality of Life Research*, **9**, 603–15.

Johansson, C., Bodin, P. and Kreuter, M. (2009). Validity and responsiveness of the spinal cord index of function: an instrument on activity level. *Spinal Cord*, **47**, 817–21.

Juniper, E. F., Guyatt, G. H., Epstein, R. S., *et al.* (1992). Evaluation of impairment of health related quality of life in asthma: development of a questionnaire for use in clinical trials. *Thorax*, **47**, 76–83.

Juniper, E. F., Guyatt, G. H., Streiner, D. L. and King, D. R. (1997). Clinical impact versus factor analysis for quality of life questionnaire construction. *Journal of Clinical Epidemiology*, **50**, 233–8.

Kline P. (2000). *Handbook of Psychological Testing*. 2nd edition. London: Routledge.

Kopec, J. A., Esdaile, J. M., Abrahamowicz, M., *et al.* (1996). The Quebec back pain disability scale: Conceptualization and development. *Journal of Clinical Epidemiology*, **49**, 151–61.

Kosinski, M., Zhao, S. Z., Dedhiya, S., Osterhaus, J. T. and Ware, J. E., Jr. (2000). Determining minimally important changes in generic and disease-specific health-related quality of life questionnaires in clinical trials of rheumatoid arthritis. *Arthritis and Rheumatism*, **43**, 1478–87.

Krueger, R. A. (2000). *Focus Groups: A practical guide for applied research*. 3rd edition. Thousand Oaks, CA: Sage.

Landis, J. R. and Koch, G. C. (1977). The measurement of observer agreement for categorical data. *Biometrics*, **33**, 159–74.

Lehman, C. D., Gatsonis, C., Kuhl, C. K., *et al.*; ACRIN Trial 6667 Investigators Group. (2007). MRI evaluation of the contralateral breast in women with recently diagnosed breast cancer. *New England Journal of Medicine*, **356**, 1295–303.

Leung, A. S., Chan, K. K., Sykes, K. and Chan, K. S. (2006). Reliability, validity, and responsiveness of a 2-min walk test to assess exercise capacity of COPD patients. *Chest*, **130**, 119–25.

Lin J. S., Brimmer, D. J., Maloney, E. M., Nyarko, E., BeLue, R. and Reeves, W. C. (2009). Further validation of the multidimensional fatigue inventory in a US adult population sample. *Population Health Metrics*, **7**, 18.

Logghe I. H., Zeeuwe P. E., Verhagen A. P., *et al.* (2009). Lack of effect of Tai Chi Chuan in fall prevention in elderly people, living at home: a randomized clinical trial. *Journal of the American Geriatric Society*, **57**, 70–5.

Lord F. M. and Novick M. R. (1968). *Statistical Theory of Mental Test Scores*. Reading, MA: Addison-Wesley.

Marinus, J., Ramaker, C., Van Hilten, J. J. and Stiggelbout, A. M. (2002). Health related quality of life in Parkinson's disease: a systematic review of disease specific instruments. *Journal of Neurology, Neurosurgery, and Psychiatry*, **72**, 241–8.

Mazaheri, M., Salavati, M., Negahban, H., *et al.* (2010). Reliability and validity of the Persian version of Foot and Ankle Ability Measure (FAAM) to measure functional limitations in patients with foot and ankle disorders. *Osteoarthritis Cartilage*, **18**, 755–9.

McConnell, S., Kolopack, P. and Davis, A. M. (2001). The Western Ontario and McMaster Universities Osteoarthritis Index (WOMAC): a review of its utility and measurement properties. *Arthritis and Rheumatism*, **45**, 453–61.

McGraw, K. O. and Wong, S. P. (1996). Forming inferences about some intraclass correlation coefficients. *Psychological Methods*, **1**, 30–46.

McHorney, C. A. and Tarlov, A. R. (1995). Individual-patient monitoring in clinical practice: are available health status surveys adequate? *Quality of Life Research*, **4**, 293–307.

McHorney, C. A., Haley, S. M. and Ware, J. E. (1997). Evaluation of the MOS SF-36 Physical Functioning scale (PF-10): II Comparison of relative precision using Likert and Rasch scoring methods. *Journal of Clinical Epidemiology*, **50**, 451–61.

Miller, G. A. (1956). The magic number seven plus or minus two: some limits on our capacity for processing information. *Psychological Review*, **63**, 81–97.

Mokkink, L. B., Knol, D. L., Zekveld, A. A., Goverts, S. T. and Kramer, S. E. (2009). Factor structure and reliability of the Dutch version of seven scales of the Communication Profile for the Hearing Impaired (CPHI). *Journal of Speech Language and Hearing Research*, **52**, 454–64.

Mokkink, L. B., Terwee, C. B., Patrick, D. L., *et al.* (2010a). International consensus on taxonomy, terminology, and definitions of measurement properties for health-related patient-reported outcomes: results of the COSMIN study. *Journal of Clinical Epidemiology*, **63**, 737–45.

Mokkink, L. B., Terwee, C. B., Patrick, D. L., *et al.* (2010b). The COSMIN checklist for assessing the methodological quality of studies on measurement properties of health status measurement instruments: an international Delphi study. *Quality of Life Research*, **19**, 539–49.

Morgan, D. L. (1998). *The Focus Group Guidebook*. Thousand Oaks, CA: Sage.

Morris, C., Doll, H., Dabies, N., *et al.* (2009). The Oxford Ankle Foot Questionnaire for children: responsiveness and longitudinal validity. *Quality of Life Research*, **18**, 1367–76.

Nelson, E., Wasson, J., Kirk, J., *et al.* (1987). Assessment of function in routine clinical practice: description of the COOP Chart method and preliminary findings. *Journal of Chronic Diseases*, **40** (Suppl 1), 55–69.

Norman, G. R., Stratford, P. and Regehr, G. (1997). Methodological problems in the retrospective computation of responsiveness to change: The lesson of Cronbach. *Journal of Clinical Epidemiology*, **50**, 869–79.

Norman, G. R., Sloan, J. A. and Wyrwich, K. W. (2003). Interpretation of changes in health-related quality of life: the remarkable universality of half a standard deviation. *Medical Care*, **41**, 582–92.

Nunnally J. C. (1978). *Psychometric Theory*. 2nd edition. New York: McGraw-Hill.

Nunnally, J. C. and Bernstein, I. H. (1994). *Psychometric Theory*. 3rd edition. New York: McGraw-Hill.

Olson, L. K., Tan, Y., Zhao, Y., Aupperlee, M. D. and Haslam, S. Z. (2010). Pubertal exposure to high fat diet causes mouse strain-dependent alterations in mammary gland development and estrogen responsiveness. *International Journal of Obesity*, **34**, 1415–26.

Oort, F. J. (2005). Using structural equation modeling to detect response shifts and true changes. *Quality of Life Research*, **14**, 587–98.

Oort, F. J., Visser, M. R. M. and Sprangers, M. A. G. (2005). An application of structural equation modeling to detect response shifts and true change in quality of life data from cancer patients undergoing invasive surgery. *Quality of Life Research*, **14**, 599–609.

Patrick, D. L., Deyo, R. A., Atlas, S. J., *et al.* (1995). Assessing health related quality of life in patients with sciatica. *Spine*, **20**, 1899–908.

Patrick, D. L., Burke, L. B., Powers, J. H., *et al.* (2007). Patient reported outcomes to support medical product labeling claims: FDA Perspective. *Value and Health*, **10** (Suppl 2), 125–37.

Petersen, M. A., Groenvold, M., Bjorner, J. B., *et al.* for the European Organisation for Research and Treatment of Cancer Quality of Life Group. (2003). Use of differential item functioning to assess the equivalence of translations of a questionnaire. *Quality of Life Research*, **12**, 373–85.

Pool, J. J., Hiralal, S., Ostelo, R. W., *et al.* (2009). The applicability of the Tampa Scale of Kinesiophobia for patients with sub-acute neck pain: a qualitative study. *Quality and Quantity*, **43**, 773–80.

Rapkin, B. D. and Schwartz, C. E. (2004). Towards a theoretical model of quality-of-life appraisal: implications of findings from studies of response shift. *Health and Quality of Life Outcomes*, **2**, 14.

Revicki, D., Hays, R. D., Cella, D. and Sloan, J. (2008). Recommended methods for determining responsiveness and minimally important differences for patient-reported outcomes. *Journal of Clinical Epidemiology*, **61**, 102–9.

Roland, M. and Morris, R. (1983). A study of the natural history of back pain. I: Development of a reliable and sensitive measure of disability in low back pain. *Spine*, **8**, 141–4.

Romagnoli, E., Burzotta, F., Trani, C., *et al.* (2009). EuroSCORE as predictor of in-hospital mortality after percutaneous coronary intervention. *Heart*, **95**, 43–8.

Ronner, H. E., Ponten, S. C., Stam C. J. and Uitdehaag, B. M. J. (2009). Inter-observer variability of the EEG diagnosis of seizures in comatose patients. *Seizure*, **18**, 257–63.

Roorda, L. D., Jones, C. A., Waltz, M., *et al.* (2004). Satisfactory cross cultural equivalence of the Dutch WOMAC in patients with hip osteoarthritis waiting for arthroplasty. *Annals of Rheumatic Diseases*, **63**, 36–42.

Rose, M., Bjorner, J. B., Becker, J., Fries, J. F. and Ware, J. E. (2008). Evaluation of a preliminary physical function item bank supported the expected advantages of the Patient-Reported Outcomes Measurement Information System (PROMIS). *Journal of Clinical Epidemiology*, **61**, 17–33.

Rosner, B., Cook, N. R., Evans, D. R., *et al.* (1987). Reproducibility and predictive values of routine blood pressure measurements in children: comparison with adult values and implications for screening children for elevated blood pressure. *American Journal of Epidemiology*, **126**, 1115–25.

Ryan, M. and Farrar, S. (2000). Using conjoint analysis to elicit preferences for health care. *British Medical Journal*, **320**, 1530–3.

Salaffi, F., Carotti, M., Gasparini, S., Intorcia, M. and Grassi, W. (2009). The health-related quality of life in rheumatoid arthritis, ankylosing spondylitis, and psoriatic arthritis: a comparison with a selected sample of healthy people. *Health and Quality of Life Outcomes*, **7**, 2.

Scheltens, P., Barkhof, F., Valk, J., *et al.* (1992). White matter lesions on magnetic resonance imaging in clinically diagnosed Alzheimer's disease. *Brain*, **115**, 735–48.

Scheltens, P., Barkhof, F., Leys, D., *et al.* (1993). A semi-quantitative scale for the assessment of signal hypersensitivities on magnetic resonance imaging. *Journal of the Neurological Sciences*, **114**, 7–12.

Schulz, K. F., Altman, D. G., Moher, D. and the CONSORT Group. (2010). CONSORT 2010 statement: updated guidelines for reporting parallel group randomized trials. *Annals of Internal Medicine*, **152**, 726–32.

Schwartz, C. E. and Rapkin, B. D. (2004). Reconsidering the psychometrics of quality of life assessment in light of response shift and appraisal. *Health and Quality of Life Outcomes*, **2**, 16.

Schwartz, C. E. and Sprangers, M. A. G. (1999). Methodological approaches for assessing response shift in longitudinal health-related quality-of-life research. *Social Science in Medicine*, **48**, 1531–48.

Scott, N. W., Fayers, P. M., Aaronson, N. K., *et al.* (2009). Differential item functioning (DIF) in the EORTC QLQ-C30: a comparison of baseline, on-treatment and off-treatment data. *Quality of Life Research*, **18**, 381–8.

Shavelson, R. J. and Webb, N. M. (1991). *Generalizability Theory. A primer.* London: Sage.

Shrout, P. E. and Fleiss, J. L. (1979). Intraclass correlations: uses in assessing rater reliability. *Psychological Bulletin*, **86**, 420–8.

Sikkes, S. A., De Lange-De Klerk, E. S., Pijnenburg, Y. A., Scheltens, P. and Uitdehaag, B. M. (2009). A systematic review of Instrumental Activities of Daily Living scales in dementia: room for improvement. *Journal of Neurology, Neurosurgery, and Psychiatry*, **80**, 7–12.

Skrondal, A. and Rabe-Hesketh, S. (2004). *Generalized Latent Variable Modeling.* Boca Raton, FL: Chapman & Hall/CRC.

Sloan, J. A., Aaronson, N., Cappelleri, J. C., Fairclough, D. L. and Varricchio, C., and the Clinical Significance Consensus Meeting Group. (2002). Assessing clinical significance of single items relative to summated scores. *Mayo Clinics Proceedings*, **77**, 479–87.

Sloan, J. A., Cella, D. and Hays, R. D. (2005). Clinical significance of patient-reported questionnaire data: another step toward consensus. *Journal of Clinical Epidemiology*, **58**, 1217–9.

Smets, E. M., Garssen, B., Bonke, B. and De Haes, J. C. (1995). The Multidimensional Fatigue Inventory (MFI) psychometric qualities of an instrument to assess fatigue. *Journal of Psychosomatic Research*, **39**, 315–25.

Solway, S., Brooks, D., Lacasse, Y. and Thomas, S. (2001). A qualitative systematic overview of the measurement properties of functional walk tests used in the cardio-respiratory domain. *Chest*, **119**, 256–70.

Spies-Dorgelo, M. N., Terwee, C. B., Stalman, W. A. and Van der Windt, D. A. (2006). Reproducibility and responsiveness of the Symptom Severity Scale and the hand and finger function subscale of the Dutch arthritis impact measurement scales (Dutch-AIMS2-HFF) in primary care patients with wrist or hand problems. *Health and Quality of Life Outcomes*, **4**, 87.

Sprangers, M. A. G. and Schwartz, C. E. (1999). Integrating response shift into health related quality-of-life research: a theoretical model. *Social Science in Medicine*, **48**, 1507–15.

Steyerberg, E. W. (2009). *Clinical Prediction Models: A practical approach to development, validation, and updating.* New York: Springer.

Strauss, M. E. and Smith, G. T. (2009). Construct validity: advances in theory and methodology. *Annual Reviews in Clinical Psychology*, **5**, 89–113.

Streiner, D. L. (2006). Building a better model: an introduction to structural equation modelling. *Canadian Journal of Psychiatry*, **51**, 317–21.

Streiner, D. L. and Norman, G. R. (2008). *Health Measurement Scales. A practical guide to their development and use.* 4th edition. Oxford: Oxford University Press.

Swinkels, R. A., Bouter, L. M., Oostendorp, R. A., Swinkels-Meewisse, I. J., Dijkstra, P. U. and De Vet, H. C. (2006). Construct validity of instruments measuring impairments in body structures and function in rheumatic disorders: which constructs are selected for validation? A systematic review. *Clinical and Experimental Rheumatology*, **24**, 93–102.

Teresi J. A. (2006). Overview of quantitative measurement methods. Equivalence, invariance, and different item functioning in health applications. *Medical Care*, **44** (Suppl), 39–49.

Terluin, B., Van Marwijk, H. W., Adèr, H. J., et al. (2006). The Four-Dimensional Symptom Questionnaire (4DSQ): a validation study of a multidimensional self-report questionnaire to assess distress, depression, anxiety and somatization. *Biomed Central Psychiatry*, **6**, 34.

Terwee, C. B., Gerding, M. N., Dekker, F. W., Prummel, M. F. and Wiersinga, W. M. (1998). Development of a disease specific quality of life questionnaire for patients with Graves' ophthalmopathy: the GO-QOL. *British Journal of Ophthalmology*, **82**, 773–9.

Terwee, C. B., Dekker, F. W., Wiersinga, W. M., Prummel, M. F. and Bossuyt, P. M. (2003). On assessing responsiveness of health-related quality of life instruments: guidelines for instrument evaluation. *Quality of Life Research*, **12**, 349–62.

Terwee, C. B., Bot, S. D., De Boer, M. R., et al. (2007). Quality criteria were proposed for measurement properties of health status questionnaires. *Journal of Clinical Epidemiology*, **60**, 34–42.

Terwee, C. B., Jansma, E. P., Riphagen, I. I. and De Vet, H. C. W. (2009). Development of a methodological PubMed search filter for finding studies on measurement properties of measurement instruments. *Quality of Life Research*, **18**, 1115–23.

The WHOQOL HIV Group. (2003). Initial steps to developing the World Health Organisation Quality of Life instrument (WHOQOL) module for international assessment of HIV/Aids. *AIDS Care*, **15**, 347–57.

Thombs, B. D., Hudson, M., Schieir, O., Taillefer, S., Baron, M. and the Canadian Scleroderma Research Group. (2008). Reliability and validity of the Center for Epidemiological Studies Depression scale in patients with systemic sclerosis. *Arthritis & Rheumatism*, **39**, 438–43.

Tourangeau, R., Rips, L. J. and Rasinsky, K. (2000). *The Psychology of Survey Response*. New York: Cambridge University Press.

Turcot, K., Aissaoui, R., Boivin, K., et al. (2009). The responsiveness of three-dimensional knee accelerations used as an estimation of knee instability and loading transmission during gait in osteoarthritis patient's follow-up. *Osteoarthritis and Cartilage*, **17**, 213–9.

UK Beam Trial Team. (2004) United Kingdom back pain exercise and manipulation (UK BEAM) randomised trial: effectiveness of physical treatment for back pain in primary care. *British Medical Journal*, doi:10.1136/bmj.38282.669225.AE

Van den Bergh, R. C. N., Korfage, I. J., Borsboom, G. J. J. M., Steyerberg, E. W. and Essink-Bot, M. (2009). Prostate cancer-specific anxiety in Dutch patients on active surveillance: validation of the memorial anxiety scale for prostate cancer. *Quality of Life Research*, **18**, 1061–6.

Van der Veer, K., Ommundsen, R., Hak, T. and Larsen, K. S. (2003). Meaning shift of items in different language versions. A cross-national validation study of the illegal aliens scale. *Quality and Quantity*, **37**, 193–206.

Van der Velde, G., Beaton, D., Hogg-Johnston, S., Hurwitz, E. and Tennant, A. (2009). Rasch analysis provides new insights into the measurement properties of the Neck Disability Index. *Arthritis & Rheumatism*, **61**, 544–51.

Van Dijk, M., Peters, J. W., Van Deventer, P. and Tibboel D. (2005). The COMFORT behaviour scale: a tool for assessing pain and sedation in infants. *American Journal of Nursing*, **105**, 33–6.

Van Herk, R., Van Dijk, M., Baar, F. P. M., Tibboel, D. and De Wit, R. (2007). Observation scales for pain assessment in older adults with cognitive impairments or communication difficulties. *Nursing Research*, **56**, 34–43.

Veldman, P. H., Reynen, H. M., Arntz, I. E. and Goris, R. J. (1993). Signs and symptoms of reflex sympathetic dystrophy: prospective study of 829 patients. *Lancet*, **342**, 1012–6.

Verhagen, A. P., De Vet, H. C., De Bie, R. A., Boers. M. and Van den Brandt, P. A. (2001). The art of quality assessment of RCTs included in systematic reviews. *Journal of Clinical Epidemiology*, **54**, 651–4.

Wagner, A. K., Gandek, B., Aaronson, N. K., *et al.* (1998). Cross-cultural comparisons of the content of SF-36 translation across 10 countries: results from the IQOLA project. *Journal of Clinical Epidemiology*, **51**, 925–32.

Walter, S. D., Eliasziw, M. and Donner, A. (1998). Sample size and optimal designs for reliability studies. *Statistics in Medicine*, **17**, 101–10.

Westerman, M. J., Hak, T., The, A. M., *et al.* (2007). Change in what matters to palliative patients: eliciting information about adaptation with SEIQoL-DW. *Palliative Medicine*, **21**, 581–6.

Westerman, M. J., Hak, T., Sprangers, M. A. G., *et al.* (2008). Listen to their answers! Response behaviour in the measurement of physical and role functioning. *Quality of Life Research*, **17**, 549–58.

Whelan, K., Judd, P. A. and Taylor, M. A. (2004). Assessment of fecal output in patients receiving enteral tube feeding: validation of a novel chart. *European Journal of Clinical Nutrition*, **58**, 1030–7.

Whelan, K., Judd, P. A., Preedy, V. R. and Taylor, M. A. (2008). Covert assessment of concurrent and construct validity of a chart to characterize fecal output and diarrhea in patients receiving enteral nutrition. *Journal of Parenteral and Enteral Nutrition*, **32**, 160–8.

Whiting, P., Rutjes, A. W. S., Reitsma, J. B., Bossuyt, P. M. M. and Kleijnen, J. (2003). The development of QUADAS: a tool for the quality assessment of studies of diagnostic accuracy included in systematic reviews. *Biomed Central Medical Research Methodology*, **3**, 25.

WHO Multicentre Growth Reference Study Group. (2006). *WHO Child Growth Standards: length/height-for-age, weight-for-age, weight-for-length, weight-for-height and body mass index-for-age: methods and development.* Geneva, Switzerland: World Health Organization.

Wilson, I. B. and Cleary P. D. (1995). Linking clinical variables with health related quality of life. *Journal of the American Medical Association*, **273**, 59–65.

Wolfe, F., Michaud, K. and Strand, V. (2005). Expanding the definition of clinical differences: from minimally clinically important differences to really important differences. Analyses in 8931 patients with rheumatoid arthritis. *Journal of Rheumatology*, **32**, 583–9.

World Health Organization. (2001). *International Classification of Functioning, Disability and Health.* Geneva, Switzerland: World Health Organization.

Wright, J. G. (2000). Evaluating the outcome of treatment. Shouldn't we be asking patients if they are better? *Journal of Clinical Epidemiology*, **53**, 549–53.

Wright, B. D. and Linacre, J. M. (1989). Observations are always ordinal: measurements, however, must be interval. *Archives of Physical Medicine and Rehabilitation*, **70**, 857–60.

Wyrwich, K. W. (2004). Minimal important difference thresholds and the standard error of measurement: is there a connection? *Journal of Biopharmaceutical Statistics*, **14**, 97–110.

Wyrwich, K. W., Tierney, W. M. and Wolinsky, F. D. (1999). Further evidence supporting an SEM-based criterion for identifying meaningful intra-individual changes in health-related quality of life. *Journal of Clinical Epidemiology*, **52**, 861–73.

Zieky, M. (1993). Practical questions in the use of DIF statistics in test development. In: Holland, P.W. and Wainer, H., Eds. *Differential Item Functioning*. Hillsdale, NJ: Lawrence Erlbaum, pp. 337–47.

Zwakhalen, S. M., Hamers, J. P., Abu-Saad, H. H. and Berger, M. P. (2006). Pain in elderly people with severe dementia: a systematic review of behavioural pain assessment tools. *Biomed Central Geriatrics*, **6**, 3.

Index